Introduction to
Clinical Methods in
Communication Disorders

Introduction to
Clinical Methods in
Communication Disorders
Third Edition

edited by

Rhea Paul, Ph.D.

Sacred Heart University
Fairfield, Connecticut

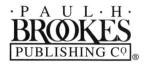

·P A U L·H·
BROOKES
PUBLISHING Cᵒ ®

Baltimore • London • Sydney

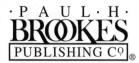

Paul H. Brookes Publishing Co.
Post Office Box 10624
Baltimore, Maryland 21285-0624
USA

www.brookespublishing.com

Typeset by Cenveo, Baltimore, Maryland.
Manufactured in the United States of America by
Sheridan Books, Chelsea, Michigan.

The case studies appearing in this book are composites based on the authors' experiences; these case studies do not represent the lives or experiences of specific individuals, and no implications should be inferred.

The reading passage on page 163 is from Fairbanks, Grant, *VOICE ARTICULATION DRILL BOOK*, *1st Edition*, © 1960. Reprinted by permission of Pearson Education, Inc., Upper Saddle River, NJ.

Library of Congress Cataloging-in-Publication Data
Paul, Rhea.
   Introduction to clinical methods in communication disorders / edited by Rhea Paul, Ph.D.—Third edition.
     pages   cm
   Includes bibliographical references and index.
   ISBN 978-1-59857-286-5 (alk. paper)
   1. Speech therapy. 2. Audiology. 3. Communication disorders. I. Title.

   RC423.I545P38 2014
   616.85′5—dc23   2013028607

British Library Cataloguing in Publication data are available from the British Library.

2018   2017   2016   2015   2014

10   9   8   7   6   5   4   3   2   1

Contents

About the Online Companion Materials

Attention instructors! PowerPoints are available to help you teach a course using *Introduction to Clinical Methods in Communication Disorders, Third Edition.* Please visit www.brookespublishing.com/paul to access customizable PowerPoint presentations for Chapters 1–13, totaling more than 150 slides.

About the Editor

Rhea Paul, Ph.D., CCC-SLP, is a professor and founding director of the speech-language pathology graduate program at Sacred Heart University in Fairfield, Connecticut, an affiliate at Haskins Laboratories and the Yale Child Study Center, and Professor Emerita at Southern Connecticut State University. She received her B.A. from Brandeis University, her master's degree in reading and learning disabilities from the Harvard Graduate School of Education, and her Ph.D. in communication disorders from the University of Wisconsin–Madison. She has been a principal investigator on research projects on language disorders and autism funded by the National Institute on Deafness and Other Communication Disorders, the National Institute of Child Health and Development, the National Alliance for Autism Research, the Meyer Memorial Trust, and the Oregon Medical Foundation. She has been a principal investigator at the Yale Autism Center of Excellence. She is also the author of more than 90 refereed journal articles, 40 book chapters, and 8 books. In 1996, she received the Editor's Award from the *American Journal of Speech-Language Pathology* and was awarded the inaugural Ritvo/Slifka Award for Innovative Clinical Research by the International Society for Autism Research in 2010. She has been a Fellow of the American Speech-Language Hearing Association since 1991.

About the Contributors

Michele A. Anderson, Ph.D., CCC-SLP, is a senior research associate at Western Michigan University. Her research interests include topics ranging from child language and literacy to working memory and adult traumatic brain injury. Currently she is Project Coordinator for an Institution of Education Sciences–grant funded national multiyear collaboration to validate a new test of child language and literacy.

Michelle S. Bourgeois, Ph.D., CCC-SLP, is a professor in the Department of Communication Sciences and Disorders at the University of South Florida and a Fellow of the American Speech Language Hearing Association at Hunter College. A clinical researcher, she investigates interventions designed to improve the quality and quantity of cognitive-communication outcomes for persons with dementia, traumatic brain injury, or aphasia and their spouses and caregivers.

Paul W. Cascella, Ph.D., CCC-SLP, is a professor and the current chair of the Department of Speech-Language Pathology and Audiology at Hunter College. His primary interests are communication services and supports for individuals with severe and low-incidence disabilities. His research specifically focuses on functional assessment and intervention strategies for individuals with intellectual disability and autism spectrum disorders. Dr. Cascella also has clinical expertise in pediatric phonology and fluency, and he is an active clinician who routinely collaborates with public school districts throughout Connecticut.

James J. Dempsey, Ph.D., is chairperson of the Department of Communication Disorders at Southern Connecticut State University. Dr. Dempsey received his doctorate from the University of Connecticut. His research interests include hearing aid fitting strategies as well as measures of functional and communicative benefits derived from hearing aid use.

Marc E. Fey, Ph.D., CCC-SLP, is a professor in the Hearing and Speech Department at the University of Kansas Medical Center. He has published numerous articles, chapters, and software programs on children's speech and language development and disorders and has written or edited three books on child-language intervention. He was editor of the *American Journal of Speech-Language Pathology* from 1996 to 1998 and chair of the American Speech-Language-Hearing Association's publications board from 2003 to 2005. He holds the Kawana Award for Lifetime Achievement in Publications and the Honors of the Association from the American Speech-Language-Hearing Association.

Elizabeth E. Galletta, Ph.D., is a speech-language pathologist and assistant professor at Hunter College, CUNY. Her research and clinical interests include fluency disorders and adult neurogenic disorders, with a focus on functional improvement poststroke. She is a visiting research scientist in the Stroke Rehabilitation Research Laboratory at the Kessler Foundation Research Center, University of Medicine and Dentistry of New Jersey in West Orange, New Jersey.

Brian A. Goldstein, Ph.D., CCC-SLP, is Dean of the School of Nursing and Health Sciences and a professor in the Speech-Language-Hearing Sciences Program at La Salle University in Philadelphia. He holds a B.A. in linguistics and cognitive science from Brandeis University and an M.A. and Ph.D. in speech-language pathology from Temple University. Dr. Goldstein is well-published in the area of communication development and disorders in Latino children. His focus is on phonological development and disorders in monolingual Spanish-speaking and Spanish–English bilingual children. He is a fellow of the American Speech-Language-Hearing Association (ASHA) and received ASHA's Certificate of Recognition for Special Contribution in Multicultural Affairs.

Monica Gordon-Pershey, Ed.D., CCC-SLP, is an associate professor in the Speech and Hearing Program, School of Health Sciences, Cleveland State University, and was formerly Program Director. She is the author of numerous articles, book chapters, and presentations on language and literacy and on the preprofessional and professional development of speech-language pathologists and literacy educators.

Jane Hindenlang, M.S., has worked as a speech-language pathologist for more than 30 years with both adults and children. In addition to her position as a clinical instructor at the Center for Communication Disorders at Southern Connecticut State University, Ms. Hindelang also coordinates the clinic for adults with neurologically based communication disorders, which includes providing educational programs and counseling for caregivers.

Aquiles Iglesias, Ph.D., Professor in the Department of Communication Sciences and Disorders at Temple University, focuses on language development of bilingual (Spanish–English) children. He is the coauthor of three assessment tools designed to assess English-language learners. His recent works focuses on factors that influence language growth in L1 and L2.

Laura M. Justice, Ph.D., is a professor at The Ohio State University, a speech-language pathologist, and researcher in early childhood language and literacy development, communication disorders, and educational interventions. She is the director of The Children's Learning Research Collaborative, a research laboratory dedicated to conducting empirical research on child development and early education.

Michelle MacRoy-Higgins, Ph.D., is a speech-language pathologist and assistant professor at Hunter College, CUNY. Her research and clinical interests include language and phonological development and disorders in children and children with autism spectrum disorders.

Kevin M. McNamara, M.A., is the director of the Center for Communication Disorders at Southern Connecticut State University, where he also serves as a clinical educator. He has presented workshops and published in the areas of communication supports for children and adults with intellectual disability and clinical education in speech-language pathology and audiology.

Gladys Millman, M.A., CCC-SLP, CAGS, is a speech-language pathologist (SLP) who also holds a degree in assistive technology and augmentative communication. She views augmentative and alternative communication (AAC) as a natural extension of her life's work because it broadens her ability to facilitate language and communication skills in others. She practices as an SLP, AAC evaluator, staff trainer, adjunct lecturer (AAC), and clinical supervisor.

Nickola W. Nelson, Ph.D., is a professor in speech pathology and audiology and the director of the Interdisciplinary Health Sciences Ph.D. program at Western Michigan University, where she also conducts research in language–literacy development and disorders. She is an American Speech-Language-Hearing Association fellow, editor of *Topics in Language Disorders*, and recipient of the 2007 Kleffner Clinical Career Award and 2011 ASHA Honors.

Mary H. Purdy, Ph.D., is a professor at Southern Connecticut State University. Her research interests are in the cognitive processes underlying aphasia and their influence on management of communication difficulty, family education and training, and interdisciplinary collaboration. She is board certified by the Academy of Neurologic Communication Disorders and Sciences.

Denise LaPrade Rini, M.A., has been a practicing clinician in pediatrics with a particular interest in children ages birth to 5 who exhibit significant communication impairments. As a member of the Department of Communication Disorders at Southern Connecticut State University, she has provided training for graduate clinicians and taught a variety of undergraduate and graduate courses for more than three decades.

Froma Roth, Ph.D., is Professor Emerita of the University of Maryland and associate director of Academic Affairs and Research Education at the American Speech-Language-Hearing Association. Her research program has been directed at specifying relationships between oral language and emergent and early literacy. She is the coauthor of a basic textbook on speech and language intervention, Treatment Resource Manual for Speech-Language Pathology (4th ed.); and the coauthor of Promoting Awareness of Speech Sounds (PASS), a published phonological awareness program for preschool and primary school settings. She serves as the Council for Exceptional Children's Division of Communication Disabilities and Deafness liaison to the National Joint Council on Learning Disabilities. Her publications emphasize issues related to the assessment and treatment of language and literacy problems from preschool through adolescence.

Mary Beth Schmitt, M.S., CCC-SLP, is a doctoral student at The Ohio State University. She has worked as a speech-language pathologist in the Texas public school system and as a clinical instructor at Texas Tech University and the University of Texas at Dallas. She is interested in evidenced-based research for preschoolers and early elementary students with language disorders.

Elizabeth S. Simmons, M.S., CCC-SLP, is a speech-language pathologist at the Yale Child Study Center, where she is a member of their multidisciplinary autism spectrum disorder assessment team. Her clinical interests include the use of technology to enhance communication in young children with autism spectrum disorders. In addition to her clinical work, she is the author of both book chapters and peer-reviewed journal articles on early speech and language development in toddlers with autism spectrum disorders.

Geralyn R. Timler, Ph.D., Assistant Professor in the Department of Speech and Language Pathology and Audiology at Miami University, focuses on social communication disorders in preschoolers, school-age children, and adolescents.

Donald A. Vogel, Au.D., has directed the Hunter College, CUNY, Center for Communication Disorders since 2003. Bridging both audiology and speech-language pathology in tasks related to the center's mission of training and service, Dr. Vogel utilizes clinical, administrative, and leadership skills learned in his years working at hospitals and clinics. He collaborates with colleagues to facilitate research on areas relating to technology and communication.

Patrick R. Walden, Ph.D., CCC-SLP, is an assistant professor in the Department of Communication Sciences and Disorders at St. John's University. His research and scholarship have focused on speech-language pathologists' workplace learning behaviors, leadership and administration in the professions, and language characteristics in children and adult clinical populations.

Acknowledgments

The completion of this book owes much to its outstanding contributors, who met deadlines and incorporated editorial suggestions with rare efficiency and grace—both of which were greatly appreciated. Our editors at Brookes also showed tremendous forbearance in helping to bring this project to fruition, and they have my deepest thanks.

To the loving memory of my husband, Charles R. Isenberg,
whose commitment to teaching endures as my constant inspiration

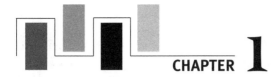
Introduction to Clinical Practice in Communication Disorders

Rhea Paul

In thinking about the message conveyed to our audience, the students reading this book, I found myself recalling some of my own clinical experiences. I remembered supervising a first-term student clinician by the name of Jane. Jane was working on articulation with Mike, a pixie-faced 3-year-old with almost completely unintelligible speech. Mike had lots to say, but Jane could understand almost none of it. He was trying to tell her something about the toy dinosaur he had brought from home and, try as she might, she just was not getting it. After attempting three or four times to get the same message across, poor little Mike burst into tears of frustration. Jane was, naturally, taken aback. Sitting behind the mirror, I saw Jane trying to "talk" the little boy into feeling better. Finally, unable to contain my own distress at seeing Mike so miserable, I went into the room and held him, rocking him until he finished crying. Mike was soon able to resume his work. In our conference following this incident, Jane remarked, "I was so glad when you came in and held him. I didn't think I was allowed to do that; it didn't seem like the kind of thing a clinician is supposed to do."

CLINICAL ART AND SCIENCE

This book is all about the kinds of things that clinicians are supposed to do and think about. In this example, Jane learned something essential about clinical practice: Even the clinician with the highest level of technical training and the most scientific outlook sometimes has to remember that our clients are first and foremost people—people with complicated, sometimes conflicting feelings and needs; people who sometimes do not use their clinical time efficiently; people whose motivation to learn better communication skills is sometimes overwhelmed by their emotions or the broader circumstances of their lives. The example shows that a good clinician must be part scientist, humanist, and philosopher, someone who is willing to carefully evaluate what professionals do (and do not do) as part of the clinical services.

But, you may be thinking, how can I learn to be a scientist, a humanist, a philosopher, and an expert on normal and disordered communication before I see my first client next semester? Well, fortunately for all of us, there is one more thing that every clinician needs to be, and that is a human being. Neither your supervisor, your client, nor anyone else will expect you to be a fully evolved clinician your first term. With your first client, and probably with some of your later ones, too, you will make mistakes. Like any other human being you will have to make amends for these mistakes, try to learn from them, and do better the next time. Competent clinicians recognize and learn from their own mistakes. Still, the purpose of this book is to help you begin to make the transition from a student of communication disorders to a speech, language, and/or hearing clinician.

Being a clinician entails some qualities that probably cannot be taught by your professors. These are the qualities we identify with the humanist, and to some extent they arise out of your own beliefs, needs, desires, and personality. It is these qualities that probably brought you to consider a career in communication disorders. These qualities include the following:

- A desire to help others

- Strengths in social interactions

- Enjoyment of close contact with people

- Strong communication skills

- The ability to take pleasure in "just talking"

- An interest in the various processes by which communication takes place

- A level of comfort with people with disabilities

These qualities are not present in everyone, but as a starting point for becoming a clinician they are essential. As you must know by now, although these qualities contribute to making you a good clinician, more is needed. You need an in-depth knowledge of the normal processes and development of communication and the characteristics, causes, and correlates of the various kinds of communication disorders. You also need knowledge of the information introduced in this book. Here you will learn about the kinds of behaviors and activities in which a clinician engages and about the contexts in which these behaviors and activities take place. The goal is that when you are through, you will have a better sense of what it is a clinician does; where he or she does it; and what general principles of ethics, public policy, cultural sensitivity, and respect for clients and families guide our behaviors and activities.

SCOPE OF PRACTICE

What do speech-language pathologists (SLPs) and audiologists do? Where do they do it? With and for whom? Why do they take this approach and not that one? These are the questions that define our scope of practice. Audiologists and SLPs work with clients from birth through old age. Audiologists screen newborns for hearing loss; SLPs work with premature infants to develop feeding, swallowing, and early parent–child communication skills. Audiologists and SLPs work with infants and toddlers with a variety of developmental disabilities, including hearing impairment, intellectual disability, autism spectrum disorders, congenital anomalies such as cleft palate, congenital disorders such as cerebral palsy or fetal alcohol syndrome, and feeding and swallowing problems. We work with children with cochlear implants. Clinicians who work with very young children are often engaged in *secondary prevention* assessment and intervention aimed at limiting the impact of disorders on communication and development. Audiologists and SLPs also work with preschool children who have these kinds of problems and hearing and/or language delays that surface in early childhood. These include articulation disorders, fluency disorders, and specific language delays. We also, unfortunately, see children in this age range whose communication has been affected by abuse or neglect or whose development has been influenced by parental substance abuse.

Audiologists and SLPs often work with school-age populations. In this age range, we see children such as those already described, as well as children who abuse their voices, have trouble producing fluent speech, or endanger their hearing through noise exposure. A large part of an SLP's practice in schools deals with students who have language-based learning disorders that affect their ability to master the academic curriculum. These students require support to enhance their language so that they can use it more effectively to succeed in school. With impetus from the No Child Left Behind Act of 2001 (PL 107-110) and the Individuals with Disabilities Education Improvement Act of 2004 (PL 108-446), school-based SLPs provide communication intervention within the context of academic instruction. They also sometimes provide management for students with emotional or social disorders that affect communication, such as Asperger syndrome, selective mutism, or children diagnosed with mental illness.

Many SLPs and audiologists work with adult clients as well. Adults with various developmental disabilities continue to require the services of communication specialists. Some young and middle-age adults experience communication disabilities as a result of illnesses or traumatic brain injury. Older adults are especially vulnerable to acquiring communication disorders. Many audiologists work with older adults experiencing age-related hearing loss. SLPs also serve older clients who may lose speech and language skills due to neurological diseases such as strokes, Parkinson's disease, and amyotrophic lateral sclerosis (Lou Gehrig's disease).

Recommended practice for clients all along the spectrum of development includes the clinician's close collaboration with their families and with other professionals involved in their care. When a client receives services from several professionals, it serves the client best if these professionals are aware of each other's goals and methods and can coordinate services for the client. Many professionals collaborate closely on teams with professionals from a range of other disciplines to help deliver services in a more integrated manner, so the client receives consistent feedback and reinforcement and has more opportunities for generalization. Clinical practice in communication disorders often involves collaboration with teachers and special educators; physical and occupational therapists; psychologists and social workers; recreational and vocational counselors; nurses and physicians; as well as with the staff of schools, residential centers, group homes, rehabilitation facilities, hospitals, and skilled nursing facilities.

SCOPE OF TEXT

The purpose of this book is to introduce you to the processes, settings, and issues involved in clinical practice in communication disorders. In Chapter 2, you will be introduced to the codes of ethics disseminated by the American Speech-Language-Hearing Association (ASHA) and the American Academy of Audiology (AAA). These codes are central to the practice of our professions because they lay out our obligations to our clients, our payers, and our colleagues and provide guidelines to help us in making sometimes difficult ethical decisions. In Chapter 3, issues of evidence-based practice are discussed, and the steps a clinician can take to find support for specific assessment protocols and intervention strategies are introduced. In Chapter 4, you learn about basic principles of assessment and the properties that make standardized tests fair and accurate. You will be encouraged to think about the times when it is appropriate to use tests and when other methods of assessment come to the fore. Audiologists and SLPs are the only professionals who do this examination, so it is especially important to be confident and capable in this aspect of our work. Chapter 5 addresses the issue of the assessment of samples of communicative behavior, including speech and language as well as nonverbal communication. One of the most important functions of an SLP is the sampling of communicative behaviors in order to determine appropriate goals and methods for intervention.

Chapter 6 moves our discussion from assessment to the domain of intervention. Here we talk about the range of intervention procedures used to help people with communication disorders improve their functioning. A continuum of approaches is discussed, and you will consider how they apply across a variety of communication disorders. In Chapter 7, the communication skills needed on the part of clinicians—such as those used in interacting with clients, families, and other professionals—are described. You will learn about the various kinds of documentation that are professionally required and the importance of acquiring skills not only in conducting assessment and intervention but also in collaborating with families and colleagues to ensure our clients' progress. You will be reminded, too, of our role as, not professional counselors, but humanists: as caring individuals who listen to concerns of clients and families, even when the concerns extend beyond speech, hearing, and language issues. Chapter 8 provides information on the laws, rules, and regulations that govern SLP and audiologist practice. You will find out about clients' rights, professional responsibilities, and the emerging public policies that affect practice. In Chapter 9, the varied settings in which communication disorders professionals practice is the topic. You will be introduced to the kinds of practice options each provides, the kinds of documentation each requires, and the various roles of communication professionals in each one. This may give you a first sense of the setting in which you might like to start your own practice. Chapter 10 addresses the issues of helping clients communicate when they come from cultural and language backgrounds different from their clinician's. These issues have become increasingly important as the demographic trends in our society reflect greater numbers of citizens with cultural and linguistic differences, individuals who, like everyone else, are vulnerable to disorders of communication. But, as you can imagine, facilitating communication is complicated when the client and clinician speak different languages or have different cultural rules for communicating. Chapter 11 reviews the many ways assistive technology affects our practice. Because many of these new technologies are based on consumer electronic devices rather than specialized equipment, it is not surprising that they are having a great impact on how to deliver services. In Chapter 12 the important role that clients and families play in the clinical process is discussed. You will consider ways of including the perspectives of families at every stage of the clinical decision-making process so as to maximize the impact of treatments beyond the clinical setting and into the real, integrated lives of the clients we serve. Finally, in Chapter 13, the crucial connections between clinical practice and research are highlighted.

Our hope is that after completing your studies with this book, you will have a greater sense of what a clinician does and does not do and a greater confidence that you will be able to make the correct choices with your first client and with every client thereafter. Although mastering both the science and the art of clinical practice will take much longer than the time you spend in school, your clinical education will provide you with the tools you need to continue learning and improving your service to clients. We hope you will consider this book a useful part of that education. Yet another part, though, will be the support you receive from your colleagues after you graduate and from the national organization that represents our professions in the United States. We would like to take the opportunity at this juncture to introduce you to this organization as well.

THE AMERICAN SPEECH-LANGUAGE-HEARING ASSOCIATION AND THE CLINICIAN

The American Speech-Language-Hearing Association is the professional, scientific, and credentialing association for the nearly 118,000 communication disorders professionals around the world. Its mission is to "promote the interests of and provide the highest quality services for professionals in audiology, speech-language pathology, and speech and hearing science, and to advocate for people with communication disabilities" (see http://www.asha.org/about). The organization disseminates standards of ethical conduct, publishes original research in its journals, and provides continuing education programs to its members. It advocates for our clients by monitoring and participating in the development and implementation of education and health care reform proposals and programs at the federal and state levels. The following list highlights many of the services ASHA provides to its members and the community. These include the following:

Political advocacy: ASHA tracks issues of concern to our clients and colleagues in legislatures, courts, and regulatory agencies at state and federal levels (see http://asha.org/advocacy).

Networking: ASHA provides opportunities for its members to shape the profession and effect changes that benefit clients and colleagues (see http://www.asha.org/advocacy/state/networks).

Continuing education: ASHA sponsors state and national conferences, distance learning opportunities, newsletters, journals, and audio- and videoconferences that enable members to keep up-to-date on clinical and professional issues (see http://www.asha.org/ce).

Multicultural initiatives: ASHA provides support to members who need to deal with multicultural issues in their practice, from lists of tests and resources to educating citizens from minority groups about the importance of communicative health (see http://www.asha.org/practice/multicultural).

Research: ASHA supports basic and applied research in communication disorders, and it keeps an extensive database to help members write grants, business plans, and reports (see http://www.asha.org/research). ASHA also publishes several journals, including the *Journal of Speech, Language and Hearing Research; Language, Speech, and Hearing Services in Schools; American Journal of Audiology;* and *American Journal of Speech-Language Pathology* (see http://www.asha.org/publications).

Technical assistance: Members can receive information about funding agencies, developing proposals, and other professional issues by contacting ASHA by telephone (1-800-498-2071) or fax (301-571-0457) or online at actioncenter@asha.org (see also http://www.asha.org/about/contacts).

Referral service: ASHA maintains a referral list of clinical programs and private practitioners who have asked to be listed. It is grouped by state and available to individuals who request referrals (see http://www.asha.org/findpro).

Employment service: Members seeking new positions may use ASHA's job placement services (see http://www.asha.org/careers).

Specialty recognition: ASHA supports the credentialing of personnel with expertise in a particular disorder, such as child language or fluency disorders (see http://www.asha.org/Certification/specialty/Clinical-Specialty-Certification and http://www.asha.org/certification/specialty).

Special interest groups: ASHA maintains 18 special interest groups (SIGs) that focus on particular aspects of practice, such as language learning and education, aural rehabilitation and its instrumentation, and augmentative and alternative communication (see http://www.asha.org/SIG).

Contact the ASHA web site for further information (http://asha.org).

The organization provides the standards for earning the clinical credential in our field, the Certificate of Clinical Competence (CCC), which can be earned in either speech-language pathology, audiology, or both. The standards for ASHA certification in speech-language pathology (as of 2014) and audiology (as of 2012) are outlined in Appendices 1A and 1B at the end of this chapter and at http://www.asha.org/Certification/2014-Speech-Language-Pathology-Certification-Standards and http://www.asha.org/Certification/2012-Audiology-Certification-Standards.

You should be aware, however, that these standards change from time to time. In addition, many states require SLPs and audiologists to be licensed with the state board of health, certified with the state department of education, or both. In many cases, licensing and teacher certification requirements overlap with ASHA certification, but it is important to check on the licensing and certification requirements for the state in which you plan to practice and for the practice settings (e.g., schools, hospitals, home health agencies, birth-to-3 programs) in which you intend to participate.

MOVING FORWARD AND LOOKING BACK

We have begun to talk here about what it means to be a clinician. What it means for you personally will unfold as you consolidate your knowledge and test it in your practicum experiences. It is our hope that you will acquire some of that knowledge from your interactions with this book's authors and their chapters. But as you acquire this new knowledge, do not let yourself forget the things you have always known. When you begin to feel overwhelmed by all the new things you must learn, by all the facts you must amass, by the equipment you must master, by the papers and reports and lesson plans you must write, remember to look back. Look back to the reasons you entered into this process, and remember what motivated you to go through such a long and rigorous training program in the first place. You do not need to leave your humane instincts behind. If you find yourself faced with a situation like the one Jane encountered, trust your intuition. As you move forward in your clinical education, your newly gained knowledge will inform your actions, but it will never replace the humane motive of bringing the birthright of communication to every individual. This is the impulse that first set you on your present path, and it should continue to guide your steps through-out your career.

STUDY QUESTIONS

1. Think about what prompted you to enter the field of communication disorders. List some of the most important reasons and why it will be important to think back on them as you proceed with your clinical education.
2. List four activities within the scope of practice of an audiologist.
3. List four activities within the scope of practice of a speech-language pathologist.
4. Identify two similarities and two differences in the certification standards for audiologists and SLPs.

REFERENCES

Individuals with Disabilities Education Improvement Act of 2004, PL 108-446, 20 U.S.C. §§ 1400 *et seq.*

No Child Left Behind Act of 2001, PL 107-110, 115 Stat. 1425, 20 U.S.C. §§ 6301 *et seq.*

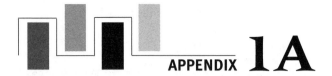

2014 Standards and Implementation Procedures for the Certificate of Clinical Competence in Speech-Language Pathology

Effective date: September 1, 2014

The Council for Clinical Certification in Audiology and Speech-Language Pathology (CFCC) is a semiautonomous credentialing body of the American Speech-Language-Hearing Association. The charges to the CFCC are to define the standards for clinical certification, to apply those standards in granting certification to individuals, to have final authority to withdraw certification in cases where certification has been granted on the basis of inaccurate information, and to administer the certification maintenance program.

A Practice and Curriculum Analysis of the Profession of Speech-Language Pathology was conducted in 2009 under the auspices of the Council on Academic Accreditation in Audiology and Speech-Language Pathology (CAA) and the CFCC. The survey analysis was reviewed by the CFCC, and the following standards were developed to better fit current practice models.

The 2014 standards and implementation procedures for the Certificate of Clinical Competence in Speech-Language Pathology will go into effect for all applications for certification received on or after September 1, 2014. View the speech-language pathology (SLP) standards crosswalk PDF at http://www.asha.org/uploadedFiles/2005-2014-SLP-Standards-Comparison.pdf for more specific information on how the standards will change from the current SLP standards to the 2014 SLP standards. Cite as follows: Council for Clinical Certification in Audiology and Speech-Language Pathology of the American Speech-Language-Hearing Association. (2012). *2014 Standards for the Certificate of Clinical Competence in Speech-Language Pathology*. Retrieved from http://www.asha.org/Certification/2014-Speech-Language-Pathology-Certification-Standards.

From Council for Clinical Certification in Audiology and Speech-Language Pathology of the American Speech-Language-Hearing Association. (2014). *2014 Standards for the certificate of clinical competence in speech-language pathology.* Retrieved from http://www.asha.org/Certification/2014-Speech-Language-Pathology-Certification-Standards

The Standards for the Certificate of Clinical Competence in Speech-Language Pathology are outlined and discussed in detail below. The Council for Clinical Certification implementation procedures follow each standard.

Standard I—Degree

Standard II—Education Program

Standard III—Program of Study

Standard IV—Knowledge Outcomes

Standard V—Skills Outcomes

Standard VI—Assessment

Standard VII—Speech-Language Pathology Clinical Fellowship

Standard VIII—Maintenance of Certification

STANDARD I: DEGREE

The applicant for certification must have a master's, doctoral, or other recognized postbaccalaureate degree.

Implementation

The CFCC has the authority to determine eligibility of all applicants for certification.

STANDARD II: EDUCATION PROGRAM

All graduate coursework and graduate clinical experience required in speech-language pathology must have been initiated and completed in a speech-language pathology program accredited by the CAA.

Implementation

If the program of graduate study is initiated and completed in a CAA-accredited program and if the program director or official designee verifies that all knowledge and skills required at that time for application have been met, approval of the application is automatic. Individuals educated outside the United States or its territories must submit documentation that coursework was completed in an institution of higher education that is regionally accredited or recognized by the appropriate regulatory authority for that country. In addition, applicants outside the United States or its territories must meet each of the standards that follow.

STANDARD III: PROGRAM OF STUDY

The applicant for certification must have completed a program of study (a minimum of 36 semester credit hours at the graduate level) that includes academic coursework and supervised clinical experience sufficient in depth and breadth to achieve the specified knowledge and skills outcomes stipulated in Standards IV-A through IV-G and Standards V-A through V-C.

Implementation

The minimum of 36 graduate semester credit hours must have been earned in a program that addresses the knowledge and skills pertinent to the ASHA Scope of Practice in Speech-Language Pathology.

STANDARD IV: KNOWLEDGE OUTCOMES

Standard IV-A

The applicant must have demonstrated knowledge of the biological sciences, physical sciences, statistics, and the social/behavioral sciences.

Implementation   Acceptable courses in biological sciences should emphasize a content area related to human or animal sciences (e.g., biology, human anatomy and physiology, neuroanatomy and neurophysiology, human genetics, veterinary science). Acceptable courses in physical sciences should include physics or chemistry. Acceptable courses in social/behavioral sciences should include psychology, sociology, anthropology, or public health. A standalone course in statistics is required. Research methodology courses in communication sciences and disorders (CSD) may not be used to satisfy the statistics requirement. A course in biological and physical sciences specifically related to CSD may not be applied for certification purposes to this category unless the course fulfills a university requirement in one of these areas.

Standard IV-B

The applicant must have demonstrated knowledge of basic human communication and swallowing processes, including the appropriate biological, neurological, acoustic, psychological, developmental, and linguistic and cultural bases. The applicant must have demonstrated the ability to integrate information pertaining to normal and abnormal human development across the lifespan.

Standard IV-C

The applicant must have demonstrated knowledge of communication and swallowing disorders and differences, including the appropriate etiologies, characteristics, anatomical/physiological, acoustic, psychological, developmental, and linguistic and cultural correlates in the following areas:

- Articulation
- Fluency
- Voice and resonance, including respiration and phonation
- Receptive and expressive language (phonology, morphology, syntax, semantics, pragmatics, prelinguistic communication and paralinguistic communication) in speaking, listening, reading, and writing
- Hearing, including the impact on speech and language

- Swallowing (oral, pharyngeal, esophageal, and related functions, including oral function for feeding; orofacial myology)
- Cognitive aspects of communication (attention, memory, sequencing, problem-solving, executive functioning)
- Social aspects of communication (including challenging behavior, ineffective social skills, and lack of communication opportunities)
- Augmentative and alternative communication modalities

Implementation It is expected that coursework addressing the professional knowledge specified in Standard IV-C will occur primarily at the graduate level.

Standard IV-D

For each of the areas specified in Standard IV-C, the applicant must have demonstrated current knowledge of the principles and methods of prevention, assessment, and intervention for people with communication and swallowing disorders, including consideration of anatomical/physiological, psychological, developmental, and linguistic and cultural correlates.

Standard IV-E

The applicant must have demonstrated knowledge of standards of ethical conduct.

Implementation The applicant must have demonstrated knowledge of the principles and rules of the current ASHA Code of Ethics.

Standard IV-F

The applicant must have demonstrated knowledge of processes used in research and of the integration of research principles into evidence-based clinical practice.

Implementation The applicant must have demonstrated knowledge of the principles of basic and applied research and research design. In addition, the applicant must have demonstrated knowledge of how to access sources of research information and relate research to clinical practice.

Standard IV-G

The applicant must have demonstrated knowledge of contemporary professional issues.

Implementation The applicant must have demonstrated knowledge of professional issues that affect speech-language pathology. Issues typically include trends in professional practice, academic program accreditation standards, ASHA practice policies and guidelines, and reimbursement procedures.

Standard IV-H

The applicant must have demonstrated knowledge of entry-level and advanced certifications, licensure, and other relevant professional credentials, as well as local, state, and national regulations and policies relevant to professional practice.

STANDARD V: SKILLS OUTCOMES

Standard V-A

The applicant must have demonstrated skills in oral and written or other forms of communication sufficient for entry into professional practice.

Implementation   The applicant must have demonstrated communication skills sufficient to achieve effective clinical and professional interaction with clients/patients and relevant others. In addition, the applicant must have demonstrated the ability to write and comprehend technical reports, diagnostic and treatment reports, treatment plans, and professional correspondence.

Standard V-B

The applicant for certification must have completed a program of study that included experiences sufficient in breadth and depth to achieve the following skills outcomes:

1. Evaluation

    a. Conduct screening and prevention procedures (including prevention activities).

    b. Collect case history information and integrate information from clients/patients, family, caregivers, teachers, and relevant others, including other professionals.

    c. Select and administer appropriate evaluation procedures, such as behavioral observations, nonstandardized and standardized tests, and instrumental procedures.

    d. Adapt evaluation procedures to meet client/patient needs.

    e. Interpret, integrate, and synthesize all information to develop diagnoses and make appropriate recommendations for intervention.

    f. Complete administrative and reporting functions necessary to support evaluation.

    g. Refer clients/patients for appropriate services.

2. Intervention

    a. Develop setting-appropriate intervention plans with measurable and achievable goals that meet clients'/patients' needs. Collaborate with clients/patients and relevant others in the planning process.

    b. Implement intervention plans (involve clients/patients and relevant others in the intervention process).

    c. Select or develop and use appropriate materials and instrumentation for prevention and intervention.

    d. Measure and evaluate clients'/patients' performance and progress.

    e. Modify intervention plans, strategies, materials, or instrumentation as appropriate to meet the needs of clients/patients.

    f. Complete administrative and reporting functions necessary to support intervention.

    g. Identify and refer clients/patients for services as appropriate.

3. Interaction and personal qualities

    a. Communicate effectively, recognizing the needs, values, preferred mode of communication, and cultural/linguistic background of the client/patient, family, caregivers, and relevant others.

    b. Collaborate with other professionals in case management.

    c. Provide counseling regarding communication and swallowing disorders to clients/patients, family, caregivers, and relevant others.

    d. Adhere to the ASHA Code of Ethics and behave professionally.

Implementation The applicant must have acquired the skills referred to in this standard applicable across the nine major areas listed in Standard IV-C. Skills may be developed and demonstrated by direct client/patient contact in clinical experiences, academic coursework, labs, simulations, examinations, and completion of independent projects.

    The applicant must have obtained a sufficient variety of supervised clinical experiences in different work settings and with different populations so that he or she can demonstrate skills across the ASHA Scope of Practice in Speech-Language Pathology. Supervised clinical experience is defined as clinical services (i.e., assessment/diagnosis/evaluation, screening, treatment, report writing, family/client consultation, and/or counseling) related to the management of populations that fit within the ASHA Scope of Practice in Speech-Language Pathology.

    Supervisors of clinical experiences must hold a current ASHA Certificate of Clinical Competence in the appropriate area of practice during the time of supervision. The supervised activities must be within the ASHA Scope of Practice in Speech-Language Pathology to count toward certification.

Standard V-C

The applicant for certification in speech-language pathology must complete a minimum of 400 clock hours of supervised clinical experience in the practice of speech-language pathology. Twenty-five hours must be spent in clinical observation, and 375 hours must be spent in direct client/patient contact.

Implementation Guided observation hours generally precede direct contact with clients/patients. The observation and direct client/patient contact hours must be within the ASHA Scope of Practice of Speech-Language Pathology and must be under the supervision of a qualified professional who holds current ASHA certification in the appropriate practice area. Such supervision may occur simultaneously with the student's observation or afterward through review and approval of written reports or summaries submitted by the student. Students may use video recordings of client services for observation purposes.

Applicants should be assigned a practicum only after they have acquired sufficient knowledge bases to qualify for such experience. Only direct contact with the client or the client's family in assessment, intervention, and/or counseling can be counted toward the practicum. Although several students may observe a clinical session at one time, clinical practicum hours should be assigned only to the student who provides direct services to the client or client's family. Typically, only one student should be working with a given client at a time in order to count the practicum hours. In rare circumstances, it is possible for several students working as a team to receive credit for the same session, depending on the specific responsibilities each student is assigned. For example, in a diagnostic session, if one student evaluates the client and another interviews the parents, both students may receive credit for the time each spent in providing the service. However, if student A works with the client for 30 minutes and student B works with the client for the next 45 minutes, each student receives credit for only the time he or she actually provided services—that is, 30 minutes for student A and 45 minutes for student B. The applicant must maintain documentation of time spent during the supervised practicum, verified by the program in accordance with Standards III and IV.

Standard V-D

At least 325 of the 400 clock hours must be completed while the applicant is engaged in graduate study in a program accredited in speech-language pathology by the CAA.

Implementation A minimum of 325 clock hours of clinical practicums must be completed at the graduate level. At the discretion of the graduate program, hours obtained at the undergraduate level may be used to satisfy the remainder of the requirement.

Standard V-E

Supervision must be provided by individuals who hold the Certificate of Clinical Competence in the appropriate profession. The amount of direct supervision must be commensurate with the student's knowledge, skills, and experience; must not be less than 25% of the student's total contact with each client/patient; and must take place periodically throughout the practicum. Supervision must be sufficient to ensure the welfare of the client/patient.

Implementation Direct supervision must be in real time. A supervisor must be available to consult with a student providing clinical services to the supervisor's client. Supervision of clinical practicums is intended to provide guidance and feedback and to facilitate the student's acquisition of essential clinical skills. The 25% supervision standard is a minimum requirement and should be adjusted upward whenever the student's level of knowledge, skills, and experience warrants.

Standard V-F

Supervised practicums must include experience with client/patient populations across the lifespan and from culturally/linguistically diverse backgrounds. Practicums must include experience with client/patient populations with various types and severities of communication and/or related disorders, differences, and disabilities.

Implementation   The applicant must demonstrate direct client/patient clinical experiences in both assessment and intervention with both children and adults from the range of disorders and differences named in Standard IV-C.

STANDARD VI: ASSESSMENT

The applicant must have passed the national examination adopted by ASHA for purposes of certification in speech-language pathology.

STANDARD VII: SPEECH-LANGUAGE PATHOLOGY CLINICAL FELLOWSHIP

The applicant must successfully complete a Speech-Language Pathology Clinical Fellowship (CF). The CF may be initiated only after completion of all academic course work and clinical experiences required to meet the knowledge and skills delineated in Standards IV and V. The CF must have been completed under the mentorship of an individual who held the ASHA Certificate of Clinical Competence in Speech-Language Pathology (CCC-SLP) throughout the duration of the fellowship.

Standard VII-A: Clinical Fellowship Experience

The CF must have consisted of clinical-service activities that foster the continued growth and integration of knowledge, skills, and tasks of clinical practice in speech-language pathology consistent with ASHA's current Scope of Practice in Speech-Language Pathology. The CF must have consisted of no less than 36 weeks of full-time professional experience or its part-time equivalent.

Implementation   No less than 80% of the Fellow's major responsibilities during the CF experience must have been in direct client/patient contact (e.g., assessment, diagnosis, evaluation, screening, treatment, clinical research activities, family/client consultations, recordkeeping, report writing, and/or counseling) related to the management process for individuals who exhibit communication and/or swallowing disabilities.

Full-time professional experience is defined as 35 hours per week, culminating in a minimum of 1,260 hours. Part-time experience of less than 5 hours per week will not meet the CF requirement and may not be counted toward completion of the experience. Similarly, work in excess of the 35 hours per week cannot be used to shorten the CF to less than 36 weeks.

Standard VII-B: Clinical Fellowship Mentorship

The Clinical Fellow must have received ongoing mentoring and formal evaluations by the CF mentor.

Implementation   Mentoring must have included on-site observations and other monitoring activities. These activities may have been executed by correspondence, review of video and/or audio recordings, evaluation of written reports, telephone conferences with the Fellow, and evaluations by professional colleagues with whom the Fellow works. The CF mentor and Clinical Fellow must have participated in regularly scheduled formal evaluations of the Fellow's progress during the CF experience.

Standard VII-C: Clinical Fellowship Outcomes

The Clinical Fellow must have demonstrated knowledge and skills consistent with the ability to practice independently.

Implementation   At the completion of the CF experience, the applicant will have acquired and demonstrated the ability to do the following:

- Integrate and apply theoretical knowledge
- Evaluate his or her strengths and identify his or her limitations
- Refine clinical skills within the Scope of Practice in Speech-Language Pathology
- Apply the ASHA Code of Ethics to independent professional practice.

In addition, upon completion of the CF, the applicant must have demonstrated the ability to perform clinical activities accurately, consistently, and independently and to seek guidance as necessary.

Standard VIII: Maintenance of Certification

Certificate holders must demonstrate continued professional development for maintenance of the CCC-SLP.

Implementation   Individuals who hold the CCC-SLP must accumulate 30 certification maintenance hours of professional development during every 3-year maintenance interval. Intervals are continuous and begin on January 1 of the year following the awarding of initial certification or reinstatement of certification. A random audit of compliance will be conducted.

Accrual of professional development hours, adherence to the ASHA Code of Ethics, submission of certification maintenance compliance documentation, and payment of annual dues and/or certification fees are required for maintenance of certification.

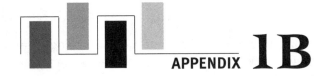

2012 Standards and Implementation Procedures for the Certificate of Clinical Competence in Audiology

Effective January 1, 2012

INTRODUCTION

A Practice and Curriculum Analysis of the Profession of Audiology was conducted in 2007 under the auspices of the Council on Academic Accreditation in Audiology and Speech-Language Pathology (CAA) and the Council For Clinical Certification in Audiology and Speech-Language Pathology (CFCC). Respondents were asked to rate clinical activity statements and foundational knowledge areas in terms of importance and in terms of where the activity should be learned (in graduate school versus on the job). The respondents were also able to indicate whether an activity or area would not be performed by a newly graduated doctoral level audiologist.

The CFCC reviewed the survey data and determined that the standards for clinical certification and the Praxis examination blueprint needed revision in order to be in line with the results of the survey. It is noteworthy that because there is no longer a period of supervised practice following the completion of graduate school, activities that are an essential part of clinical practice must be included in graduate education and in the certification standards. The Scope of Practice in Audiology and the Preferred Practice Patterns for the Profession of Audiology documents also served as resources in the development of the new standards. The proposed standards were distributed for select and widespread peer review in 2008, and all comments were considered in the final version of the document. The CFCC approved the new standards in July 2009 and set an implementation date of January 1, 2012. Cite as follows: Council For Clinical Certification in Audiology and Speech-Language Pathology of the American Speech-Language-Hearing Association. (2012). *2012 Standards for the Certificate of Clinical Competence in Audiology.* Retrieved from http://www.asha.org/Certification/2012-Audiology-Certification-Standards.

From Council For Clinical Certification in Audiology and Speech-Language Pathology of the American Speech-Language-Hearing Association. (2012). *2012 Standards for the certificate of clinical competence in audiology.* Retrieved from http://www.asha.org/Certification/2012-Audiology-Certification-Standards

The Standards for the Certificate of Clinical Competence in Audiology are outlined and discussed in detail below. The Council For Clinical Certification implementation procedures follow each standard.

Standard I—Degree

Standard II—Education Program

Standard III—Program of Study

Standard IV—Knowledge and Skills Outcomes

Standard V—Assessment

Standard VI—Maintenance of Certification

STANDARD I: DEGREE

Applicants for certification must have a doctoral degree. The course of study must address the knowledge and skills necessary to independently practice audiology.

Implementation

Verification of the graduate degree is required of the applicant before the certificate is awarded. Degree verification is accomplished by submitting 1) an application signed by the director of the graduate program, indicating the degree date, and 2) an official transcript showing that the degree has been awarded, or a letter from the university registrar verifying completion of requirements for the degree.

Individuals educated outside the United States or its territories must submit official transcripts and evaluations of their degrees and courses to verify equivalency. These evaluations are typically conducted by credential evaluation services agencies recognized by the National Association of Credential Evaluation Services (NACES). Information that must be provided is 1) confirmation that the degree earned is equivalent to a U.S. doctoral degree, 2) translation of academic coursework into the American semester hour system, and 3) indication as to which courses were completed at the graduate level.

The CFCC has the authority to determine eligibility of all applicants for certification.

STANDARD II: EDUCATION PROGRAM

The graduate degree must be granted by a program accredited by the CAA.

Implementation

Applicants whose graduate degree was awarded by a U.S. institution of higher education must have graduated from a program holding CAA accreditation in audiology. Satisfactory completion of academic coursework, clinical practicums, and knowledge and skills requirements must be verified by the signature of the program director or official designee of a CAA-accredited program or a program admitted to CAA candidacy.

STANDARD III: PROGRAM OF STUDY

Applicants for certification must complete a program of study that includes academic coursework and a minimum of 1,820 hours of supervised clinical practicums sufficient in depth and breadth to achieve the knowledge and skills outcomes stipulated in Standard IV. The supervision must be provided by individuals who hold the ASHA Certificate of Clinical Competence (CCC) in Audiology.

Implementation

The program of study must address the knowledge and skills pertinent to the field of audiology. Clinical practicums must be approved by the academic program from which the student intends to graduate. The student must maintain documentation of time spent in supervised practicums, which the academic program verifies in accordance with Standard IV.

Students shall participate in practicums only after they have had sufficient preparation to qualify for such experience. Students must obtain a variety of clinical practicum experiences in different work settings and with different populations so that they can demonstrate skills across the scope of practice in audiology. Acceptable clinical practicum experience includes clinical and administrative activities directly related to patient care. *Clinical practicum* is defined as direct patient/client contact, consultation, record keeping, and administrative duties relevant to audiology service delivery. Time spent in clinical practicum experiences should occur throughout the graduate program.

Supervision must be sufficient to ensure the welfare of the patient and the student in accordance with the ASHA Code of Ethics. Supervision of clinical practicums must include direct observation, guidance, and feedback to permit the student to monitor, evaluate, and improve performance and to develop clinical competence. The amount of supervision must also be appropriate to the student's level of training, education, experience, and competence.

Supervisors must hold a current ASHA CCC in the appropriate area of practice. The supervised activities must be within the scope of practice of audiology to count toward certification.

STANDARD IV: KNOWLEDGE AND SKILLS OUTCOMES

Applicants for certification must have acquired knowledge and developed skills in six areas: foundations of practice, prevention/identification, assessment, (re)habilitation, advocacy/consultation, and education/research/administration.

This standard distinguishes between the acquisition of knowledge for Standards IV-A.1–21 and IV-C.1 and the acquisition of knowledge and skills for Standards IV-A.22–29, IV-B, IV-C.2–11, IV-D, IV-E, and IV-F. The applicant must submit a completed application for certification signed by the academic program director verifying successful completion of all knowledge and skills in all six areas of Standard IV. The applicant must maintain copies of transcripts and documentation of academic coursework and clinical practicums.

Standard IV-A: Foundations of Practice

The applicant must have knowledge of the following:

A1. Embryology and development of the auditory and vestibular systems, anatomy and physiology, neuroanatomy and neurophysiology, and pathophysiology

A2. Genetics and associated syndromes related to hearing and balance

A3. Normal aspects of auditory physiology and behavior over the lifespan

A4. Normal development of speech and language

A5. Language and speech characteristics and their development across the lifespan

A6. Phonologic, morphologic, syntactic, and pragmatic aspects of human communication associated with hearing impairment

A7. Effects of hearing loss on communication and educational, vocational, social, and psychological functioning

A8. Effects of pharmacologic and teratogenic agents on the auditory and vestibular systems

A9. Patient characteristics (e.g., age, demographics, cultural and linguistic diversity, medical history and status, cognitive status, and physical and sensory abilities) and how they relate to clinical services

A10. Pathologies related to hearing and balance and their medical diagnosis and treatment

A11. Principles, methods, and applications of psychometrics

A12. Principles, methods, and applications of psychoacoustics

A13. Instrumentation and bioelectrical hazards

A14. Physical characteristics and measurement of electric and other nonacoustic stimuli

A15. Assistive technology

A16. Effects of cultural diversity and family systems on professional practice

A17. American Sign Language and other visual communication systems

A18. Principles and practices of research, including experimental design, statistical methods, and application to clinical populations

A19. Legal and ethical practices (e.g., standards for professional conduct, patient rights, credentialing, and legislative and regulatory mandates)

A20. Health care and educational delivery systems

A21. Universal precautions and infectious/contagious diseases

The applicant must have knowledge of and skills in the following:

A22. Oral and written forms of communication

A23. Principles, methods, and applications of acoustics (e.g., basic parameters of sound, principles of acoustics as related to speech sounds, sound/noise measurement and analysis, and calibration of audiometric equipment), as applicable to:

    a.   Occupational and industrial environments

    b.   Community noise

    c.   Classroom and other educational environments

    d.   Workplace environments

A24. The use of instrumentation according to manufacturer's specifications and recommendations

A25. Determining whether instrumentation is in calibration according to accepted standards

A26. Principles and applications of counseling

A27. Use of interpreters and translators for both spoken and visual communication

A28. Management and business practices, including but not limited to cost analysis, budgeting, coding and reimbursement, and patient management

A29. Consultation with professionals in related and/or allied service areas

Standard IV-B: Prevention and Identification

The applicant must have the knowledge and skills necessary to do the following:

B1.   Implement activities that prevent and identify dysfunction in hearing and communication, balance, and other auditory-related systems

B2.   Promote hearing wellness, as well as the prevention of hearing loss and protection of hearing function by designing, implementing, and coordinating universal newborn hearing screening, school screening, community hearing, and occupational conservation and identification programs

B3.   Screen individuals for hearing impairment and disability/handicap using clinically appropriate, culturally sensitive, and age- and site-specific screening measures

B4.   Screen individuals for speech and language impairments and other factors affecting communication function using clinically appropriate, culturally sensitive, and age- and site-specific screening measures

B5.   Educate individuals on potential causes and effects of vestibular loss

B6.   Identify individuals at risk for balance problems and falls who require further vestibular assessment and/or treatment or referral for other professional services

Standard IV-C: Assessment

The applicant must have knowledge of and skills in the following:

C1. Measuring and interpreting sensory and motor evoked potentials, electromyography, and other electrodiagnostic tests for purposes of neurophysiologic intraoperative monitoring and cranial nerve assessment

C2. Assessing individuals with suspected disorders of hearing, communication, balance, and related systems

C3. Evaluating information from appropriate sources and obtaining a case history to facilitate assessment planning

C4. Performing otoscopy for appropriate audiological assessment/management decisions, determining the need for cerumen removal, and providing a basis for medical referral

C5. Conducting and interpreting behavioral and/or electrophysiological methods to assess hearing thresholds and auditory neural function

C6. Conducting and interpreting behavioral and/or electrophysiological methods to assess balance and related systems

C7. Conducting and interpreting otoacoustic emissions and acoustic immitance (reflexes)

C8. Evaluating auditory-related processing disorders

C9. Evaluating functional use of hearing

C10. Preparing a report, including interpreting data, summarizing findings, generating recommendations, and developing an audiological treatment/management plan

C11. Referring to other professions, agencies, and/or consumer organizations

Standard IV-D: Intervention (Treatment)

The applicant must have knowledge of and skills in the following:

D1. The provision of intervention services (treatment) to individuals with hearing loss, balance disorders, and other auditory dysfunction that compromises receptive and expressive communication

D2. Development of a culturally appropriate, audiological rehabilitative management plan that includes, when appropriate, the following:

   a. Evaluation, selection, verification, validation, and dispensing of hearing aids, sensory aids, hearing-assistive devices, alerting systems, and captioning devices, and educating the consumer and family/caregivers in the use of and adjustment to such technology

   b. Determination of candidacy of persons with hearing loss for cochlear implants and other implantable sensory devices and provision of fitting, mapping, and audiological rehabilitation to optimize device use

   c. Counseling relating to psychosocial aspects of hearing loss and other auditory dysfunction and processes to enhance communication competence

    d. Provision of comprehensive audiological treatment for persons with hearing loss or other auditory dysfunction, including but not exclusive to communication strategies, auditory training, speech reading, and visual communication systems

D3. Determination of candidacy for vestibular and balance rehabilitation therapy to persons with vestibular and balance impairments

D4. Treatment and audiological management of tinnitus

D5. Provision of treatment services for infants and children with hearing loss; collaboration/consultation with early interventionists, school-based professionals, and other service providers regarding development of intervention plans (i.e., individualized education programs and/or individualized family service plans)

D6. Management of the selection, purchase, installation, and evaluation of large-area amplification systems

D7. Evaluation of the efficacy of intervention (treatment) services

Standard IV-E: Advocacy/Consultation

The applicant must have knowledge of and skills in the following:

E1. Educating and advocating for communication needs of all individuals that may include advocating for the programmatic needs, rights, and funding of services for those with hearing loss, other auditory dysfunction, or vestibular disorders

E2. Consulting about accessibility for persons with hearing loss and other auditory dysfunction in public and private buildings, programs, and services

E3. Identifying underserved populations and promoting access to care

Standard IV-F: Education/Research/Administration

The applicant must have knowledge of and skills in the following:

F1. Measuring functional outcomes, consumer satisfaction, efficacy, effectiveness, and efficiency of practices and programs to maintain and improve the quality of audiological services

F2. Applying research findings in the provision of patient care (evidence-based practice)

F3. Critically evaluating and appropriately implementing new techniques and technologies supported by research-based evidence

F4. Administering clinical programs and providing supervision of professionals as well as support personnel

F5. Identifying internal programmatic needs and developing new programs

F6. Maintaining or establishing links with external programs, including but not limited to education programs, government programs, and philanthropic agencies

STANDARD V: ASSESSMENT

Applicants for certification must demonstrate successful achievement of the knowledge and skills delineated in Standard IV by means of both formative and summative assessments.

Standard V-A: Formative Assessment

The applicant must meet the education program's requirements for demonstrating satisfactory performance through ongoing formative assessment of knowledge and skills.

Implementation   Applicants and program faculties should use the ongoing assessment to help the applicant achieve requisite knowledge and skills. Thus, assessments should be followed by implementation strategies for acquisition of knowledge and skills.

Standard V-B: Summative Assessment

The applicant must pass the national examination adopted by ASHA for purposes of certification in audiology.

Implementation   Evidence of a passing score on the ASHA-approved national examination in audiology must be submitted to the ASHA National Office by the testing agency administering the examination. Acceptable exam results are those submitted for initial certification in audiology that have been obtained no more than 5 years prior to the submission of the certification application and no more than 2 years after the application for certification is received by the Certification Unit of the ASHA National Office.

STANDARD VI: MAINTENANCE OF CERTIFICATION

Demonstration of continued professional development is mandated for maintenance of the CCC in audiology. The renewal period will be 3 years. This standard will apply to all certificate holders, regardless of the date of initial certification.

Once certification is awarded, maintenance of that certification is dependent upon accumulation of the requisite professional development hours every 3 years. Payment of annual dues and/or certification fees is also a requirement of certification maintenance. A certificate holder whose dues and/or fees are in arrears on August 31 will have allowed their certification to expire on that date.

Individuals who hold the CCC in audiology must accumulate 30 contact hours of professional development over the 3-year period and must submit a compliance form in order to meet this standard. Individuals will be subject to random review of their professional development activities.

If certification maintenance requirements are not met, certification will lapse. Reinstatement of certification will be required, and certification reinstatement standards in effect at the time of submission of the reinstatement application must be met.

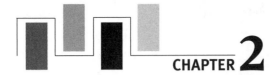

CHAPTER 2

Ethical Practice in Communication Disorders

Rhea Paul and Paul W. Cascella

CHAPTER OBJECTIVES

After reading this chapter, students will be able to

- Discuss ethical issues in communication disorders
- List statements of principles for ethical practice
- Describe infection control procedures
- Define *conflicts of interest* and *misrepresentation*

CASE EXAMPLE 1

Michelle is a speech-language pathologist (SLP) at a local rehabilitation center in a busy urban New England community. Because of ongoing expansion by the rehabilitation agency over the past 5 years, the speech-language pathology department has employed speech therapy assistants to help manage the clinical caseload. As a supervisor, Michelle has found that these assistants are dedicated and able to implement treatment plans and procedures that she has taught them. Of late, Michelle has found that her own job has spread her thin across agency committees, task forces, and the new satellite birth-to-3 program across town. As a result, she finds that she is less often able to directly supervise the speech assistants and she relies on telephone and e-mail consultation to review client data sheets and case notes. After talking with Nicole, one of her especially talented speech assistants, Michelle has allowed Nicole to modify a treatment plan for three adults with aphasia even though Michelle has not directly seen these patients in the past 4 weeks.

CASE EXAMPLE 2

Tom is an audiologist who works at a local teaching hospital that contracts with four skilled nursing facilities. In this contract, residents participate in audiological evaluations and follow-up, usually the first and third Tuesdays of every month. On any of these days, Tom may see up to 20 people from any or all of the four nursing facilities. On one particularly busy day, Tom has a list of residents who are scheduled for appointments, but he loses track of which patients kept their appointments, which residents canceled, and who was added at the last minute. At the end of the day, Tom sits down to write his case notes on the residents. Unfortunately, because the day was so busy, Tom cannot be sure which residents were seen and which had canceled. When he goes to complete billing, he accidentally bills for services for two residents who were not actually seen that day.

CASE EXAMPLE 3

Adam is an SLP who works for a local public preschool. Whenever a new student is seen for a speech-language evaluation, Adam collects case history information, including medical information about the child. During a recent evaluation, Adam learned that Jasmine, a 3-year-old girl with specific language impairment, was born prematurely and had prenatal exposure to alcohol and cocaine. Adam is also an assistant coach for the high school baseball team in the same public school district. That afternoon, he mentions Jasmine's name to one of the other coaches and comments on her prenatal exposure to substances.

As a beginning clinician in speech-language pathology or audiology, you may confront ethical situations not unlike the ones described for Michelle, Tom, and Adam. Each of us has our own personal standards and perceptions of ethical behavior. When thinking about the term **ethics,** it is common to consider the moral and/or civil codes of conduct for a particular person, situation, community, religious group, organization, or society. These codes evolve from a philosophy of human interaction that values behaviors that are personally or collectively regarded as good, honest, proper, and respectable. Each of us has a set of personal ethics that have been formed from our upbringing, acculturation, life experiences, personal choices, and education. As children, we likely heard our parents stress that certain behaviors were right or wrong. Some of us were taught to follow the Golden Rule (i.e., "Do unto others..."), to treat older people

Table 2.1. Reasons for a professional code of ethics

Consumer protection and client welfare are safeguarded.
The professional reputation of the discipline is maintained.
Professional behavior is regulated.
Objective guidance is available for ethical dilemmas and deliberation.
Practitioners can rely on an external code in addition to their own values.
Clients have an objective standard against which to evaluate their clinician's actions.

with respect, to tell the truth, to play fairly in sports competitions, and to never cheat on exams. As adults, we consciously choose our own individual ethics and values. These guide us to interact with our families and friends in what we personally consider the right way to behave; we are motivated also by our sense of duty, responsibility, and obligation. Personal ethics are important because they enable us to make choices about our own behavior. Personal ethics differ from person to person, and not everyone with similar ethical tenets applies them in the same way. Therefore, many professions abide by a set of **professional ethics** that establish right and wrong actions in serving clients in the workplace. Professional ethics publicly state the common core values and collective obligation shared by people in a particular discipline. Though we each bring our personal ethics to clinical practice, the American Speech-Language-Hearing Association (ASHA) and the American Academy of Audiology (AAA) have codified a set of standards for ethical behavior. Each organization has its own **code of ethics** that includes tangible expectations that define acceptable conduct and conscientious judgment in the practice of speech-language pathology and audiology. As members of the communication disorders discipline, each of us is expected to accept these tenets and apply them to clinical settings. A professional code of ethics enables us to look toward a common set of core values when confronted with ethical dilemmas in the workplace. Table 2.1 gives a list of reasons for a professional code of ethics.

This chapter introduces you to the ethical standards that are the foundation of clinical practice in communication disorders. Ethical principles are presented and case situations that may raise ethical dilemmas are described. As you read the examples of ethical dilemmas, take a moment to pause to consider your personal response. Both the ASHA Code of Ethics and the AAA Code of Ethics are reprinted in the appendixes at the end of this chapter (see Appendix 2A and 2B, respectively). An overview of the two codes of ethics follows.

THE AMERICAN SPEECH-LANGUAGE-HEARING ASSOCIATION CODE OF ETHICS

The ASHA Code of Ethics (ASHA, 2010) applies to people who are already credentialed (i.e., the Certificate of Clinical Competence–Speech-Language Pathology, CCC-SLP; the Certificate of Clinical Competence–Audiology, CCC-A), candidates in the process of earning credentials (i.e., students; Clinical Fellowship [CF] participants), and members of the organization. The ASHA Code of Ethics consists of three parts: the Preamble, Principles of Ethics, and Rules of Ethics. The Preamble introduces the philosophy of ethical service delivery and the overall content, principles, and structure of the ASHA Code of Ethics. The Principles of Ethics section is divided into four parts, each of which provides a broad statement about ethical conduct. Principle of Ethics I focuses on the professional's responsibility to safeguard the welfare of clients and research participants. Principle of Ethics II relates to the responsibility of providing the highest level of service possible. Principle of Ethics III outlines standards related to interaction with the public, and Principle of Ethics IV outlines standards and responsibilities to the profession. Within each principle, Rules of Ethics articulate acceptable and restricted actions. In matters where ethical violations may occur, ASHA has a Board of Ethics that handles the adjudication of alleged violations (http://www.asha.org/About/governance/committees/Board-of-Ethics).

THE AMERICAN ACADEMY OF AUDIOLOGY CODE OF ETHICS

The AAA Code of Ethics (AAA, 2011) applies to current and potential members of this organization. The AAA Code of Ethics consists of two parts:

- Statements of principles and rules

- Procedures for management of alleged violations

The Statements of Principles and Rules section highlights specific actions deemed ethically acceptable to audiology practice. The Procedures for the Management of Alleged Violations section outlines the due process format when violations are suspected and identifies the penalties that can be assigned. This section also outlines record keeping, confidentiality, and public disclosure.

ETHICAL PRINCIPLES IN PROFESSIONAL PRACTICE

To begin our discussion of ethics, we start by considering some of the common core principles shared by AAA and ASHA.

The Principle of Safeguarding Client Welfare

At the core of ethical practice is a guarantee that clinicians will act to ensure the rights, dignity, protection, and autonomy of clients and participants in research. Let's look at some concrete examples of how clinicians can guarantee client welfare.

Beneficence and Nonmaleficence *Beneficence* means that professionals promote the interests and welfare of others, whereas *nonmaleficence* means that professionals deliberately avoid inflicting potential or actual harm (e.g., emotional harm, physical harm) on clients. These principles compel professionals to monitor their own behavior as well as that of caregivers who interact with clients. For example, we are expected to report situations in which we perceive that children, adults, or elders may be victims of physical, emotional, and/or sexual abuse, as well as neglect by their caregivers.

Nondiscrimination How would you feel at parent–teacher night when you learn that Timothy, a 7-year-old boy who stutters, has two mothers for parents? Or, how would you react when another child's parent asks, "Have you accepted Jesus as your personal savior?" How might you feel when you are assigned to work with a class of preschoolers, one of whom is being raised by her grandparents because her mother is incarcerated? Or, maybe one of your hospital outpatient clients is a transgender woman who wants speech therapy so that her voice sounds more like that of a female. These may be difficult situations for you based on your own personal values; nonetheless, every client's right to quality services is guaranteed because clinicians must practice nondiscrimination. This means that clinicians do not exclude clients from their professional practice for reasons other than the person's potential to benefit from our services. Ethical practice is compromised when a clinician discriminates by making a clinical decision based on a client's race, gender, ethnicity, religion, age, national origin, sexual orientation, or disability status.

Referral   Another example of securing a client's welfare is the use of referral. This occurs when an SLP or audiologist feels that a client presents a communication disorder beyond the clinician's level of expertise. Professional referrals safeguard a client's right to appropriate clinical services. Let us take our example of the transgendered client. A referral would be appropriate if a clinician has no experience in gender-appropriate voice treatment approaches and thus would be unable to provide that person with competent voice services. In contrast, when we receive a referral, we are expected to exercise independent judgment about the content, frequency, and duration of services that may be recommended. In other words, outside influences should not interfere with evaluation and treatment decisions. For example, an audiologist may receive a physician referral to fit a client with a hearing aid because the physician noted that client had some difficulty hearing case history questions during a physical exam. Before proceeding with a hearing aid, the audiologist should first complete an independent hearing evaluation to assess client need and/or potential to benefit from such equipment. For either type of referral (i.e., by the clinician or to the clinician), we are prohibited from receiving a commission or gift that could influence our professional practice and decision making.

Informed Consent   Informed consent means that clients are told about their speech-language or hearing condition and are informed about the relative strengths, weaknesses, and risks (i.e., side effects) associated with a recommended plan of action or inaction. For people who are unable to authorize legal consent (i.e., children, people with an intellectual disability), this must be obtained from family members or legal guardians. With informed consent, the clinician enables the client to exercise autonomy during the course of treatment. This principle also guarantees that clients can voluntarily withdraw from a treatment protocol at any point during its course. For example, think about how you would react to a middle school child who decides that he no longer wants stuttering therapy even though his speech continues to include blocks, prolongations, and repetitions? How might you attempt to guarantee his welfare if he voluntarily withdraws from treatment?

Confidentiality   In daily practice, we often hear clinical and personal information about clients (e.g., health status, medical history, educational background, cognitive status, financial status, family structure). Sometimes, it may be very tempting to share this information with people not affiliated with the client's treatment protocol. The principle of confidentiality means that professionals share privileged information only with people directly responsible for client management and/or care and only for purposes related to the client's welfare. As professionals, we are bound to neither use privileged information for gossip within a work setting nor repeat any confidential information outside of the clinical environment. This requires some self-control on the clinician's part because it is too easy to slip into talking about clients in the teacher's lounge or hospital elevator when others, who should not be privy to the information discussed, may be within earshot. In addition, a federal law (the Health Insurance Portability and Accountability Act [HIPAA] of 1996, PL 104-191) mandates that clients have rights and protections regarding how and to whom their health information is shared. This information includes medical records and conversations between clients and health care providers. Client confidentiality may become an ethical dilemma when precedents override the client's right to confidentiality in law or other compelling circumstances. This might arise, for example, if you are working with an adult with aphasia who expresses in therapy that he wants to kill himself. It might come up too, if a mother confides to you that her child's stepfather has repeatedly hit the child. Should these statements compel you to breach your client's right to confidentiality?

Prognosis and Cures   Implicit in ethical practice is that professionals must not imply or guarantee cures. Instead, clinicians are expected to make a reasonable prognosis, or a statement that describes the likelihood that a benefit will be gained from treatment. If a person is not likely to benefit from initial or ongoing treatment, intervention should not be recommended or continued. In practice, this means that we do not recommend treatment for every person who has a speech-language or hearing disorder. Instead we exercise professional judgment about the likelihood that treatment will yield a client benefit. For example, how would you handle a situation in which family members insist on speech therapy services for a person with advanced dementia residing in a nursing facility?

Infection Control   Clinicians are expected to safeguard their clients and themselves from infectious diseases by maintaining infection control and prevention procedures. Hygienic precautions usually include hand washing and the use of barriers (e.g., gloves, masks). In addition, clinicians are expected to disinfect equipment and know the proper procedures for the disposal of bodily fluids (e.g., saliva, blood). All clinicians are expected to practice universal precautions, even if the clinicians do not work in a medical setting. In other words, universal precautions apply to preschools and schools, child care settings, home health, university clinics, birth-to-3 programs, group homes, and private practices. For example, it would not be remarkable for you to handle bodily fluids if you are working with an infant-and-toddler early intervention group. Table 2.2 shows a list of common infection control procedures.

Table 2.2.　Infection control procedures

Hand washing	You must vigorously lather and rub your hands, wrists, and forearms with warm water and liquid antibacterial soap before and after each clinical session.
Disposable gloves	You must wear disposable gloves when you have contact with clients' bodily fluids or substances (e.g., saliva, blood, cerumen, vomit).
Contaminated items	Consumable items (e.g., gloves, tongue depressors) that come into contact with clients' bodily fluids or substances must be disposed of into a plastic bag and tied securely. Nonconsumable items (e.g., eartips, specula) must be decontaminated.
Decontamination/disinfecting	Disinfectant must be thoroughly applied to all nonconsumable items, clinical materials, and clinical furniture. A solution of one-tenth bleach and nine-tenths water is recommended.
Illness	Clinical sessions should be rescheduled when either the clinician or the client has an infectious illness or condition.
Vaccinations	Clinicians should seriously consider vaccination for hepatitis B, rubella, and the mumps. Clinicians are also encouraged to have a yearly tuberculosis test.

The Principle of Competence

Another core ethical principle for audiologists and SLPs is **competent practice.** This occurs when a clinician provides effective diagnostic procedures, accurate prognosis, and appropriate therapy strategies for the particular disorder, as well as an ongoing monitoring of client progress and outcomes. Both ASHA and AAA have several practice guidelines that enable clinicians to evaluate their own professional competence. For example, ASHA has preferred practice documents for specific populations—including assessment and intervention for infants and toddlers—as well as for swallowing, preschool speech-language and communication, autism, assessment and intervention, and speech-language screenings for children and adults (http://www.asha.org/Practice-Portal). Clinicians can refer to these documents for guidance about competent practice.

Ethical practice obligates each of us to understand clearly our own strengths and limitations and dictates that we practice only in those areas in which we regard ourselves as competent. For example, how can you address the communication needs of a child with autism spectrum disorder if you have no previous experience working with this condition? Or, what if you find yourself in a situation in which you have been laid off from your hospital adult neurogenics position and find that the only local job openings are in home-based birth-to-3 services? Is it ethical to provide services when you do not have prior experience in a particular clinical setting? Many audiologists and SLPs become specialists for a particular population, disorder, and/or service delivery model. Specialization occurs with in-depth experience, advanced knowledge, and training beyond the initial credential. Whether a specialist or a generalist, each of us is expected to be a lifelong learner who maintains clinical competency through continuing education. **Continuing education** enables clinicians to update their skills by keeping up with the latest trends and advances in their discipline. This can be achieved by reading textbooks and journal articles, attending workshops, taking a course at a local university, shadowing professional colleagues, and participating in research activities.

Table 2.3.   Contemporary issues that may influence ethical competence

Competition	Clinicians must balance ethics with competition for employment and the market share (i.e., competitive bidding, marketing, advertising).
Service eligibility	Clinicians must balance client-specific data (i.e., prognosis) with federal and state education and health care regulations to decide who is likely to benefit from clinical services and how services should be provided.
Discharge	Clinicians must be able to carefully balance the ethical issues surrounding client discharge, especially when the clinician's judgment disagrees with the client's judgment, organizational policies, and/or funding resources.
Resources	When resources are lacking in public education (e.g., budget, shortage of personnel), clinicians must continue to act competently.
Managed care	Clinicians must balance ongoing changes in medical reimbursement and the cost of health care with the needs presented by clients.
Scope of practice	Clinicians must stay current on and be judicious of the latest technologies within clinical practice.
Paraprofessionals	Clinicians must be able to carefully judge the utilization of speech assistants and aides in service delivery.

Ethical clinicians judge their own fitness for providing services and withdraw from practice if their own professional conduct is influenced by substance abuse or related health conditions. Similarly, it is expected that clinicians will monitor the ethical compliance of other SLPs and audiologists. Ethical compliance relies on clinicians who keep up-to-date on contemporary issues that influence clinical practice. Table 2.3 provides examples of several issues that uniquely challenge us to balance our ethics and competency.

The Principle of Acting without a Conflict of Interest

A **conflict of interest** occurs when an SLP or audiologist receives personal or financial gain from clients or manufacturers that compromises professional judgment because there are strings and/or expectations attached. When a conflict of interest arises, clinicians can lose their sense of objectivity and their decision making becomes clouded. Examples of potential conflicts of interest include self-dealing (utilizing commercial enterprises in which you have a financial stake) and self-referral (referring patients between two work settings, both of which employ the same clinician). A conflict of interest might also occur when a clinician draws cases for private practice from his or her primary place of employment. This can occur especially when school-based clinicians provide private services to children during the summer recess. In and of itself, doing so is not a conflict of interest so long as the school administration is aware of these services and clients are fully informed about service options and costs.

The Principle of Acting without Misrepresentation

 CASE EXAMPLE 4

Adele is an SLP at a local community hospital whose staff are developing a marketing plan to attract more business. Because there are many community-based speech-language-hearing providers, an advertising strategy that "catches the eye" is being sought. After a morning meeting, it has been decided that more clients will be drawn to this hospital if Adele's social skills program for children with autism is advertised as one of the best in the state. Adele does not feel right about this decision even though she believes the program is effective. Adele knows that she has not done efficacy research or published her results for professional review.

Later that day, Adele participates in a meeting with hospital administration where it is noted that patient billable hours have decreased with the implementation of a new insurance reimbursement system. At the meeting, Adele is informed that without this reimbursement, the speech pathology staff are likely to lose personnel. Adele also learns that particular diagnoses are guaranteed reimbursement, as are persons for whom the prognosis for improvement is rated "good." Although it is never directly stated, Adele feels as though she is encouraged to reconsider the diagnostic criteria for particular diagnoses, as well as the factors that relate to prognosis. (*Source*: American Speech-Language-Hearing Association.)

How would you respond if you were Adele? Because of her morning meeting, she is concerned that the hospital advertising strategy may be a form of misrepresentation. **Misrepresentation** is a type of dishonesty that occurs when truth is distorted or falsified. In this case, misrepresentation occurs because there is an exaggerated description of Adele's social skills program. Another example of misrepresentation can occur if clinicians exaggerate their own personal levels of training, experience, and expertise or that of persons who provide clinical services (e.g., CF participants, graduate students, speech assistants, aides). Clients should be specifically informed about the educational level of the person providing services.

Because of her afternoon meeting, Adele continues to be concerned about misrepresentation. Here, she is being asked to ignore competent clinical diagnostic procedures (i.e., criteria, prognosis) to secure insurance reimbursement. In effect, Adele would be misrepresenting the client's status by making a diagnosis and a prognosis solely to maintain the financial solvency of her employer.

Finally, another form of misrepresentation occurs when a clinician unfairly influences client decisions by "stacking the deck" a particular way, such as by deliberately leading the client to a decision in the clinician's, not the client's, best interest. Ethically, clients are guaranteed access to all the information necessary for making decisions about their care and rehabilitation. We are not supposed to mislead a client by omitting information that would otherwise be helpful in client decision making. For example, for clients with a hearing loss, audiologists should provide information about the variety of hearing aids (e.g., brand, type, cost, size) that might be beneficial to a particular client.

Ethical Practice within Professional Supervision and Instruction

Audiologists and SLPs often supervise other people as part of their job description. We may supervise people who are already credentialed (i.e., persons with a CCC, teaching certification, or state license), CF participants, student clinicians, or speech assistants and aides. Clinical supervisors should model ethical behavior, and they are expected to monitor the ethical compliance of the persons they supervise. When an unethical behavior is suspected or observed, the supervisor must take specific action to prevent violation of ethical standards, whether or not the person supervised is credentialed or an ASHA or AAA member.

For CF participants, it is expected that the supervisor will make a good-faith effort to meet the terms (i.e., expectations, follow-up) outlined in the contract (e.g., http://www.asha.org/Certification/Certification-Standards-for-SLP–Clinical-Fellowship). For student clinicians, ASHA guidelines require that supervisors hold the appropriate CCC credential, provide an appropriate amount and type of diagnostic and clinical supervision, and provide ongoing written and oral feedback to the student. ASHA also has practice guidelines that outline the supervision requirements of speech-language pathology assistants (http://www.asha.org/Practice-Portal/Professional-Issues/Speech-Language-Pathology-Assistants).

Our code of ethics also tells us that although certain tasks may be delegated to students, clinical fellows, assistants, and paraprofessionals, responsibility for care of the client remains with the certified professional. As SLPs and audiologists, it is incumbent upon us to delegate only tasks for which support personnel are adequately trained and credentialed. Moreover, even when doing appropriate levels of assessment and treatment, support personnel must be adequately supervised to ensure client welfare.

Ethical Behavior within Professional Relationships

Clinicians are expected to maintain **professional relationships** with other communication specialists, as well as with personnel from other professions. There are many ways to demonstrate collegial behavior. First, we can work to understand the nature of related disciplines and the particular job functions of our teaching, medical, and allied health colleagues. Second, professional behavior includes a give-and-take open communication style so that all team members have the opportunity to discuss pertinent issues in a client's treatment plan. Third, education and rehabilitation professionals are expected to work in a climate of mutual respect and cooperation by avoiding personal conflict. This is especially true given recent efforts in interprofessional service provision, inclusive education, and team teaching models.

THE IMPLEMENTATION OF ETHICAL PRACTICE FOR CLINICIANS

With a foundation in ethical principles, it is important that practicing and future clinicians have an understanding of how to judge their own compliance with ethical practice standards. All clinicians benefit from having a framework in which ethical situations can be discussed and debated. One such approach is the **Ethics Calibration Quick Test** (ECQT; Lubinki & Frattali, 1994; see Figure 2.1). Using the ECQT, we are able to analyze the ethical propriety of a situation by considering the ethical conflict, the values that are involved, the evidence, the possible plans of action, and the decision-making process. After you review the ECQT, return to Case Examples 1, 2, and 3 at the beginning of the chapter to make a judgment about Michelle's, Tom's, and Adam's ethical compliance. In Case Example 1, you should be concerned about the degree of supervision Michelle provides to the speech assistants and whether she should

1. What is the problem/conflict/dilemma?
   Is it a professional violation, a legal violation, or both?

2. What values are in conflict?
   Under these circumstances, what do I value the most?
   Will my feelings interfere with my judgment?

3. What evidence is provided by the parties involved?
   Whose evidence is most convincing?
   Is there a consistency in the facts?
   Have I heard all of the facts?
   What is acceptable practice in this situation?
   Who is most believable?
   Have I considered other viewpoints?

4. What courses of action can I take or recommend?
   Do I need outside consultation?
   Have I considered the social, cultural, and political impact of the consequences?
   Have I considered the short-term and long-term impact of the consequences?

5. In whose best interest is the decision?
   Will the decision be fair to all parties concerned?
   If yes, why? If not, why?

6. How will the decision make me feel about myself today and tomorrow?

Figure 2.1. Using the Ethics Calibration Quick Test, clinicians are able to analyze the ethical propriety of a situation by considering the ethical conflict, the values that are involved, the evidence, the possible plans of action, and the decision-making process. (From Lubinski/Hudson. *Professional issues in speech-language pathology and audiology*, 4E. © 2013 Delmar Learning, a part of Cengage Learning, Inc. Reproduced by permission. http://www.cengage.com/permissions)

allow a speech assistant, even a talented one, to modify a treatment program. For Michelle, this situation calls for the hiring of another SLP and a review of ASHA's guidelines about the supervision of speech-language pathology assistants (ASHA, 2004b). In Case Example 2, Tom has billed for services not rendered and has unintentionally committed fraud. Also, because Tom cannot be certain about which clients received which services, his ability to keep accurate records should be questioned. Tom needs to develop a more accurate and reliable system for keeping records. In Case Example 3, Adam needs to be careful about client confidentiality and privileged information. Even though other baseball coaches are employed by the school district, there is no reason for them to be told privileged information about a child. Adam needs to review the school district's policy on educational confidentiality.

Another model for ethical decision making comes from Chabon and Morris (2004; see Figure 2.2), who proposed a consensus model for ethical decisions. In this model, the clinician is encouraged to evaluate the specific facts and values so as to specifically state the ethical dilemma. Then, the analysis includes the possible courses of action and the degree to which these are consistent with professional standards, social rules, and self-interests.

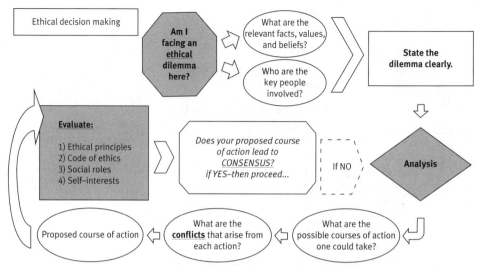

Figure 2.2. A consensus model for ethical decisions. (Reprinted by permission from Chabon, S., & Morris, J.F. [2004, February 17]. A consensus model for making ethical decisions in a less-than-ideal world. *The ASHA Leader.* Copyright 2004 by American Speech-Language-Hearing Association. All rights reserved.)

Ethical Practice Review by the American Academy of Audiology and the American Speech-Language-Hearing Association

In addition to our own evaluation of ethical scenarios, both AAA and ASHA have centralized committees that address ethical situations. The AAA committee is called the Ethical Practice Board, and the ASHA committee is called the Board

CASE EXAMPLE 5

Ms. Robertson, a 78-year-old, is hospitalized after a hip fracture. A speech-language consultation is requested because her physician is concerned about her cognitive abilities. Scott, a student clinician, conducts the evaluation. He observes mild cognitive deficits, but he also notes that Ms. Robertson coughs immediately after taking sips of water and that she has a wet voice quality for several minutes after drinking. From the medical record, Scott notes that she had pneumonia on admission to the hospital and has been treated for pneumonia at least three times in the past 9 months.

Scott discusses his observations with his supervisor and recommends a swallowing evaluation. His supervisor suggests Ms. Robertson coughs because she is recovering from pneumonia. Furthermore, the supervisor says they were consulted for a cognitive assessment, and thus his observations about her swallowing are inappropriate to include in his report. Scott is concerned about the patient but unsure of his role as a student and questions how to interpret his own observations.[1]

---

[1] From Blake, A. (1999). When student and supervisor disagree about patient care. *ASHA, 41*(6), 65. © 1999 American Speech-Language-Hearing Association. Reprinted by permission.

of Ethics. One role of these groups is to develop position statements that further define particular ethical rules already cited in each code. A second role of these committees is to handle the adjudication process when violations are alleged. Through a due process format, complaints are heard, evidence can be admitted, sanctions or penalties are applied, and appeals are processed. A third role of these committees is to educate ASHA and AAA members about ethics. One way the ASHA committee educates its members is by placing teaching situations in a periodic column in *The ASHA Leader* that discusses case situations that highlight specific ethical actions, for example, Case Example 5. As a final task, try using the ECQT or the consensus model to analyze this case example.

CONCLUSION

By introducing you to ethical practice, this chapter may lead you to think about your own personal ethics and the degree to which they are consistent with the professional ethics set by ASHA and AAA. Ethical guidelines will enable you to protect the rights and welfare of your clients and participants in research. Professional codes of ethics provide you with an objective set of standards against which to compare your daily professional actions. By adhering to standards and ethical principles, we are collectively able to promote our clients' welfare, as well as safeguard our own professional reputations and those of the professions of speech-language pathology and audiology.

STUDY QUESTIONS

1. Why is it important to have ethical standards in professional practice?
2. Give three examples of how an SLP or audiologist can safeguard a client's welfare.
3. Identify at least two ways in which a clinician can maintain his or her competence.
4. Describe at least three external factors that influence clinical competence. Why is it important that a clinician understand the influence of these factors?
5. Define and give an example of each of the following terms: *misrepresentation, conflict of interest, nondiscrimination, infection control, informed consent,* and *referral.*
6. What is the role of the clinical supervisor in ethical practice?
7. Why is it necessary for ASHA and AAA to have committees that review ethical standards and actions?
8. What revisions might your recommend to the ASHA or AAA Code of Ethics? Why?

REFERENCES

American Academy of Audiology. (2011). *Code of ethics.* Houston, TX: Author.

American Speech-Language-Hearing Association. (2010). *Code of ethics* [Ethics]. Retrieved from http://www.asha.org/policy

American Speech-Language-Hearing Association. (1993). *Ethics: Resources for*

professional preparation and practice. Rockville, MD: Author.

Blake, A. (1999). When student and supervisor disagree about patient care. *ASHA, 41*(6), 65.

Chabon, S., & Morris, J.F. (2004, February 17). A consensus model for making ethical decisions in a less-than-ideal world. *The ASHA Leader.* Retrieved from http://www.asha.org/Publications/leader/2004/040217/040217e.htm

Health Insurance Portability and Accountability Act (HIPAA) of 1996, PL 104-191, 42 U.S.C. §§ 201 *et seq.*

Lubinki, R., & Frattali, C. (Eds.). (1994). *Professional issues in speech-language pathology and audiology* (1st ed.). Clifton Park, NY: Thomson Delmar Learning.

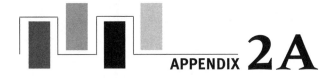

APPENDIX 2A

ASHA Code of Ethics (ASHA, 2010)

Preamble

The preservation of the highest standards of integrity and ethical principles is vital to the responsible discharge of obligations by speech-language pathologists, audiologists, and speech, language, and hearing scientists. This Code of Ethics sets forth the fundamental principles and rules considered essential to this purpose.

Every individual who is (a) a member of the American Speech-Language-Hearing Association, whether certified or not, (b) a nonmember holding the Certificate of Clinical Competence from the Association, (c) an applicant for membership or certification, or (d) a Clinical Fellow seeking to fulfill standards for certification shall abide by this Code of Ethics.

Any violation of the spirit and purpose of this Code shall be considered unethical. Failure to specify any particular responsibility or practice in this Code of Ethics shall not be construed as denial of the existence of such responsibilities or practices.

The fundamentals of ethical conduct are described by Principles of Ethics and by Rules of Ethics as they relate to the responsibility to persons served, the public, speech-language pathologists, audiologists, and speech, language, and hearing scientists, and to the conduct of research and scholarly activities.

Principles of Ethics, aspirational and inspirational in nature, form the underlying moral basis for the Code of Ethics. Individuals shall observe these principles as affirmative obligations under all conditions of professional activity.

Rules of Ethics are specific statements of minimally acceptable professional conduct or of prohibitions and are applicable to all individuals.

Principle of Ethics I

Individuals shall honor their responsibility to hold paramount the welfare of persons they serve professionally or who are participants in research and scholarly activities, and they shall treat animals involved in research in a humane manner.

From American Speech-Language-Hearing Association. (2010). *Code of ethics* [Ethics]. Retrieved from http://www.asha.org/policy; reprinted by permission. © 2010 American Speech-Language-Hearing Association.

Rules of Ethics

1. Individuals shall provide all services competently.

2. Individuals shall use every resource, including referral when appropriate, to ensure that high-quality service is provided.

3. Individuals shall not discriminate in the delivery of professional services or the conduct of research and scholarly activities on the basis of race or ethnicity, gender, gender identity/gender expression, age, religion, national origin, sexual orientation, or disability.

4. Individuals shall not misrepresent the credentials of assistants, technicians, support personnel, students, Clinical Fellows, or any others under their supervision, and they shall inform those they serve professionally of the name and professional credentials of persons providing services.

5. Individuals who hold the Certificate of Clinical Competence shall not delegate tasks that require the unique skills, knowledge, and judgment that are within the scope of their profession to assistants, technicians, support personnel, or any nonprofessionals over whom they have supervisory responsibility.

6. Individuals who hold the Certificate of Clinical Competence may delegate tasks related to provision of clinical services to assistants, technicians, support personnel, or any other persons only if those services are appropriately supervised, realizing that the responsibility for client welfare remains with the certified individual.

7. Individuals who hold the Certificate of Clinical Competence may delegate tasks related to provision of clinical services that require the unique skills, knowledge, and judgment that are within the scope of practice of their profession to students only if those services are appropriately supervised. The responsibility for client welfare remains with the certified individual.

8. Individuals shall fully inform the persons they serve of the nature and possible effects of services rendered and products dispensed, and they shall inform participants in research about the possible effects of their participation in research conducted.

9. Individuals shall evaluate the effectiveness of services rendered and of products dispensed, and they shall provide services or dispense products only when benefit can reasonably be expected.

10. Individuals shall not guarantee the results of any treatment or procedure, directly or by implication; however, they may make a reasonable statement of prognosis.

11. Individuals shall not provide clinical services solely by correspondence.

12. Individuals may practice by telecommunication (e.g., telehealth/e-health), where not prohibited by law.

13. Individuals shall adequately maintain and appropriately secure records of professional services rendered, research and scholarly activities conducted, and products dispensed, and they shall allow access to these records only when authorized or when required by law.

14. Individuals shall not reveal, without authorization, any professional or personal information about identified persons served professionally or identified participants involved in research and scholarly activities unless doing so is necessary to protect the welfare of the person or of the community or is otherwise required by law.

15. Individuals shall not charge for services not rendered, nor shall they misrepresent services rendered, products dispensed, or research and scholarly activities conducted.

16. Individuals shall enroll and include persons as participants in research or teaching demonstrations only if their participation is voluntary, without coercion, and with their informed consent.

17. Individuals whose professional services are adversely affected by substance abuse or other health-related conditions shall seek professional assistance and, where appropriate, withdraw from the affected areas of practice.

18. Individuals shall not discontinue service to those they are serving without providing reasonable notice.

Principle of Ethics II

Individuals shall honor their responsibility to achieve and maintain the highest level of professional competence and performance.

Rules of Ethics

1. Individuals shall engage in the provision of clinical services only when they hold the appropriate Certificate of Clinical Competence or when they are in the certification process and are supervised by an individual who holds the appropriate Certificate of Clinical Competence.

2. Individuals shall engage in only those aspects of the professions that are within the scope of their professional practice and competence, considering their level of education, training, and experience.

3. Individuals shall engage in lifelong learning to maintain and enhance professional competence and performance.

4. Individuals shall not require or permit their professional staff to provide services or conduct research activities that exceed the staff member's competence, level of education, training, and experience.

5. Individuals shall ensure that all equipment used to provide services or to conduct research and scholarly activities is in proper working order and is properly calibrated.

Principle of Ethics III

Individuals shall honor their responsibility to the public by promoting public understanding of the professions, by supporting the development of services designed to fulfill the unmet needs of the public, and by providing accurate information in all communications involving any aspect of the professions, including the dissemination of research findings and scholarly activities, and the promotion, marketing, and advertising of products and services.

Rules of Ethics

1. Individuals shall not misrepresent their credentials, competence, education, training, experience, or scholarly or research contributions.

2. Individuals shall not participate in professional activities that constitute a conflict of interest.

3. Individuals shall refer those served professionally solely on the basis of the interest of those being referred and not on any personal interest, financial or otherwise.

4. Individuals shall not misrepresent research, diagnostic information, services rendered, results of services rendered, products dispensed, or the effects of products dispensed.

5. Individuals shall not defraud or engage in any scheme to defraud in connection with obtaining payment, reimbursement, or grants for services rendered, research conducted, or products dispensed.

6. Individuals' statements to the public shall provide accurate information about the nature and management of communication disorders, about the professions, about professional services, about products for sale, and about research and scholarly activities.

7. Individuals' statements to the public when advertising, announcing, and marketing their professional services; reporting research results; and

promoting products shall adhere to professional standards and shall not contain misrepresentations.

Principle of Ethics IV

Individuals shall honor their responsibilities to the professions and their relationships with colleagues, students, and members of other professions and disciplines.

Rules of Ethics

1. Individuals shall uphold the dignity and autonomy of the professions, maintain harmonious interprofessional and intraprofessional relationships, and accept the professions' self-imposed standards.

2. Individuals shall prohibit anyone under their supervision from engaging in any practice that violates the Code of Ethics.

3. Individuals shall not engage in dishonesty, fraud, deceit, or misrepresentation.

4. Individuals shall not engage in any form of unlawful harassment, including sexual harassment or power abuse.

5. Individuals shall not engage in any other form of conduct that adversely reflects on the professions or on the individual's fitness to serve persons professionally.

6. Individuals shall not engage in sexual activities with clients, students, or research participants over whom they exercise professional authority or power.

7. Individuals shall assign credit only to those who have contributed to a publication, presentation, or product. Credit shall be assigned in proportion to the contribution and only with the contributor's consent.

8. Individuals shall reference the source when using other persons' ideas, research, presentations, or products in written, oral, or any other media presentation or summary.

9. Individuals' statements to colleagues about professional services, research results, and products shall adhere to prevailing professional standards and shall contain no misrepresentations.

10. Individuals shall not provide professional services without exercising independent professional judgment, regardless of referral source or prescription.

11. Individuals shall not discriminate in their relationships with colleagues, students, and members of other professions and disciplines on the basis of

race or ethnicity, gender, gender identity/gender expression, age, religion, national origin, sexual orientation, or disability.

12. Individuals shall not file or encourage others to file complaints that disregard or ignore facts that would disprove the allegation, nor should the Code of Ethics be used for personal reprisal, as a means of addressing personal animosity, or as a vehicle for retaliation.

13. Individuals who have reason to believe that the Code of Ethics has been violated shall inform the Board of Ethics.

14. Individuals shall comply fully with the policies of the Board of Ethics in its consideration and adjudication of complaints of violations of the Code of Ethics.

American Academy
of Audiology Code of Ethics

PREAMBLE

The Code of Ethics of the American Academy of Audiology specifies professional standards that allow for the proper discharge of audiologists' responsibilities to those served and that protect the integrity of the profession. The Code of Ethics consists of two parts. The first part, the Statement of Principles and Rules, presents precepts that members (all categories of members, including student members) of the Academy agree to uphold. The second part, the Procedures, provides the process that enables enforcement of the Principles and Rules.

PART I. STATEMENT OF PRINCIPLES AND RULES

Principle 1

Members shall provide professional services and conduct research with honesty and compassion, and shall respect the dignity, worth, and rights of those served.

Rule 1a: Individuals shall not limit the delivery of professional services on any basis that is unjustifiable or irrelevant to the need for the potential benefit from such services.

Rule 1b: Individuals shall not provide services except in a professional relationship and shall not discriminate in the provision of services to individuals on the basis of sex, race, religion, national origin, sexual orientation, or general health.

Principle 2

Members shall maintain high standards of professional competence in rendering services.

Rule 2a: Members shall provide only those professional services for which they are qualified by education and experience.

From American Academy of Audiology. (2011). Code of ethics. Retrieved from http://www.audiology.org/resources/documentlibrary/Pages/codeofethics.aspx; reprinted by permission.

Rule 2b: Individuals shall use available resources, including referrals to other specialists, and shall not give or accept benefits or items of value for receiving or making referrals.

Rule 2c: Individuals shall exercise all reasonable precautions to avoid injury to persons in the delivery of professional services or execution of research.

Rule 2d: Individuals shall provide appropriate supervision and assume full responsibility for services delegated to supportive personnel. Individuals shall not delegate any service requiring professional competence to unqualified persons.

Rule 2e: Individuals shall not knowingly permit personnel under their direct or indirect supervision to engage in any practice that is a violation of the Code of Ethics.

Rule 2f: Individuals shall maintain professional competence, including participation in continuing education.

Principle 3

Members shall maintain the confidentiality of the information and records of those receiving services or involved in research.

Rule 3a: Individuals shall not reveal to unauthorized persons any professional or personal information obtained from the person served professionally, unless required by law.

Principle 4

Members shall provide only services and products that are in the best interest of those served.

Rule 4a: Individuals shall not exploit persons in the delivery of professional services.

Rule 4b: Individuals shall not charge for services not rendered.

Rule 4c: Individuals shall not participate in activities that constitute a conflict of professional interest.

Rule 4d: Individuals using investigational procedures with human participants or prospectively collecting research data from human participants shall obtain full informed consent from the participants or legal representatives. Members conducting research with human participants or animals shall follow accepted standards, such as those promulgated in the current Responsible Conduct of Research (current edition, 2009) by the U.S. Office of Research Integrity.

Principle 5

Members shall provide accurate information about the nature and management of communicative disorders and about the services and products offered.

Rule 5a: Individuals shall provide persons served with the information a reasonable person would want to know about the nature and possible effects of services rendered or products provided or research being conducted.

Rule 5b: Individuals may make a statement of prognosis but shall not guarantee results, mislead, or misinform persons served or studied.

Rule 5c: Individuals shall conduct and report product-related research only according to accepted standards of research practice.

Rule 5d: Individuals shall not carry out teaching or research activities in a manner that constitutes an invasion of privacy or that fails to inform persons fully about the nature and possible effects of these activities, affording all persons informed free choice of participation.

Rule 5e: Individuals shall maintain accurate documentation of services rendered according to accepted medical, legal, and professional standards and requirements.

Principle 6

Members shall comply with the ethical standards of the Academy with regard to public statements or publication.

Rule 6a: Individuals shall not misrepresent their educational degrees, training, credentials, or competence. Only degrees earned from regionally accredited institutions in which training was obtained in audiology, or a directly related discipline, may be used in public statements concerning professional services.

Rule 6b: Individuals' public statements about professional services, products, or research results shall not contain representations or claims that are false, misleading, or deceptive.

Principle 7

Members shall honor their responsibilities to the public and to professional colleagues.

Rule 7a: Individuals shall not use professional or commercial affiliations in any way that would limit services to or mislead patients or colleagues.

Rule 7b: Individuals shall inform colleagues and the public in an objective manner consistent with professional standards about products and services they have developed or research they have conducted.

Principle 8

Members shall uphold the dignity of the profession and freely accept the Academy's self-imposed standards.

Rule 8a: Individuals shall not violate these Principles and Rules or attempt to circumvent them.

Rule 8b: Individuals shall not engage in dishonesty or illegal conduct that adversely reflects on the profession.

Rule 8c: Individuals shall inform the Ethical Practices Committee when there are reasons to believe that a member of the Academy may have violated the Code of Ethics.

Rule 8d: Individuals shall fully cooperate with reviews being conducted by the Ethical Practices Committee in any matter related to the Code of Ethics.

PART II. PROCEDURES FOR THE MANAGEMENT OF ALLEGED VIOLATIONS

Introduction

Members of the American Academy of Audiology are obligated to uphold the Code of Ethics of the Academy in their personal conduct and in the performance of their professional duties. To this end it is the responsibility of each Academy member to inform the Ethical Practices Committee of possible Code of Ethics violations. The processing of alleged violations of the Code of Ethics will follow the procedures specified below in an expeditious manner to ensure that violations of ethical conduct by members of the Academy are halted in the shortest time possible.

Procedures

1. Suspected violations of the Code of Ethics shall be reported in letter format giving documentation sufficient to support the alleged violation. Letters must be addressed to

    Chair, Ethical Practices Committee
    c/o Executive Director
    American Academy of Audiology
    11480 Commerce Park Dr., Suite 220
    Reston, VA 20191

2. Following receipt of a report of a suspected violation, at the discretion of the Chair, the Ethical Practices Committee will request a signed Waiver of Confidentiality from the complainant indicating that the complainant will allow the Ethical Practices Committee to disclose his or her name should this become necessary during investigation of the allegation.

a. The Ethical Practices Committee may, under special circumstances, act in the absence of a signed Waiver of Confidentiality. For example, in cases where the Ethical Practices Committee has received information from a state licensure or registration board of a member having his or her license or registration suspended or revoked, then the Ethical Practices Committee will proceed without a complainant.

b. The Chair may communicate with other individuals, agencies, and/or programs for additional information as may be required for review at any time during the deliberation.

3. The Ethical Practices Committee will convene to review the merit of the alleged violation as it relates to the Code of Ethics

a. The Ethical Practices Committee shall meet to discuss the case, either in person or by electronic means or teleconference. The meeting will occur within 60 days of receipt of the waiver of confidentiality or of notification by the complainant of refusal to sign the waiver. In cases where another form of notification brings the complaint to the attention of the Ethical Practices Committee, the Committee will convene within 60 days of notification.

b. If the alleged violation has a high probability of being legally actionable, the case may be referred to the appropriate agency. The Ethical Practices Committee may postpone member notification and further deliberation until the legal process has been completed.

4. If there is sufficient evidence that indicates a violation of the Code of Ethics has occurred, upon majority vote, the member will be forwarded a Notification of Potential Ethics Concern.

a. The circumstances of the alleged violation will be described.

b. The member will be informed of the specific Code of Ethics rule that may conflict with member behavior.

c. Supporting Academy documents that may serve to further educate the member about the ethical implications will be included as appropriate.

d. The member will be asked to respond fully to the allegation and submit all supporting evidence within 30 calendar days.

5. The Ethical Practices Committee will meet either in person or by teleconference either (a) within 60 calendar days of receiving a response from the member to the Notification of Potential Ethics Concern to review the response and all information pertaining to the alleged violation, or (b) within 60 calendar days of notification to member if no response is received from the member to review the information received from the complainant.

6. If the Ethical Practices Committee determines that the evidence supports the allegation of an ethical violation, then the member will be provided written notice containing the following information:

    a. The right to a hearing in person or by teleconference before the Ethical Practices Committee

    b. The date, time and place of the hearing

    c. The ethical violation being charged and the potential sanction

    d. The right to present a defense to the charges

At this time the member should provide any additional relevant information. As this is the final opportunity for a member to provide new information, the member should carefully prepare all documentation.

7. Potential rulings

    a. When the Ethical Practices Committee determines there is insufficient evidence of an ethical violation, the parties to the complaint will be notified that the case will be closed.

    b. If the evidence supports the allegation of a Code violation, the rules(s) of the Code violated will be cited and sanction(s) will be specified.

8. The Committee shall sanction members based on the severity of the violation and history of prior ethical violations. A simple majority of voting members is required to institute a sanction unless otherwise noted. Sanctions may include one or more of the following:

    a. Educative letter. This sanction alone is appropriate when:

        1. The ethics violation appears to have been inadvertent.

        2. The member's response to Notification of Potential Ethics Concern indicates a new awareness of the problem and the member resolves to refrain from future ethical violations.

    b. Cease and desist order. The member signs a consent agreement to immediately halt the practice(s) that were found to be in violation of the Code of Ethics.

    c. Reprimand. The member will be formally reprimanded for the violation of the Code of Ethics.

    d. Mandatory continuing education.

        1. The Ethical Practices Committee will determine the type of education needed to reduce chances of recurrence of violations.

        2. The member will be responsible for submitting documentation of continuing education within the period of time designated by the Ethical Practices Committee.

        3. All costs associated with compliance will be borne by the member.

e. Probation of suspension. The member signs a consent agreement in acknowledgement of the Ethical Practices Committee's decision and is allowed to retain membership benefits during a defined probationary period.

   1. The duration of probation and the terms for avoiding suspension will be determined by the Ethical Practices Committee.

   2. Failure of the member to meet the terms for probation will result in the suspension of membership.

f. Suspension of membership.

   1. The duration of suspension will be determined by the Ethical Practices Committee.

   2. The member may not receive membership benefits during the period of suspension.

   3. Members suspended are not entitled to a refund of dues or fees.

g. Revocation of membership. Revocation of membership is considered the maximum punishment for a violation of the Code of Ethics.

   1. Revocation requires a two-thirds majority of the voting members of the Ethical Practices Committee.

   2. Individuals whose memberships are revoked are not entitled to a refund of dues or fees.

   3. One year following the date of membership revocation the individual may reapply for, but is not guaranteed, membership through normal channels and must meet the membership qualifications in effect at the time of application.

9. The member may appeal the Final Finding and Decision of the Ethical Practices Committee to the Academy Board of Directors. The route of appeal is by letter format through the Ethical Practices Committee to the Board of Directors of the Academy. Requests for appeal must (a) be received by the Chair of the Ethical Practices Committee within 30 days of the Ethical Practices Committee's notification of the Final Finding and Decision; (b) state the basis for the appeal and the reason(s) that the Final Finding and Decision of the Ethical Practices Committee should be changed; and (c) not offer new documentation.

   The Ethical Practices Committee Chair will communicate with the Executive Director of the Association to schedule the appeal at the earliest feasible Board of Director's meeting.

   The Board of Directors will review the documents and written summaries and deliberate the case.

The decision of the Board of Directors regarding the member's appeal shall be final.

10. In order to educate the membership, the Ethical Practices Committee, upon majority vote, shall present the circumstances and nature of the cases in *Audiology Today* and in the Professional Resource area of the Academy website. The member's identity will not be made public.

11. No Ethical Practices Committee member shall give access to records or act or speak independently or on behalf of the Ethical Practices Committee without the expressed permission of the members then active. No member may impose the sanction of the Ethical Practices Committee or interpret the findings of the Ethical Practices Committee in any manner that may place members of the Ethical Practices Committee or Board of Directors, collectively or singly, at financial, professional, or personal risk.

12. The Ethical Practices Committee Chair shall maintain a Book of Precedents that shall form the basis for future findings of the Committee.

Confidentiality and Records

Confidentiality shall be maintained in all Ethical Practices Committee discussion, correspondence, communication, deliberation, and records pertaining to members reviewed by the Ethical Practices Committee.

1. Complaints and suspected violations are assigned a case number.

2. Identity of members involved in complaints and suspected violations and access to Ethical Practices Committee files is restricted to the following:

    a. Ethical Practices Committee Chair

    b. Ethical Practices Committee member designated by Ethical Practices Committee Chair when the Chair recuses him- or herself from a case.

    c. Executive Director

    d. Agent/s of the Executive Director

    e. Other/s, following majority vote of the Ethical Practices Committee

3. Original records shall be maintained at the Central Records Repository at the Academy office in a locked cabinet.

    a. One copy will be sent to the Ethical Practices Committee Chair or member designated by the Chair.

    b. Copies will be sent to members.

4. Communications shall be sent to the members involved in complaints by the Academy office via certified or registered mail, after review by legal counsel.

5. When a case is closed, (a) the Chair will forward all documentation to the Academy Central Records Repository, and (b) members shall destroy all material pertaining to the case.

6. Complete records generally shall be maintained at the Academy Central Records Repository for a period of 5 years.

   a. Records will be destroyed 5 years after a member receives a sanction less than suspension, 5 years after the end of a suspension, or after membership is reinstated.

   b. Records of membership revocations for persons who have not returned to membership status will be maintained indefinitely.

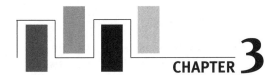

CHAPTER 3

Evidence-Based Decision Making in Communication Intervention

Marc E. Fey, Laura M. Justice, and Mary Beth Schmitt

CHAPTER OBJECTIVES

After reading this chapter, students will be able to

- Define evidence-based practice (EBP)
- Explain the difference between internal and external evidence and how each contributes to evidence-based decisions
- List and explain the six steps in making EBP decisions
- List and define three critical features of external evidence that EBP clinicians should critically appraise
- Describe the different forms of research designs and the level of evidence each one provides

You are a speech-language pathologist (SLP) working in a public school when Pamela, the parent of one of your clients, comes to you demanding that her child, Adam, receive a new intervention that she has just read about. You have been working with Pamela and Adam for the previous 2 years to address a significant impairment of language. Pamela reports that she read about this intervention in a popular parenting magazine. The article provided data from the intervention developer showing the effectiveness of the new intervention for children such as Adam. The article also included several testimonials from parents regarding the extraordinary benefits of the intervention. Thus, from Pamela's perspective, the intervention not only is appropriate for Adam but also represents a cure for Adam's language impairment. You tell Pamela that you are unfamiliar with this new intervention but that you are willing to investigate its merits and the appropriateness of delivering it to Adam. Pamela agrees that you should investigate the intervention, but she indicates that she is not willing to negotiate on its appropriateness. She wants Adam to undergo the desired intervention, even though it is very costly because of the intensity it requires. She informs you that she will not authorize a new individualized education plan (IEP) that does not include the new intervention.

The above example is not intended to portray parents as the "bad guys" in cases in which clinicians must make difficult decisions regarding the provision of new or controversial speech and language interventions. Similar situations that do not involve parents arise all the time:

- What if a supervisor endorses a new technique and believes you and other SLPs should apply it to all clients with certain specific characteristics?

- What if you receive a handout detailing dramatic improvements as a function of a particular intervention at a booth at a professional conference?

- What if you attend a workshop by an international expert at a conference that details an "innovative" and "state-of-the-art" technique designed for clients like many on your caseload?

- What if you read about the results of a clinical trial in a prominent journal that shows a technique to work extremely well for some clients with a particular communicative impairment, albeit not all?

When considering scenarios such as these, it is important to ask: what conditions would prompt you to discontinue an intervention procedure you currently provide for a particular client or group of clients in favor of a new technique? As important, under what conditions would you *not* be willing to change your technique?

Answering questions such as these requires a level of clinical expertise that clinicians develop during graduate training and beyond. This expertise allows clinicians to make knowledgeable and conscientious choices when faced with critical decisions presented by experts, supervisors, clients, and caregivers. Expertise develops not only through clinical experience and theoretical understanding of communication development and disorders, but also through the accumulation of knowledge and understanding of a constantly evolving scientific literature relevant to clinical practice. The conscientious integration of clinical experience, theoretical knowledge, and knowledge of the scientific literature is termed **evidence-based practice** (EBP).

This chapter focuses primarily on EBP as it applies to intervention decisions for clients for whom communication services have been deemed necessary. The first part of the chapter offers a comprehensive definition of EBP, various forms of evidence, and how that evidence can inform clinical decisions. Then, a six-step process on how to implement EBP is outlined and illustrated using a case example.

WHAT IS EVIDENCE-BASED PRACTICE?

In many ways, EBP is what its name suggests; it involves solving clinical problems by going to the published literature to find the best available scientific evidence to support the use or disuse of specific speech and language intervention approaches, intensities, procedures, activities, goal attack strategies, and so forth. Nonetheless, integration of evidence from the scientific literature is not as simple as it sounds, because not all evidence is created equal. Just like researchers, clinicians must know what types of studies provide the strongest (and weakest) evidence to support or reject a particular clinical approach. They must also be able to recognize examples of these stronger and weaker types of evidence when they find them in the literature.

It is important, however, to note that published studies are not the only form of evidence to be considered in EBP decisions. An evidence-based decision can be made confidently only when three types of evidence have been carefully considered (American Speech-Language-Hearing Association [ASHA], 2004, 2005; Porzsolt et al., 2003; Sackett, Straus, Richardson, Rosenberg, & Haynes, 2000):

- External evidence from published research

- Internal evidence from careful evaluation of client and family characteristics, their willingness to participate, and their preferences

- Internal evidence from examination of clinician preferences; professional competencies and values; and workplace values, policies, and culture

In short, EBP involves a careful process of decision making that specifies the types of evidence that warrant consideration and types of evidence that do not.

EXTERNAL EVIDENCE IN EVIDENCE-BASED PRACTICE DECISIONS

In EBP, the clinical professional consults the available *external evidence* regarding the impact of specific intervention techniques and tools. Some evidence available in published research, however, should have little bearing on decision making, whereas other evidence should be wholly discounted. Dollaghan (2004, 2007) identified three propositions concerning how to approach external evidence for use in evidence-based decision making:

1. The opinions of expert authorities (including consensus groups) should be viewed with skepticism and even discounted when they contradict evidence from rigorous scientific research.

2. Not all research is a suitable basis for informing decisions made in clinical practice.

3. Clinicians must be meticulously judgmental about the quality of evidence used to inform clinical practices.

These propositions provide guidelines for considering how to tackle situations such as those posed at the beginning of this chapter.

External Evidence from Experts

The first of Dollaghan's propositions (2004, 2007) notes that the opinions of expert authorities can and should be viewed with skepticism. This proposition makes it clear how to respond to the parent, supervisor, colleague, or designated expert who cites another expert, an authoritative textbook, or even a panel of experts as support for some new or existing approach. These authoritative viewpoints deserve consideration, but history shows that they are often wrong. A good example of this from speech-language pathology is a recommendation by Fey (1986) regarding how clinicians might teach early object words to children for the purpose of commenting, based on the principle of informativeness. According to the principle of informativeness, children are expected to be most likely to imitate and label the names for objects that are novel, or informative, in the context (Greenfield &

Zukow, 1978; Leonard, Cole, & Steckol, 1979; Schwartz & Leonard, 1985; Snyder, 1978). In an application of this principle to language intervention, Fey suggested that clinicians might first engage the child in some repetitive activity, such as putting puzzle pieces into their slots. Then, when the child develops accurate expectations of what is coming next (e.g., another puzzle piece), the clinician could present an object or attribute that is new and unexpected (i.e., informative) in the context (e.g., a cup), and say its name. According to Fey, this approach could be used to accelerate object–word learning in young children (Greenfield & Zukow, 1978; Leonard et al., 1979; Schwartz & Leonard, 1985; Snyder, 1978).

The suggestion Fey (1986) offered, presented in an authoritative textbook, might have seemed useful for evidence-based decision making; but unfortunately, the merits of the suggestion as described did not hold up when the procedure was subjected to rigorous empirical testing. When Sorensen and Fey (1992) tested the approach, they found no evidence that it helped children learn words more quickly than another approach that paired the object name with a redundant, and therefore noninformative, object. In fact, the informativeness approach failed as a word-teaching procedure possibly because when the activities were performed repeatedly (as was called for in the approach), the children learned to expect the unexpected. This effectively rendered objects redundant and noninformative when they were presented in contexts designed to make them novel and informative.

The principle of informativeness may still be generally valid and highly useful in language intervention. Clinical implementation of the principle, however, is complex and introduces many factors not present in the experiments and assessment protocols in which it has been used so successfully. And this is the point of the first proposition. Until suggestions proposed by expert authorities are tested clinically under rigorous conditions, clinicians cannot know what effects an expert's recommendation can be expected to have on a client's learning and use of language. Consequently, it is preferable to have direct evidence of the effects of a new intervention instead of an expert's opinion that the new intervention should have desirable effects. Thus, when confronted with expert opinion, clinicians should seek further substantiation of these opinions from more rigorous and preferably experimental evidence, should it be available. If rigorously tested evidence is not available, then such opinions should be greeted with healthy skepticism.

External Evidence from Basic Research

The second of Dollaghan's propositions (2004, 2007) states that not all research is relevant to decisions about clinical practice. Research is essentially of two varieties: basic and applied (Stokes, 1997). Basic research attempts to further knowledge of fundamental processes, and in the field of clinical communication, it is vital for furthering the understanding of how children develop speech and language. Applied research is designed to address specific societal needs, and in the field of communication disorders, it addresses the needs concerning the impact of various intervention approaches. The latter type of research is particularly relevant to informing EBP, whereas evidence from basic research is less relevant. This is not to say that basic research does not have value; on the contrary, discoveries from basic research often lead to important clinical hypotheses. Clinicians knowledgeable of relevant basic science are likely to have a better understanding of the theoretical principles upon which their interventions are based than do clinicians who have not read the basic literature. With such an understanding, these clinicians are likely to be highly creative and principled when making decisions when evidence from high-level, high-quality clinical trials is not available. Conversely, EBP practitioners realize that clinical conclusions stemming from basic research are tentative and often incorrect and that clinical practice is best informed by applied research designed to test specific interventions, including their processes and their impacts. Consider an example:

Suppose that a clinician and members of her clinical staff are looking for new ways to teach young children to use object labels in acts of commenting that lead to frequent and consistent spontaneous use in meaningful contexts. A colleague suggests that the clinician try a new approach to teaching object labels that features repetition through picture cards. The clinician points out correctly that the evidence base supplied for the new approach (i.e., the opinions and limited clinical experiences of an expert) is weak and that alternative sources of evidence should be sought. She then counters with evidence from basic research investigations that supports the use of the informativeness technique, as recommended by Fey (1986). In fact, there is considerable support from studies of typical and impaired language development on the principle of informativeness (Greenfield & Zukow, 1978; Leonard et al., 1979; Schwartz & Leonard, 1985; Snyder, 1978). Nonetheless, the only experimental examination of informativeness as an intervention principle that is available is the study of Sorensen and Fey (1992), which failed to support the Fey (1986) recommendation. The clinician who advocates for the informativeness approach may still be in a stronger position than her colleague who supports the new picture technique. This is because the informativeness technique is advocated on the grounds of underlying theory and projections from basic research whereas the picture card procedure is recommended on the basis of the opinion of an expert. The clinician, however, must realize the tenuous foundation of her argument, unless she can augment the evidence from basic research with other forms of clinical evidence.

Level and Quality of External Evidence

The third of Dollaghan's propositions (2004, 2007) makes clear that it is the responsibility of the EBP clinician not just to look for external evidence relevant to clinical decisions but also to evaluate and question the level and quality of that evidence. This proposition contends that clinicians must be knowledgeable concerning what constitutes high-level evidence. For example, consider the example of Pamela and Adam from the beginning of the chapter. Suppose that there are two studies reported in the literature indicating that the intervention Pamela requests appears to lead to positive outcomes. One of the studies is a case study of a single child, whereas the other is a pretest–posttest research design with no control group. As a knowledgeable clinician, you note to Pamela that as encouraging as these reports are, the level of evidence they provide must be viewed as weak. Both case studies and pretest–posttest designs that lack a control group show little certainty of the findings, as they do not control for effects unrelated to the intervention such as maturation. Consequently, even if these types of studies are executed with rigorous attention to measurement and implementation fidelity, they constitute very weak evidence of a cause–effect relationship between the intervention and the observed outcomes. In short, they provide an inadequate rationale for the costly approach demanded by Pamela.

There is an important conundrum in this case, however, in which Pamela asks, "What evidence do *you* have to support continuation of the approach you are now providing to my child?" This is a valid question expressing an important point, and it should always be anticipated by practitioners. The EBP mindset requires not only rigorous evaluation of new approaches; it also requires careful self-evaluation of existing approaches that many consider to reflect best practice. In situations such as Pamela's case, you would need to know whether there is equally strong or stronger research evidence supporting your own current methods over the approach advocated by Pamela. In addition, you would need to consider other sources of evidence to determine whether Pamela's desired approach has sufficient merit to warrant a change in programs.

Limitations of the External Evidence

The SLPs who accept Dollaghan's three propositions (2004, 2007) have adopted an EBP attitude or perspective that will serve them well. This is true even if at present these SLPs are unable to search for and find strong evidence to support all their intervention decisions, which will often be the case. The SLPs who have a healthy skepticism toward their own clinical practices recognize that the successes they observe often are due to factors outside their control rather than due to their clinical procedures. Consequently, they keep careful records about the clients they treat, the intervention options they exercise, and the outcomes they observe. They seek and evaluate external evidence from the research literature that can help them to be more certain about the potential effectiveness of their clinical practices. They question the authors of the articles they read and the experts whose presentations they attend to determine the amount and quality of evidence underlying these individuals' recommendations. They are honest and explicit about the evidentiary bases for their practices when they discuss clinical options with caregivers and other professionals. Finally, they adopt or reject new approaches based on their integration of the best available scientific and clinical evidence following their critical examinations of their own experiences and of the available external evidence.

A concern of many practitioners is that EBP will make them slaves to external research evidence, forcing them to follow certain paths when their experience, expertise, and particular child and family circumstances dictate otherwise. Although the risk of this misrepresentation of EBP is real, it is important to note that even the most ardent evidence-based practitioners in medicine recognize the importance of internal evidence. Evidence-based practitioners acknowledge that the client's and the family's values, preferences, and willingness to participate when making evidence-based decisions (e.g., Sackett et al., 2000), as well as the clinician's expertise, experience, and preferences, must be taken into consideration.

INTERNAL EVIDENCE REGARDING THE CHILD AND FAMILY IN EVIDENCE-BASED PRACTICE DECISIONS

Any intervention decision that is based on evidence must be based minimally on the client's speech and language status as well as any other characteristics that might influence the response to intervention, such as social, attentional, cognitive, and educational performance. Thus, in any application of EBP to clinical decisions, the clinician must ask, "Does the available research evidence even apply to this particular client?" The clinician answers this question first by examining whether the target client and family resembles the populations sampled in the studies from which support for intervention is based. If the answer to this question is "No," the support for the use of the target approach is weakened on the basis of internal evidence, and the approach may not be applicable. For example, the results from a set of studies demonstrating the efficacy of an intervention approach that improves the language comprehension of children with primary language impairment may not be relevant for a clinician working with a child with a cognitive delay and a mild hearing loss. Similarly, a single good study demonstrating the efficacy of a parent-administered intervention may not be useful to a clinician working with a family in which the caregivers have indicated an unwillingness or inability to deliver the intervention to their child.

In considering the internal evidence regarding a client and the client's family, the clinician must also consider the following questions: What do the client and family see as the client's greatest needs? Are the client's and family's goals consistent with those targeted in the published studies? Are the attitudes of the client and family consistent with the target intervention when considering 1) the level and type of family involvement, 2) the nature of the communication problem, or 3) the intervention intensity and approaches?

Evidence-based practitioners must be cognizant of the potential mismatch between a research-supported, targeted intervention approach and the client's and family's values or willingness to participate in the approach (e.g., van Kleeck, 1994). There are four possible responses to a mismatch. First, clinicians can apply the target intervention approach in spite of their awareness of the dissonance between the intervention and family values. Clinicians who neglect client and family desires in this way, however, are likely following a path of greatest resistance. Implementation of and success with the new approach in these cases will likely be limited, even if the evidence in support of the target intervention approach is very strong. Such neglect is inconsistent with EBP principles and, therefore is not recommended.

Second, clinicians can adopt an alternative intervention approach judged to be more consonant with the client's and family's perspectives. This option may often be reasonable and justifiable, even when there is strong research evidence in support of the target intervention approach. This option is strongest, however, when there is similarly strong research evidence supporting the alternative intervention approach. Clinicians can strengthen this decision if they have a documented record of success in administering the alternative intervention approach to other clients.

Third, clinicians can attempt to modify the target intervention approach to reduce the mismatch. Of course, when clinicians modify approaches that have demonstrated efficacy, they could be altering the very components responsible for the effects observed in the published studies. Consequently, clinicians will need to carefully document intervention outcomes, even when the modified intervention approach has a strong foundation in experimental evidence.

Fourth, clinicians can attempt to conference with the client or family so that a research-supported approach not consonant with them can be implemented. Some clients and families may be willing to participate in intervention programs that conflict somewhat with their individual values and cultural perspectives. This is especially true if clinicians objectively and unemotionally present evidence that the target intervention approach is the one most likely to bring about the greatest change in the client's performance over the shortest period of time. When clinicians choose to counsel the family, however, they must be extremely careful to respect the family's perspectives.

INTERNAL EVIDENCE REGARDING THE CLINICIAN AND SCHOOL IN EVIDENCE-BASED PRACTICE DECISIONS

Internal evidence can also be derived from a clinician's expertise and experience, or clinical craft, as well as from the resources and culture present in the clinician's work environment. This evidence must be weighed carefully in any valid EBP decisions. When considering their own expertise and experience, the most important questions that clinicians must ask are these:

- What intervention approach would you normally apply in a case *without* the assistance of external research-based evidence?

- Why would you use this approach?

- What level of success have you had with this approach?

- Did you document your results when you applied this approach in other, similar cases?

Consideration of these questions early in the decision-making process can help clinicians better understand their own clinical biases as well as the foundations of those biases. In some cases, for example, a bias may be based on a long history of success that has been well documented in a clinician's records. In these cases, this internal evidence might well outweigh available external evidence for an alternative approach provided in one or more well-implemented clinical trials. Such a decision would be consistent with EBP as long as the clinician has sought out the appropriate external evidence and carefully and fairly weighed it against existing internal evidence. In other cases, a clinician might recognize that his or her standard care is based primarily on the opinions of past instructors and clinical supervisors and from his or her uncontrolled case reports, which are weak forms of evidence for supporting decision making. The clinician should consider changing his or her clinical practice if new evidence from strong clinical trials supporting a new approach is discovered.

A SIX-STEP APPROACH TO INTERVENTION DECISIONS USING EVIDENCE-BASED PRACTICE

Although much has been written recently about EBP in speech-language pathology (ASHA, 2004, 2005; Justice & Fey, 2004), most of the literature on this topic has described the process in broad strokes, focusing primarily on what EBP is and providing rationales for its adoption. Relatively little has been written about what EBP practitioners actually should do. A general six-step model of EBP decision making is provided in this section (see Table 3.1) and illustrated with a case example.

Table 3.1.   Six steps crucial to every evidence-based practice decision about intervention

1. Develop a four-part clinical question that explicitly focuses on PICO (i.e., P = the*patient*, *patient group*, or *problem*; I = *intervention* being considered; C = *comparison* treatment; O = desired *outcome*).

2. Find the internal evidence and answer the question based solely on this evidence, to include 1) attention to client–family values, desires, and circumstances; and 2) the clinician's knowledge of the condition, the clinician's knowledge of the client, the clinician's clinical experience, the clinician's theoretical knowledge, and the school's attitudes regarding the need for change.

3. Find the external or published research evidence.

4. Critically evaluate the external evidence.

5. Integrate the internal and external evidence.

6. Apply and evaluate the outcome of the decision.

Source: Porszolt et al. (2003).

A CASE EXAMPLE ILLUSTRATING SIX STEPS TO FOLLOW WHEN USING EBP

Aaron, who is 5 years and 9 months old, is a kindergartener being evaluated by an EBP clinician, Phyllis. Aaron's kindergarten teacher referred Aaron to Phyllis because his language, social, and prereading skills are not as well developed as those of his peers. Classroom and therapy room evaluations reveal that Aaron rarely communicates with his peers but that he converses with his mother and Phyllis during playtime and shared-storybook reading. In the classroom, Phyllis observes that Aaron uses a lot of pantomime to repair communication breakdowns.

Aaron receives a standard score of 87 on the Peabody Picture Vocabulary Test–3 (Dunn & Dunn, 2007) and a listening quotient of 80 on the Test of Language Development-Primary–3 (Newcomer & Hammill, 2008). His mean length of utterance (MLU) in the richest sample, which was obtained when he was playing with his mother, is 2.5. Language sample analysis shows that Aaron's sentences are simple (i.e., one verb) and often incomplete (e.g., omission of subject, verb, or object), and they typically omit grammatical functors (e.g., articles, auxiliary verbs, bound morphemes), especially those associated with verbs. Aaron's speech is particularly hard for adults to understand, but some of his peers in the classroom seem to follow his messages, especially when they are accompanied by pantomime. According to his teacher, however, none of his peers interacts consistently with Aaron during play- or work times in the classroom.

Based on these results, Phyllis decides to initiate a program of speech and language intervention for Aaron. She selects the basic goals of enhancing Aaron's expressive grammar and his expressive phonology (intelligibility) but does not know which of the two goals to prioritize. Phyllis asks herself, "Do I focus intervention on both areas the whole time, as I usually do in such cases? Or, should I focus solely on grammar, to achieve greater changes in this domain but possibly influencing phonology indirectly? Alternatively, what if I placed my full attention on the intelligibility issue? What would happen to Aaron's grammar? Are there other alternatives I'm not considering?" These are questions often asked by clinicians working with children who simultaneously exhibit significant impairments of both speech sound production and language. This is the type of clinical problem that is tractable using EBP procedures. Although Phyllis has extremely limited time to search for the necessary literature, she decides to follow the six-step EBP decision-making process.

Step 1: Develop a Four-Part Clinical Question

Evidence-based practitioners uniformly agree that the first step in making an EBP decision is careful delineation of a clinical question. The system for developing an appropriate question follows the acronym **PICO** (Centre for Evidence-Based Medicine, 2001a, 2001b; Sackett et al., 2000; see also Table 3.1). In this acronym, *P* represents Patient, Patient group, or Problem; *I* represents the Intervention being considered; *C* represents the Comparison intervention (such as the current practice or no treatment); and *O* represents the desired Outcome. In Aaron's case, Phyllis follows the PICO acronym to formulate this question: "Would a 5-year-old kindergartner with primarily expressive specific language impairment affecting grammar and speech (*P*) show improvement with an intervention that targets both phonology and grammar simultaneously (*I*) or one that targets phonology and grammar through sequential blocks (*C*), for example, a block of phonology followed by a block of grammar, as shown by improvements in grammar and phonology in spontaneous production probes and/or conversational contexts (*O*)?"

Step 2: Find the Internal Evidence and Answer
the Clinical Question Based Solely on This Evidence

In most EBP decision-making schemes, the step following the identification of the question is a search for external research evidence. Porzsolt and colleagues (2003), however, suggested that the insertion of another step prior to examining the external research seemed to help clinicians to better understand the effect of their efforts to identify relevant external research. In this step, the clinician examines the internal evidence to determine what would be his or her typical intervention approach based solely on that evidence without examining the latest research. In effect, the clinician develops his or her own non-EBP solution as the target intervention for the clinical question. In addition, the clinician identifies any client or family factors that would influence intervention decisions.

In the example of Aaron, it is useful to consider two possible child–family and clinician–school scenarios and the ways they could affect Aaron's response to intervention. In the first scenario, Aaron is alert and cooperative and transitions easily from one task to another. The teacher indicates that Aaron's peers are having difficulty understanding him, and he is starting to show signs of embarrassment. His parents show a clear understanding of Aaron's speech and language difficulties and their potential effect on his educational performance. They also understand the various options for goal attack strategies (e.g., targeting grammar and phonology simultaneously, alternating targets in blocks), and they have indicated in the Planning and Placement Team (PPT) meeting that they would endorse any approach that shows a clear recognition of Aaron's needs in both grammar and phonology. Phyllis is relatively comfortable with intervention for children with concomitant problems in grammar and phonology. When working with previous clients, Phyllis typically has first targeted the child's intelligibility problem and then has moved on to grammatical problems, if necessary, as the child becomes easier to understand. Phyllis has records from numerous previous clients to document the positive outcomes in grammar and phonology experienced with this sequential blocking of phonology followed by grammar. Given her track record for this approach and Aaron's growing level of embarrassment, Phyllis plans to address phonology first and then move to grammar targets once the phonology has resolved.

In the second scenario, although Aaron is cooperative, he is easily distracted. His teacher reports that he does not change smoothly from one task to the next. His parents do not seem to understand the part of Aaron's problems related to language, and they emphasize that their greatest concern is his speech intelligibility. Furthermore, Phyllis is relatively comfortable with intervention for children with concomitant problems in grammar and phonology. When working with previous clients, Phyllis has simultaneously addressed both intelligibility and grammatical concerns. Her approach targets speech sounds that are difficult for Aaron but that are also important for marking morphosyntactic forms—such as those for plurals, possessives, subject–verb agreement, regular verb tense—such as [s] and [z]; and final word clusters, such as [kt] (e.g., *walked*) and [st] (e.g., *passed*). Phyllis has records from numerous clients to document the positive outcomes in both grammar and phonology experienced with this simultaneous approach. In Aaron's case, she decides to target both domains simultaneously to incorporate the parents' interest in addressing phonology and because of her previous, positive experience with this approach.

Step 3: Find the External Research Evidence

If Phyllis were practicing from an EBP perspective, she would have to admit that the decision-making processes exemplified in the two scenarios is not evidence-based. To make it evidence-based, she should be prepared to examine the existing evidence to help resolve the clinical question of what intervention approach would be best for Aaron. In medicine, clinicians might search for studies relevant to their PICO-based questions in specialized databases, which are highly accessible. Furthermore, clinicians might find one or more systematic reviews or meta-analyses of studies (primarily randomized controlled trials) related to their clinical questions via Internet-based database projects, such as the Cochrane Collaboration's health care database (http://www.cochrane.org); the Campbell Collaboration's database in social, behavioral, and educational domains (http://www.campbellcollaboration.org); or the What Works Clearinghouse, which focuses on practices in education (http://ies.ed.gov/ncee). These databases also provide critical appraisals (i.e., study reports) of individual clinical trials that enable clinicians to quickly and efficiently ascertain the results and validity of a particular study. In some areas of health care, clinical practice guidelines based on systematic reviews and meta-analyses are available. The Scottish Intercollegiate Guidelines Network (http://www.sign.ac.uk/guidelines) exists primarily to produce such guidelines for clinicians. In these cases, a panel of experts would already have systematically reviewed the experimental literature, made recommendations concerning the clinical problem, and graded those recommendations to specify the level of confidence clinicians might have in putting them into practice.

Unfortunately, the database of studies that evaluate intervention objectively is not nearly as large in speech-language pathology as it is in medicine, nor is it as well organized. The Academy of Neurologic Communication Disorders and Stroke has a project with the goals of producing intervention and diagnostic guidelines and delineating research needs (http://www.ancds.org/practice.html). Several guidelines have been produced and are available for use by EBP clinicians working with adults with neurogenic speech, language, and cognitive disorders. This work illustrates how much progress can be made, but it also shows how far the field of speech-language pathology has to go in developing guidelines for clinicians working with a range of disorders and age groups, if EBP is to become standard clinical practice.

Given this state of affairs, it is reasonable for you to ask, "What can clinicians do now to make use of external evidence as they implement EBP principles to their clients' benefit?" Some of the reasonable answers to this question can be illustrated by returning to the hypothetical case of Phyllis and Aaron and by assuming that Phyllis is interested in making an evidence-based decision.

Phyllis decides to begin her search at Highwire Press (http://highwire.org), which hosts many frequently cited journals on speech and language, including all ASHA journals. Highwire Press not only provides a large repository of articles for Phyllis's search, it also provides easy and free access to articles in all ASHA journals for ASHA members and for individuals at subscribing institutions.

Phyllis uses the Highwire Press's search capability to locate articles containing three relevant key words: *phonology, grammar,* and *intervention*. The first 40 results of this search provide a number of encouraging possibilities. After Phyllis reads the titles and brief summaries of these articles, she finds that seven articles seem most pertinent to her question. She reads the abstracts of these articles to determine which are most likely to be useful. Based on the information provided in the abstracts on the participants' ages, the problems, the types of interventions provided, and the type of research design used, the following six articles appear highly relevant to Phyllis's clinical question:

1. Tyler, Lewis, Haskill, and Tolbert (2003): "Outcomes of Different Speech and Language Goal Attack Strategies"

2. Tyler, Lewis, Haskill, and Tolbert (2002): "Efficacy and Cross-Domain Effects of a Morphosyntax and a Phonology Intervention"

3. Fey and colleagues (1994): "Effects of Grammar Facilitation on the Phonological Performance of Children with Speech and Language Impairments"

4. Tyler and Sandoval (1994): "Preschoolers with Phonological and Language Disorders: Treating Different Linguistic Domains"

5. Seeff-Gabriel, Chiat, and Pring (2012): "Intervention for Co-occurring Speech and Language Difficulties: Addressing the Relationship Between the Two Domains"

6. Tyler, Lewis, and Welch (2003): "Predictors of Phonological Change Following Intervention"

Because she is pressed for time, Phyllis decides to focus on the one article most relevant to her clinical problem, at least at first. The most recent of the short-listed articles by Seeff-Gabriel et al. (2012) is filled with important insights, but she recognizes from the abstract that it is a report of an uncontrolled case study that cannot provide information on cause-and-effect relationships. The article that appears best to suit her immediate needs is Tyler, Lewis, Haskill, et al. (2003). Thus, she decides to seek information relevant to the clinical question by critically evaluating the Tyler, Lewis, Haskell, et al. (2003) article.

It is important to note that Phyllis's EBP approach is far from ideal. Her review of the external evidence would examine only a single database. A much broader literature needs to be searched. In addition, Phyllis's plan to read and evaluate a single article may be questioned. Ultimately, she should examine all the experimental literature that is available and relevant to the clinical question. An exhaustive literature review may be practical, however, only when groups of clinicians focus on common problems and work together. This is not always possible, though, and it can be assumed that this is not possible in Phyllis's present situation. Phyllis realizes that her literature review and critical appraisal will be incomplete. Despite this fact, her review of the external evidence in this example reflects an important first step in integrating external evidence into clinical decisions.

Step 4: Critically Appraise the External Evidence

Any research publication identified as a potential candidate for addressing PICO-inspired questions must be carefully evaluated. This evaluation, or critical appraisal of the topic (CAT; Sackett et al., 2000), grades the article for 1) its relevance to the clinical question; 2) the level of evidence provided by the study in the article based on the study's design and quality; and 3) the direction, strength, and consistency of the study's observed outcomes.

The Tyler, Lewis, Haskill, et al. (2003) article, which Phyllis chose, describes a study in which 47 children participated. The children's ages ranged from 3–0 to 5–11, and the children had concomitant speech and language impairment. Forty children were randomly assigned to one of four intervention groups. These children all received a 30-minute individual session and a 45-minute group session every week for 24 weeks. The same approach to speech-language intervention was used in all intervention groups, but the sequencing of intervention targets varied. The first group, which targeted phonology first, received 12 weeks of phonological intervention followed by 12 weeks of morphosyntactic intervention. The second group, which targeted morphosyntax first, received 12 weeks of morphosyntactic intervention followed by 12 weeks of phonological intervention. The third group received alternating cycles of 1 week of phonological intervention and 1 week of morphosyntactic intervention for 24 weeks. The fourth group received intervention that simultaneously addressed both phonology and morphosyntax for 24 weeks. The children's phonological and morphosyntactic gains were measured using percentage of consonants correct on the Bankson-Bernthal Test of Phonology (Bankson & Bernthal, 1990) and percentage of correct use of a small set of verb morphemes used to mark tense and agreement as measured from a spontaneous language sample.

Relevance to the Clinical Question Critical appraisal of external evidence begins by examining the relevance of the study to the clinical question. Clinicians determine the relevance by examining the study for its description of the individuals who participated, its intervention methods, and its outcome measures.

	Yes	Unclear	No
Are the participants clearly described and does the sample include patients like the target client?	X	Xª	—
Is the intervention sufficiently well described that it could be put into practice?	X	—	—
Is the intervention feasible for your practice and client?	X	—	—
Are the outcome measures valid and reliable indicators of clinical significance?	X	—	—

Figure 3.1.   Some questions addressing the relevance of clinical questions raised for Aaron. Note that answers apply to the study by Tyler, Lewis, Haskill, et al. (2003). ªThe clinician in Scenario 1 rated this question as "Yes," but the clinician in Scenario 2 rated this question as "Unclear." In Scenario 2, Aaron was distractible and had difficulty moving to new tasks. The description of the participants in the research report provides no information on participants' attention and ability to transition from one task to another. (*Source*: Scottish Intercollegiate Guidelines Network, 2004.)

A study found irrelevant for a particular problem or a particular case might not be further considered at all. Clinicians also consider whether the intervention is feasible to implement in a particular setting or with a particular client. For instance, an intervention might not be feasible if it involves a computer program that is not yet commercially available.

Figure 3.1 presents specific questions that can be used for determining the relevance of a study, and it provides answers to these questions as they relate to Aaron and the Tyler, Lewis, Haskill, et al. (2003) article. The sample of participants in the study appears to include children such as Aaron in age and speech-language profile, although the article provided little information regarding additional features that could potentially influence intervention outcomes. For example, Phyllis does not know if any of the children in the study had attentional or transitional problems as Aaron has in the second scenario. Likewise, the article provides no information on the family characteristics of the children, such as parental education and socioeconomic status. In other respects, the study is clearly relevant to Aaron's case, particularly the speech-language characteristics of the sample participants. Also, the intervention approach is well described, especially for a research report; the intensity and structure of the interventions seem feasible for use in Phyllis's school system; and the outcome measures appear valid, reliable, and clinically meaningful. Thus, with some reservations, Phyllis regards the study as relevant to the clinical question in both scenarios.

Level of Evidence Represented by the Study Design and Quality   Critical appraisal of the external evidence involves not only establishing the relevance of professional literature to a particular population or problem but also judging the level of the evidence, as determined by the study design and the methodological rigor employed. Although there are numerous ranking systems available, the one developed by the Oxford Centre for Evidence-Based Medicine (CEBM; Centre for Evidence-Based Medicine, 2001b) is perhaps most frequently used or adapted. Table 3.2 provides an adaptation of this system, which shows how different forms of evidence (e.g., systematic review, randomized controlled trial, expert opinion) are ranked for the level of evidence provided. There are four levels of evidence: 1, 2, 3, and 4, ranging from highest to lowest with several further sublevels.

Table 3.2. Levels of evidence

Level	Type(s) of evidence
1a	A systematic review of randomized controlled trials with consistent study outcomes
1b	A well-conducted single randomized controlled trial (RCT) with a narrow confidence interval
2a	A systematic review of nonrandomized quasi-experimental trials or a systematic review of single-subject experiments that document consistent study outcomes
2b	A high-quality quasi-experimental trial or a lower quality RCT or a single-subject experiment with consistent outcomes across replications
3	A case series or a poor-quality quasi-experimental study
4	An expert opinion that originated without ongoing critical appraisal or based on theoretical knowledge or basic research

Source: Centre for Evidence-Based Medicine (2001b).

Categorization of a study involves consideration of three critical features: research design (e.g., case study, clinical trial), methodological quality, and the consistency or strength of observed effects.

Research Design Each research study is designed in a particular way to answer a specific question or set of questions. For example, a study that determines the validity of a measure of speech intelligibility in children is designed very differently than a study that determines the effects of a parent-implemented speech intervention for preschool children. In evidence-based decision making, the strongest evidence on which an intervention decision can be based is derived from studies featuring **experimental designs.** In true experimental designs, the researcher assigns participants randomly to two or more treatment groups and places rigorous control on all known additional variables that might affect a **dependent variable.** With other variables controlled, the direct influence of the intervention (the **independent variable**) on a particular outcome (the dependent variable) can be assessed.

Experimental designs that involve groups of participants to estimate the relationship between a clinical intervention and an outcome are called **randomized control trials (RCTs).** In an RCT, the researcher assigns participants randomly to two or more groups. Each group then receives a systematic intervention (or, in some cases, no intervention), and the outcomes for each group are compared. In an RCT, all groups are treated identically with the exception of the intervention variable(s) being tested. Because participants are randomly assigned to groups, any differences between groups at the outset of the study are unlikely to be systematic and do not reflect the biases of the researcher. Thus, when one group outperforms another over the course of the intervention, a causal inference connecting the outcome with the intervention is appropriate. High-quality RCTs provide clinicians with the highest level of evidence available from a single study (Level 1b; see Table 3.2). Level 1b evidence is superseded only by the outcomes of systematic reviews that aggregate the findings from two or more RCTs (Level 1a; see Table 3.2).

Other research designs are also pertinent to evidence-based decision making. These designs include quasi-experimental designs, single-case designs, and case studies. Although **quasi-experimental studies** attempt to estimate the relationship between independent and dependent variables, these designs are not truly experimental because the researcher does not randomly assign participants to different intervention groups. For example, control groups may be formed out of convenience (e.g., participants could not attend all the intervention sessions), or a new intervention may be compared with one tried in the past, using the performance of some previous group as a historical control. Many of these designs are logically similar to RCTs, but because participants are not assigned to groups at random, there are more opportunities for selection bias to influence the outcomes. Conclusions from quasi-experimental studies about the effects of intervention are generally assumed to be riskier than are conclusions drawn from an RCT. Therefore, the results of even high-quality quasi-experimental studies constitute weaker levels of evidence (Level 2b; see Table 3.2) than do those of high-quality RCTs.

Single-case experimental designs are also informative to EBP. Unlike the typical RCT when the researcher focuses on inferences about group performance, single-case experiments provide a great deal of specific information about the individual participants. These designs are experimental because the researchers systematically manipulate variables so that a relationship between the intervention and the outcome can be inferred. Single-case designs have an advantage over group experimental designs in that they allow in-depth monitoring of how individuals respond to interventions over time. Thus, in these designs, causal inferences about the intervention may be applied to specific individuals. In addition, single-case designs require fewer participants than do group experimental designs, which is a significant advantage for clinical research focused on low-incidence disabilities. The greatest liability of these studies is that it is difficult to generalize the results of one or more single-case studies to a broader population of intervention candidates.

One single-case research design, called the **multiple baselines across behaviors design,** is commonly used. In this design, intervention begins on a subset of goals, while performance on nontreated goals is monitored. After a criterion is reached on treated targets, intervention begins on another subset of goals, while any remaining untreated goals are still monitored. This pattern may continue over a long period of time. If the gains in a participant's performance for each behavior coincide with the initiation of intervention for that behavior, a causal inference associating the intervention and the improvements becomes appropriate. The Oxford CEBM system does not include single-case experiments in its strategies for determining levels of evidence. Because these designs are so important in communication disorders, however, strong single-case experiments can be placed at Level 2b (see Table 3.2). This is consistent with high-quality quasi-experimental studies and lower-quality RCTs, and it is similar to the level assigned to single-case experiments by the Section 1 Task Force of the Division of Clinical Psychology of the American Psychological Association (Lonigan, Elber, & Johnson, 1998). Nonetheless, it is important to note that not all intervention researchers would agree that the level of evidence provided by well-controlled single-case experiments should be so high.

An additional research design used to inform evidence-based decision making is the **case study design.** In a case study, a single individual, event, or context is intensively studied using both qualitative (e.g., interviews, field observations) and quantitative data (e.g., test scores). Case studies can be used to determine how easy or difficult it is to implement an intervention; how well clients tolerate the procedures and intensity of intervention; and whether the intervention has sufficient promise to warrant the planning and execution of additional, more rigorous studies of the intervention's effects. Despite being a type of clinical trial, this design provides a very weak form of evidence for intervention effects because it is impossible to causally link any observed outcomes to the intervention, even if the intervention is expertly implemented and outcomes are rigorously monitored.

A **case series** is simply a collection of case studies in which several participants receive the same intervention and their outcomes are measured following the intervention. Even when a case series involves many participants who all respond similarly, the evidence the series produces can be no higher than Level 3 (see Table 3.2) because the researcher exerts no controls over factors that may be influencing intervention outcomes, and causal inferences of intervention impact are impossible.

To determine the research design used in a relevant study, clinicians must ask a set of questions such as those presented in Figure 3.2. As Phyllis critically appraises the Tyler, Lewis, Haskill, et al. (2003) article, she finds that the study is not a systematic review of a particular research design and answers the first two questions in Figure 3.2, "No." This means that the evidence from the article cannot be Level 1a or 2a (see Table 3.2). Groups were compared in the article, however, pre and post measures were obtained, and participants were randomly assigned to four intervention groups. These are defining characteristics of RCTs. Phyllis recognizes that the study is an RCT but wonders whether to characterize it as Level 1b (single high-quality RCT) or Level 2b (lower quality RCT). To make this determination, she must evaluate the methodological quality of the study.

Methodological Quality   The level of evidence provided by a study is based not solely on its research design but also on its methodological quality. Examinations of the quality of published studies, even those designs providing the highest level of evidence, show that quality is highly variable (e.g., Troia, 1999), even in highly respected journals. Thus, once clinicians identify a study relevant to an evidence-based question and its research design, they must evaluate its quality. Although it

	Yes	Unclear	No
Does the study systematically review randomized controlled trials?	—	—	X
Does the study systematically review quasi-experimental or single-subject experimental studies?	—	—	X
Are two or more groups compared?	X	—	—
Are measures collected before and after therapy?	X	—	—
Are participants randomly assigned to groups?	X	—	—
Are there controls within or across individual participants?	—	—	X

Figure 3.2.   Some useful questions for determining the design of a clinical trial. Note that answers apply to the study by Tyler, Lewis, Haskill, et al. (2003). (*Source*: Scottish Intercollegiate Guidelines Network, 2004.)

	Yes	Unclear	No
Are the participant groups equivalent in regard to dependent variables and other key variables at pretest, or are differences accounted for statistically?	X	—	—
Are assessors blind to group assignments?	—	—	X
Are coders blind to group assignments?	—	X	—
Is the implementation of the intervention conditions monitored for fidelity?	—	—	X
Are outcome measures reliable and valid?	X	—	—
Are dropouts in all intervention conditions accounted for?	X	—	—

Figure 3.3.   Some useful questions for determining the quality of a clinical trial. Note that answers evaluate the quality of the study reported by Tyler, Lewis, Haskill, et al. (2003). (*Source*: Scottish Intercollegiate Guidelines Network, 2004.)

is beyond the scope of this chapter to characterize the quality of different research designs by means of a thorough examination of approaches, several published articles provide excellent descriptions of quality indicators for true experimental and quasi-experimental designs (Gersten et al., 2005), as well as single-case designs (Horner et al., 2005).

The basic process of appraising methodological quality can be illustrated by posing questions such as those that appear in Figure 3.3. These questions provide means for a more in-depth examination of the quality of the evidence provided by RCT studies. The main concern at this stage is to determine whether the researcher has taken sufficient steps to avoid bias and subjectivity. Researchers generally avoid bias and subjectivity by 1) ensuring that before intervention begins, the participant groups are equivalent or arrangements have been made to minimize the effects of group inequalities; 2) individuals who either collect, transcribe, code, or record test data are blind to the participants' group assignments; 3) outcome measures have demonstrated reliability and validity; and 4) either few participants leave the intervention groups before the study has been completed or careful analyses have been conducted to determine that the study results have not been influenced by any changes in group membership. Failures to take these steps make it possible for bias and subjectivity to enter into the results, thus limiting confidence in any conclusions about causal relationships between the intervention and the observed outcomes.

Figure 3.3 shows that the Tyler, Lewis, Haskill, et al. (2003) study fares reasonably well on these variables, except that the testers, and perhaps also some transcribers, were aware of the participants' group assignments. The concern is not necessarily

	Yes	Unclear	No
Were experimental effects statistically significant?	X	—	—
If more than one measure was used, were the effects across measures consistent?	—	—	X
Is the magnitude of the observed effects (i.e., effect size) reported and interpreted?	X	—	—
Were the effects clinically meaningful?	X	—	—

Figure 3.4.   Useful questions for determining the strength and consistency of observed effects. Note that answers apply to the study by Tyler, Lewis, Haskill, et al. (2003). (*Source*: Scottish Intercollegiate Guidelines Network, 2004.)

that the testers and transcribers intentionally favored one participant group over another; rather, the fear is that biases can affect outcomes even when research personnel make strong and conscious efforts *not* to show any kind of favoritism. On the positive side, all participants completed the study, and each group had similarly high proportions of the total number of scheduled sessions. The interventions were well described and the number of sound and morpheme elicitations was reported to have been consistent across groups. Still, there was only limited monitoring of the interventions to ensure that they were delivered as described. Because of those factors, Phyllis rates this study as "Unclear" on this dimension. Although the study was generally well conducted, there is the possibility that bias and subjectivity could have influenced its results to undermine causal inferences. Phyllis ultimately rates the level of evidence for this study as Level 2b (see Table 3.2).

Consistency and Strength of Observed Effects   An available study may implement the most rigorous research design, and it may also exhibit strong methodological quality; nonetheless, it is possible that the effects of the intervention are weak or inconsistent. For example, a well-conducted RCT may find that group intervention for people with aphasia has little advantage over an individual intervention program, or it may find that the group intervention influences one area of language, such as word finding, but not sentence length, suggesting that the effects of the intervention are small or inconsistent. It is important to consider the strength and consistency of observed outcomes across dependent measures. The strength of the intervention effect is typically examined by studying **statistical significance** and **effect-size estimates.** In experimental and quasi-experimental designs, statistical significance is the probability that differences between groups observed over a course of intervention resulted from the manipulation of the independent variable. Researchers typically use a probability threshold of .05 to differentiate results attributable to chance (>.05) from those attributable to experimental manipulation (<.05).

An intervention effect that is statistically reliable, however, is not necessarily clinically meaningful. For example, a listening intervention for clients with hearing loss may have a statistical advantage over a control condition because the members of the intervention group show more consistent change on the dependent variable over time than the members of the control group. At the same time, the actual improvement in listening performance of participants in the intervention group could be very small, suggesting that in reality the interventions are similar in their effect or that the small advantage attributed to the intervention is not worth the costs of implementing it. To estimate the magnitude of intervention effects, researchers calculate the *size of the effect*. The most common measures of the size of the effect estimate the magnitude of an intervention's effect in standard deviation units.

To thoroughly appraise the Tyler, Lewis, Haskill, et al. (2003) study for their EBP purposes, Phyllis must answer the questions as shown in Figure 3.4, which review the size and consistency of the observed effects in the study. Phyllis's answers indicate that the study yielded some significant differences between groups. After 24 weeks, the participants in the alternating group made greater gains in morphosyntax than did the participants in the other three groups. These differences were statistically reliable and the effects were large. In fact, after 24 weeks of intervention, the mean correct use of finite verb morphemes for participants in the alternating group was approximately one full standard deviation higher than the gains made by the participants in the other groups (i.e., size of effect = 1). In contrast, although the study provided some evidence that the participants in each group made gains in the percentage of target and generalization sounds produced correctly, there were no differences between group gains in phonology at 24 weeks when comparing the phonology-first and the morphosyntax-first groups. Thus, Tyler, Lewis, Haskill, et al. (2003) appropriately concluded that their study supported the use of a strategy that alternates morphosyntactic and grammatical goals on a weekly basis compared to the tested alternatives. Tyler, Lewis, Haskill, et al. (2003) also noted that their study needs to be replicated by other researchers.

To summarize Phyllis's critical appraisal of the Tyler, Lewis, Haskill, et al. (2003) study, the study is a Level 2b RCT that, although generally well implemented, had some characteristics that might have allowed bias and subjectivity to influence the results. The observed effects in favor of the alternating sequence approach, however, were large and clinically meaningful. This Level 2b evidence surpasses a number of other types of evidence (e.g., expert opinion, theory, basic research, case study, poor quality quasi-experimental research). After determining this, Phyllis must ask herself, "How should the evidence influence what I do in my management of Aaron's speech and language problems?" Answering this question requires her to merge the external evidence with the internal evidence.

Step 5: Integrate the Internal and External Evidence

The extent to which the results of the Tyler, Lewis, Haskill, et al. (2003) study should influence Phyllis's intervention decision cannot be determined solely by ascertaining the level and quality of the external evidence. An evidence-based decision depends on the way in which a clinician consolidates the available internal and external evidence. For example, in the first scenario, Aaron is alert and cooperative, and his parents have advocated the use of any approach that targets their son's phonological and grammatical difficulties. Although Phyllis has identified her own preference in addressing each area of concern separately, she is intrigued by this study's findings. Since Aaron should be able to handle either approach and his parents are supportive of any method that will help Aaron, the Level 2b evidence provided by Tyler and colleagues' study convinces Phyllis to adopt the alternative goal attack approach with Aaron.

Now consider Phyllis's approach in the second scenario. She is much more comfortable with her current intervention approach in that she frequently targets intelligibility simultaneously with grammar, identifying targets that are relevant to both areas of concern. Although she recognizes it as a relatively weak form of evidence, Phyllis has pre and post information in her own treatment records that documents the success of this approach with children similar to Aaron. Perhaps more important, Aaron in this scenario is arguably not as good a fit to the alternating strategy as he is in the first scenario, because it is not clear that the evidence from Tyler, Lewis, Haskill, et al. (2003) is applicable to children with Aaron's attentional challenges. Phyllis must ask herself, "Would Aaron's attentional difficulties and problems moving from one task to another complicate the application of the alternating intervention? Would his parents' desire for the intervention to focus on intelligibility negatively influence attempts to employ the alternating strategy?" Based on her clinical experience, Phyllis argues that the answer to both of these questions is yes. Taking all these factors into consideration, she decides to recommend her typical approach with an emphasis on simultaneously addressing phonology and grammar, despite her awareness of the Level 2b evidence available to support an alternating approach. In Aaron's PPT meeting, she tells the parents about the evidence from Tyler and colleagues' study that supported the alternating strategy and explains her rationale for adopting a strategy other than the alternating approach. After discussing issues, the parents concur with this strategy and sign Aaron's IEP.

These two scenarios illustrate how an evaluation of the same external evidence may not always result in the same clinical decision. Actions that might be recommended based on the results of a review of external evidence may be deemed less suitable or even inappropriate after a careful integration of the external and internal evidence.

Step 6: Evaluate the Decision by Documenting Outcomes

There are very few studies in which all members of a treatment group completing an intervention study responded precisely to the same extent and in the same positive manner. In the same way, some clients enrolled in clinical interventions can be expected to show little or no progress despite receiving the same intervention as those who make dramatic gains. Consequently, inferences based on evidence from research must be questioned, even when the external and internal evidence is uncharacteristically supportive of a particular intervention option. Clinicians must carefully measure participant outcomes during interventions selected through evidence-based decision making. When intervention outcomes support evidence-based decisions, clinicians should continue to implement them, and they may even attempt to apply the decision to a broader set of intervention candidates. When outcomes do not measure up to the evidence-based predictions, EBP clinicians must ask why, and they must seek the answers to this question from their own internally generated evidence as well as from new and extant findings provided in the research literature.

CONCLUSION

This chapter has introduced many important concepts related to EBP in speech-language intervention. In addition, guidelines for what clinicians might do to begin their EBP initiatives in the short term have been recommended. This presentation should lead readers to three broad conclusions.

1. EBP principles do *not* limit SLPs to the use of clinical practices shown by the external evidence to be efficacious and effective. At this stage of the profession's development, the evidence that clinicians need to support their clinical decisions often is simply unavailable. In these cases, principled decisions based on a comprehensive understanding of relevant theory and basic research and careful attention to available internal evidence are likely to be of greatest benefit to the clients and families served. In fact, new ideas concerning intervention possibilities are most likely to emanate from such understanding.

2. EBP principles *do* require SLPs to critically examine their own practices to determine what types and what amounts of evidence support current practices. Recognizing situations in which extant practices are *not* supported by strong clinical studies is equally as important as identifying those practices that are well grounded in research.

3. EBP principles *do* require SLPs to be skeptical about the use of all intervention practices. This conclusion is especially true when practices in speech-language pathology generally do not have a strong body of evidentiary support. In such cases, clinicians must be particularly vigilant with respect to monitoring the outcomes of their interventions, they should actively seek evidence in the literature that is relevant to their clinical questions, and they should encourage members of the research community to design studies that address their most important and pressing clinical questions. This conclusion is most especially true when there is less external evidence for a selected approach relative to some alternative. In all cases, knowledge and understanding of the literature relevant to clinical decisions put clinicians in the best position to make and defend their decisions, to evaluate the outcomes of those decisions, and to deal effectively with parents, professionals, and policy makers who have a vested interest in ensuring that SLPs are accountable for what they do.

STUDY QUESTIONS

1. Define *evidence-based practice* in your own words.

2. A clinician in the public school chooses a new treatment approach for a child on her caseload based on a recent publication in *LSHSS*. This clinician has

    a. Used EBP practice to guide her clinical decisions
    b. Considered external evidence to make her decision
    c. Considered internal evidence to make her decision
    d. a and b

3. What does the acronym PICO stand for? How is it used in evidence-based decision making?

4. List the six steps used to make evidence-based clinical decisions.

5. Name and describe three critical features that must be considered when critically appraising external evidence to assist in a decision about the use of a new speech-language intervention approach.

FURTHER READING

Justice, L.M., & Fey, M.E. (2004). Evidence-based practice in schools: Integrating craft and theory with science and data. *The ASHA Leader*, 4–5, 30–32.
Sackett, D.L., Straus, S.E., Richardson, W.S., Rosenberg, W., & Haynes, R.B. (2000). *Evidence-based medicine: How to practice and teach EBM*. New York, NY: Churchill Livingstone.

REFERENCES

American Speech-Language-Hearing Association (ASHA). (2004). *Evidence-based practice in communication disorders: An introduction.* [Technical report]. Retrieved from http://www.asha.org/NR/rdonlyres/B36BF8F8-C4C3-4E86-8FAD-26D76F130CBF/0/ebpTR.pdf

American Speech-Language-Hearing Association (ASHA). (2005). *Evidence-based practice in communication disorders* [Position statement]. Retrieved from http://www.asha.org/NR/rdonlyres/4837FDFC-576B-4D84-BDD6-8BFF2A803AD3/0/v4PS_EBP.pdf

Bankson, N., & Bernthal, J. E. (1990). *Bankson-Bernthal Test of Phonology.* Austin, TX: PRO-ED.

Centre for Evidence-Based Medicine. (2001a). *Focusing clinical questions.* Retrieved from http://www.cebm.net/focus_quest.asp

Centre for Evidence-Based Medicine. (2001b). *Levels of evidence and grades of recommendation.* Retrieved from http://www.cebm.net/levels_of_evidence.asp

Dollaghan, C.A. (2004). Evidence-based practice in communication disorders: What do we know, and when do we know it? *Journal of Communication Disorders, 37,* 391–400.

Dollaghan, C.A. (2007). *The handbook for evidence-based practice in communication disorders.* Baltimore, MD: Paul H. Brookes Publishing Co.

Dunn, L.M., & Dunn, L.M. (2007). *Peabody Picture Vocabulary Test* (4th ed.). San Antonio, TX: PsychCorp.

Fey, M. (1986). *Language intervention with young children.* Boston, MA: Allyn & Bacon.

Fey, M., Cleave, P.L., Ravida, A.I., Long, S.H., Dejmal, A.E., & Easton, D.L. (1994). Effects of grammar facilitation on the phonological performance of children with speech and language impairments. *Journal of Speech and Hearing Research, 37,* 594–607.

Gersten, R., Fuchs, L.S., Compton, D., Coyne, M., Greenwood, C., & Innocenti, M.S. (2005). Quality indicators for group experimental and quasi-experimental research in special education. *Exceptional Children, 71,* 149–164.

Greenfield, P., & Zukow, P. (1978). Why do children say what they say when they say it? An experimental approach to the psychogenesis of presupposition. In K.E. Nelson (Ed.), *Children's language* (Vol. 1, pp. 287–336). New York, NY: Gardner Press.

Horner, R.H., Carr, E.G., Halle, J., McGee, G., Odom, S., & Wolery, M. (2005). The use of single-subject research to identify evidence-based practice in special education. *Exceptional Children, 71,* 165–179.

Justice, L.M., & Fey, M.E. (2004). Evidence-based practice in schools: Integrating craft and theory with science and data. *The ASHA Leader, 4–5,* 30–32.

Leonard, L., Cole, B., & Steckol, K. (1979). Lexical usage of retarded children: An examination of informativeness. *American Journal of Mental Deficiency, 84,* 49–54.

Lonigan, C., Elber, J., & Johnson, S. (1998). Empirically supported interventions for children: An overview. *Journal of Clinical Child Psychology, 27,* 138–145.

Newcomer, P.L., & Hammill, D.D. (2008). *Test of language development—primary* (4th ed.). San Antonio, TX: PRO-ED.

Porzsolt, F., Ohletz, A., Thim, A., Gardner, D., Ruatti, H., Meier, H., ... Schott, L. (2003). Evidence-based decision making: The six-step approach. *EBM Notebook, 8* (November-December), 165–166.

Sackett, D.L., Straus, S.E., Richardson, W.S., Rosenberg, W., & Haynes, R.B. (2000). *Evidence-based medicine: How to practice and teach EBM.* New York, NY: Churchill Livingstone.

Schwartz, R., & Leonard, L. (1985). Lexical imitation and acquisition in language-impaired children. *Journal of Speech and Hearing Disorders, 50,* 141–149.

Scottish Intercollegiate Guidelines Network. (2004). *Sign 50: A guideline developers' handbook. Annex C.* Retrieved from http://www.sign.ac.uk/guidelines/fulltext/50/annexc.html

Seeff-Gabriel, B., Chiat, S., & Pring, T. (2012) Intervention for co-occurring speech and language difficulties: Addressing the relationship between the two domains. *Child Language Teaching and Therapy, 28,* 123–135.

Snyder, L. (1978). Communicative and cognitive abilities and disabilities in the sensorimotor period. *Merrill-Palmer Quarterly, 24,* 161–180.

Sorensen, P., & Fey, M.E. (1992). Informativeness as a clinical principle: What's really new? *Language, Speech, and Hearing Services in Schools, 23*, 320–328.

Stokes, D.E. (1997). *Pasteur's quadrant.* Washington, DC: Brookings Institution Press.

Troia, G. (1999). Phonological awareness intervention research: A critical review of the experimental methodology. *Reading Research Quarterly, 34*, 28–53.

Tyler, A.A., Lewis, K.E., Haskill, A., & Tolbert, L.C. (2002). Efficacy and cross-domain effects of a morphosyntax and a phonology intervention. *Language, Speech, and Hearing Services in Schools, 33*, 52–66.

Tyler, A.A., Lewis, K.E., Haskill, A., & Tolbert, L.C. (2003). Outcomes of different speech and language goal attack strategies. *Journal of Speech, Language, and Hearing Research, 46*, 1077–1094.

Tyler, A., Lewis, K.E., & Welch, C.M. (2003) Predictors of phonological change following intervention. *American Journal of Speech Language Pathology, 12*, 289–298.

Tyler, A.A., & Sandoval, K.T. (1994). Preschoolers with phonological and language disorders: Treating different linguistic domains. *Language, Speech, and Hearing Services in Schools, 25*, 215–234.

van Kleeck, A. (1994). Potential cultural bias in training parents as conversational partners with their children who have delP it is zays in language development. *American Journal of Speech-Language Pathology, 3*(1), 67–78.

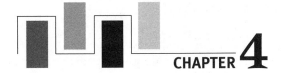

CHAPTER 4

Principles of Communication Assessment

Michelle MacRoy-Higgins and Elizabeth E. Galletta

CHAPTER OBJECTIVES

After reading this chapter, students will be able to

- State three purposes for assessment
- Compare and contrast formal and informal testing procedures
- Discuss the psychometric principles of reliability and validity, as they relate to testing procedures
- Define standardization as it relates to formal and informal tests
- Describe procedures when assessing clients' language, speech, fluency, voice, oral mechanism, and initial considerations for alternative and augmentative communication (AAC)

When a Speech-Language Pathologist (SLP) performs an assessment, it involves gathering information from a variety of sources, interpreting this information to make decisions, and presenting this information to clients, caregivers, and other professionals. The term **assessment** is synonymous with the term **evaluation;** both terms refer to the process of gathering and interpreting information for the purpose of making decisions. The outcome of assessment is typically the determination of the presence or absence of a communication disorder. When a communication disorder exists, a **diagnosis** or diagnostic label is established. Prior to visiting a SLP for an evaluation, a client may have been given a medical diagnosis (e.g., traumatic brain injury, myasthenia gravis, multiple sclerosis) from a physician, or a psychological (e.g., autism spectrum disorder) or educational (learning disability) diagnosis from a psychologist. The diagnosis that an SLP provides describes the client's swallowing or communication disorder (e.g., nonfluent aphasia, dysarthria, pragmatic language impairment). Speech-language pathologists provide diagnoses because many times a diagnostic label is required for billing, reimbursement, or special education eligibility. An assessment will also result in recommendations that describe whether speech and language therapy is warranted and if so, the frequency of therapy (e.g., once weekly, daily) and the type of therapy (e.g., group, individual). The evaluation should also help the SLP determine **prognosis,** which is a prediction of future communication skills, either with or without intervention. Some factors that may influence a client's prognosis are age, severity of communication disorder, family support, and co-occurring medical conditions.

Speech-language pathologists work as a part of an **interdisciplinary** team. This means that we work with and/or collaborate with other professionals (e.g., audiologists, physicians, nurses, physical therapists, occupational therapists, social workers, psychologists, dentists, regular education teachers, special education teachers) to meet the needs of the clients with whom we work. As a member of an interdisciplinary team, we may receive **referrals** from other professionals to perform speech-language, swallowing and/or feeding evaluations. Other sources of referral include the client's family members and caregivers, or an individual may refer him- or herself for an evaluation. This is most often seen in adults but may be observed in adolescent clients as well.

The use of **evidenced-based practice** (EBP) has been established by the American Speech-Language-Hearing Association (ASHA) as the gold standard for SLPs. That is, when making decisions about evaluation procedures and materials, it is crucial that we use research-based evidence, in addition to our expertise and experience as an SLP, while also considering each client's preferences and values (ASHA, 2005). The use of EBP in our evaluation process will guide us in selecting the most sensitive, specific, and diagnostically accurate assessment instruments for assigning diagnoses and will guide the development of appropriate prognostic statements and treatment recommendations. See Chapter 3 for detailed information about EBP.

PURPOSES OF ASSESSMENT

There are several distinct reasons for conducting an assessment, and depending on the particular purpose, procedures or instruments may vary. As we consider these, let us use the following examples to illustrate some of our assessment principles.

 CASE EXAMPLES

1. Sam is a 2-year, 6-month-old boy who has delayed expressive language. He started babbling at 12 months of age, and his current vocabulary consists of 20 intelligible words. He has shown some frustration with his lack of communication skills both at home and at child care, where he has been observed to hit other children to obtain a desired toy.

2. Molly is a 4-year-old girl with Down syndrome. She demonstrates delays in all developmental areas (speech; receptive language; expressive language and gross motor, fine motor, adaptive behavior, and cognitive skills). Molly's strengths include her social skills.

3. John is an 8-year-old boy with spastic cerebral palsy (CP). John's fine motor and gross motor skills are impaired; he is not ambulatory and uses a wheelchair. His speech is highly unintelligible, and he is not understood many times by his family, teachers, and peers, causing John to withdraw from conversations.

4. Sally is a 13-year-old girl with high-functioning autism spectrum disorder. She is in the eighth grade in a general education setting. Her syntax, morphology, phonology, and semantics are grossly within normal limits. Sally has particular difficulty with classroom discourse skills, pragmatics, and social communication with her peers.

5. James is a 65-year-old male who is recently retired. His wife encouraged him to see an SLP because, she reports, James "talks too loud" and responds inappropriately during conversation. James reports that he is also having difficulty understanding conversations in restaurants and in noisy situations such as parties.

6. Alexa is a 14-year-old girl who stutters. She attends a public high school in an urban setting. She had speech therapy as a younger child and is self-referred due to increased pressure to speak in high school. Socially, she is confident and aspires to be a physician.

7. Eddie is a 72-year-old stroke survivor with no overt physical disability. He experienced a CVA 2 years ago and received speech therapy while he was hospitalized. He lives independently and travels to senior citizen groups and stroke support groups in his community.

8. Mary is a 59-year-old woman with Parkinson's disease. She was a third-grade teacher but retired due to difficulties maintaining her stamina in the classroom setting. She is experiencing some difficulty with people understanding her and some difficulty with what she describes as *residue* in her throat when she swallows.

Let us examine the main purposes of assessment and how they might apply to clients like these.

Screening

A **screening** is a brief procedure used to determine the presence of a disorder. The results from a screening inform the clinician whether a comprehensive evaluation is indicated. If a client fails a screening, then an in-depth evaluation is necessary. Typically, a screening will result in a *pass* or *fail* determination based on various predetermined criteria. For example, a screening procedure for adults that are in an inpatient facility can involve asking a patient to name common objects, (e.g., a pen, a watch, glasses), follow simple and complex directions, and/or describe a picture. When working with a client like James, we might do a language screening to determine whether his problems in understanding conversation have a language component, in addition to providing an in-depth audiological assessment. A school-based SLP may be involved with annual kindergarten screenings or in annual hearing screenings in collaboration with the school nurse in elementary school settings. An SLP working in a birth-to-3 agency might do a screening for both hearing and language to determine the next steps in evaluating a toddler like Sam. For James, an audiologist may screen his hearing in order to decide whether a comprehensive audiological examination is indicated.

Screening may focus on one particular area; for example, we might do a language comprehension screening for John to determine whether his understanding of language is affected, in addition to his limitations in speech production as a result of his spastic CP. For James, we would most likely focus on hearing

Table 4.1. Examples of screening instruments used in speech, language, and communication assessments

Child		
Name	Age	Assessment area
Adolescent Language Screening Test (ALST; Morgan & Guilford, 1984)	11–17 years	Language: pragmatics, receptive and expressive vocabulary, concepts, sentence formulation, morphology, phonology
Bankson-Bernthal Test of Phonology (BBTOP; Bankson & Bernthal, 1990)	3–9 years	Articulation, phonological processes
Boone Voice Program for Children–Second Edition (Boone, 1993)	Grades K–8	Voice
Clinical Evaluation of Language Fundamentals–Fifth Edition (CELF-5; Semel, Wiig, & Secord, 2013)	5–21 years	Language: receptive and expressive morphology, syntax, semantics
Early Language Milestones Scale–Second Edition (ELM Scale-2; Coplan, 1993)	Birth–3 years	Language: receptive and expressive semantics, syntax; phonology
Fluharty Preschool Speech and Language Screening Test–Second Edition (FPSLST-2; Fluharty, 2000)	3–6 years	Language: vocabulary, articulation, syntax
Kindergarten Language Screening Test–Second Edition (KLST-2; Gauthier & Madison, 1998)	3.5–6 years	Language: receptive and expressive semantics, syntax
Screening Test for Developmental Apraxia of Speech–Second Edition (STDAS-2; Blakeley, 2000)	4–12 years	Apraxia

Adult		
Name	Age	Assessment area
Bedside Evaluation Screening Test–Second Edition (BEST-2; West, Sands, & Ross-Swain, 1998)	Adult	Aphasia: speaking, comprehension, reading
Brief Test of Head Injury (BTHI; Helm-Estabrooks & Hotz, 1991)	14 years–adult	Cognition, linguistic, and communicative abilities
Oral Speech Mechanism Screening Examination–Third Edition (OSMSE-3; St. Louis & Ruscello, 2000)	5–78 years	Oral-motor mechanism

screening. For other cases, we may need to screen several areas of function. A child referred to a school-based SLP by the classroom teacher for speech dysfluencies might need screening that will address not only fluency but also articulation and language. Table 4.1 presents examples of some screening instruments that can be used with a variety of clients.

Determining Eligibility for Services

In many cases speech-language therapy is supported by public funding (e.g., school district) or by third-party sources (e.g., health insurance). Each funding source may have specific guidelines to determine if a client is eligible for services. Therefore, it is typically necessary to document, by means of assessment, the type and severity of each client's communication disorder in order to establish the client's eligibility for services. For example, some school districts indicate that a child must perform 1.5 or 2 standard deviations (*SDs*) below the mean on a standardized test battery when compared with children who are the same age; others may require performance below a certain level on a test as well as documentation of disability based on a language sample or parent or teacher report.

As mentioned before, the evaluation allows the clinician to make a diagnosis that describes a client's particular communication disorder. For example, Sally, the client with high-functioning autism, may not have received any diagnosis until she reached eighth grade because she is generally quiet and withdrawn and has well-developed formal language skills. As an adolescent, though, her social communication disorder may become more obvious because schoolwork requires more social understanding to comprehend complex narratives and to participate in academically focused group assignments. She may now need to have a diagnosis that entitles her to services that will assist her in developing better pragmatic skills. The diagnosis not only establishes eligibility for services but also helps the SLP to determine the goals and methods of intervention that are appropriate for each client. Sally's SLP will need not only to provide a diagnosis but also to describe the specific kinds of communication problems Sally displays in order to set objectives for her intervention program.

Documenting Progress

When clinicians assess a client and describe the client's communication in detail, they are establishing the client's **baseline** performance. A baseline describes a client's current level of communicative functioning, including both strengths and weaknesses. The baseline is used both to determine the starting point for intervention and to serve as a point of comparison against assessment data collected after some intervention has taken place. This comparison allows clinicians to show that the time and money spent on therapy resulted in some meaningful change. For example, public schools require annual eligibility determination. With a student like Sally, it will be necessary to assess her conversational ability before beginning intervention and again after intervention has been delivered in order to show growth in her pragmatic skills. For adults like Mary with Parkinson's disease, who may be in outpatient or inpatient rehabilitation, third-party payers, such as insurance companies or Medicare, may require documentation of progress in order to justify continued care. The result of ongoing assessment is documented not only to provide accountability for services but also to adjust therapy goals and methods to maximize progress or to decide when therapy is no longer achieving the targeted outcomes.

METHODS OF ASSESSMENT

Four main types of assessment tools are used in our field. They include **case history questionnaires, norm-referenced tests** (also called *formal tests*), **criterion-referenced tests,** and observational tools. A comprehensive evaluation typically utilizes all four types of tools in order to get the best understanding of a particular client's communication skills.

Case History Interviews

Each assessment begins with gathering information about the client and his or her communication disorder. This information is used to focus the assessment on presenting problems, investigate contributing factors, and understand the social context of the client's communication. Detailed information about case history gathering can be found in Chapter 7.

Norm-Referenced Tests

Norm-referenced tests involve comparing a client's performance to a sample of individuals who are similar to the client. These tests conform to certain properties that make them fair, or valid, comparison tools. These properties include representative samples, standard scores, standardization, validity, and reliability. Let us examine each of these properties in turn.

Representative Samples   The norming sample, or group of individuals to whom a client taking a test is being compared, should meet certain standards in order to ensure that the comparison is a fair one. The sample should be big (most authorities on test construction set a minimum of 100 subjects per age group as a lower limit; see Paul & Norbury, 2012). It should also be representative, or contain individuals who represent the typical range of performance. This usually means that the norming sample will include people of all the ages the test will be used to assess, from more than one geographic region, both genders, and a range of socio-economic and ethnic backgrounds. Here is why: Suppose the norming sample for a driving test consisted only of people from Louisiana. These people would probably have little knowledge about driving in snow, ice, or hail, so their knowledge of this area would be very limited. But a driver from Minnesota would need to have that knowledge in order to be a successful driver. If a test normed on Louisiana drivers were given to a person who would be driving mostly in Minnesota, the test would not be a very good measure of how successful a driver that person is likely to be. Evidence-based assessment requires that clinicians examine the description of the norming sample in a standardized test carefully to make sure the sample is big and representative enough to result in a fair comparison for a given client.

Standard Scores   When a test is given to a large enough group of people, the scores on that test can be graphed so that they form a bell-shaped curve. This curve represents the **normal distribution** (see Figure 4.1), one in which most of the scores fall close to the **mean** or average for the entire group and fewer scores fall farther from the average in either direction, higher or lower. This is another reason why norming samples need to be large; if they are not, the scores will not distribute themselves into a nice bell shape and so, again, comparisons of a client's score to the norming sample may not be fair and accurate. The normal curve for a test is used to establish **standard scores.** These represent how far from the average score a particular raw score (or the number of items the individual got *correct* on a test) falls. How far is far? Distance from the average score is measured in **standard deviation units** (*SD* units); an *SD* unit is the average distance that scores fall from the average. If you remember your statistics, you may recall that the *SD* is calculated by taking the following steps:

1. Taking the score each person in the norming sample got on the test

2. Subtracting it from the average score for the norming sample

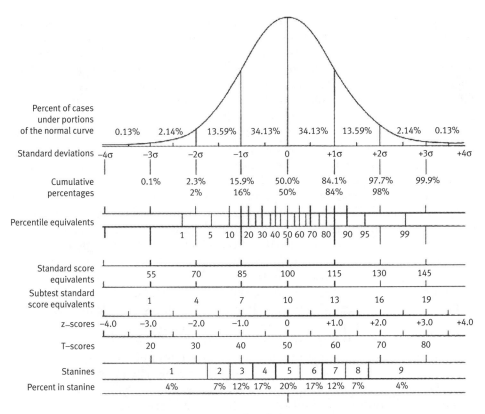

Figure 4.1. Bell-shaped curve representing different types of standard scores.

3.   Adding up all those differences, then

4.   Dividing that sum by the number of people in the norming sample

Norm-referenced tests convert raw scores to scores that show how many *SD* units from the average score for the norming sample your client's score falls. There are several types of standard scores, including *z*-scores, *T*-scores, and stanines, as shown on Figure 4.1. The most common type is the standard score equivalent or quotient score. This sets the average score for the norming sample at 100 and the standard deviation at 15. IQ tests use these kinds of scores, so an IQ score of 100 means that the client's score falls just at the average for the norming sample. Scores of 85 are 1 *SD* below average, those of 115 are 1 *SD* above.

But we still do not know how far from average is too far! Unfortunately, the answer is, it depends. As the normal curve in Figure 4.1 shows, the portions of the curve in which scores fall can be divided into regions based on the number of *SD*s from average. About 34% of scores fall up to 1 *SD* above average; another 34% fall up to 1 *SD* below average. So 68% of the people taking at test will fall within 1 *SD* from the average score. These people are not significantly different from average. But as we get farther from the average, fewer and fewer scores fall within each *SD* region. About 14% fall between 1 *SD* and 2 *SD*s above average, another 14% fall between 1 *SD* and 2 *SD*s below. Do clients who score 1–2 *SD*s below average have a disability? If they do, then 14% of all people would be considered to have a disability—this is probably too many people to provide with services. What about between 2 *SD*s and 3 *SD*s below average? Only about 2% of scores fall there. Some agencies require scores more than 2 *SD*s below average in order for clients to qualify for services. Others might require only 1.5 *SD*s below average for service eligibility. So, although standard scores do not tell in and of themselves how low is low enough, they can be used to establish eligibility in the context of the eligibility requirements of the particular agency serving the client.

Percentile ranks are another way to represent where an individual score falls in comparison to the normal distribution. The percentile rank represents the percentage of people performing at or below a particular score. The 50th percentile represents the mean; therefore 50% of the norming population scored above this score and 50% score below. Percentile ranks are often used to describe scores to teachers and families because they are easy to understand. But like standard scores, they need to be interpreted in light of the eligibility requirements for disability services. Some agencies specify percentile ranks that qualify people for services. For example, children who fall in the bottom 10th percentile are considered to qualify for services in some schools.

Raw scores are sometimes converted into equivalent scores, expressed in years or grades. An age equivalent is the raw score that is average for a given age (e.g., 5 years, 0 months); a grade equivalent is the raw score that is average for a particular grade. It is important to understand that equivalent scores indicate that an individual has answered correctly the same number of items as are average for a person that age or grade, but it does not necessarily mean that the client is performing as does a person who is that age or grade. Equivalent scores also do not provide information on how far from the average the client's own age or grade a score falls, so it is difficult to use the score to determine eligibility for services.

Even though standard procedures are described for administering norm-referenced tests, there is always error in measurement simply because human behavior is variable. If I take a test before I have my coffee in the morning, my score is likely to be different than if I take the same test after lunch. Whatever score is obtained is only an estimate of an individual's "true" performance, although you may never know for sure what the "true" performance is (Maybe I would do better on the test if I take it after breakfast, when the coffee kicks in; maybe I will be a bit logy after lunch; it's hard to know!). The **standard error of measurement** (SEM) reflects this kind of uncertainty: the average degree to which the obtained score differs from the theoretical "true score." Since we can never really know the true score, we use the SEM to obtain a confidence interval, which is a range of scores that has a high probability of containing the individual's true score within it. For example, suppose Figure 4.2 were a test given to our client Molly, who has Down syndrome. Her observed standard score was 81. Information in the test manual would tell us that a 90% confidence interval around this score would range from 76 to 87. That would mean that if Molly were to take the test a lot of times, theoretically 90% of the time Molly's score would fall between 76 and 87. This information is helpful if we want to compare Molly's scores on this test before and after an intervention to improve her vocabulary. We would want to show that her score after intervention was not only higher than 81, her observed score, but that it was higher than 87, a score she would have been 90% likely to get (because

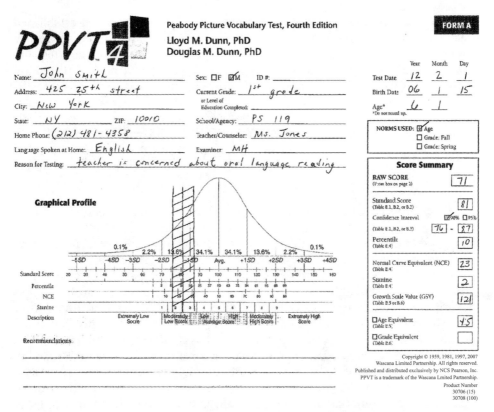

PPVT4™

Peabody Picture Vocabulary Test, Fourth Edition
Lloyd M. Dunn, PhD
Douglas M. Dunn, PhD

FORM A

Name: *John Smith*   Sex: ☐F ☑M   ID #: ____

Address: *425 25th street*   Current Grade: *1st grade*
                                  or Level of
City: *New York*   Education Completed: ____

State: *NY*   ZIP: *10010*   School/Agency: *PS 119*

Home Phone: *(212) 481-4358*   Teacher/Counselor: *Ms. Jones*

Language Spoken at Home: *English*   Examiner: *MH*

Reason for Testing: *teacher is concerned about oral language, reading*

	Year	Month	Day
Test Date	*12*	*2*	*1*
Birth Date	*06*	*1*	*15*
Age*	*6*	*1*	

*Do not round up.

NORMS USED: ☑ Age
☐ Grade: Fall
☐ Grade: Spring

Score Summary

RAW SCORE (From box on page 2)	*71*
Standard Score (Table E.1, B.2, or B.3)	*81*
Confidence Interval ☑90% ☐95%	
(Table E.1, B.2, or B.3)	*76* - *87*
Percentile (Table E.4)	*10*
Normal Curve Equivalent (NCE) (Table E.4)	*23*
Stanine (Table E.4)	*2*
Growth Scale Value (GSV) (Table B.5 or B.6)	*121*
☐ Age Equivalent (Table E.5)	*4:5*
☐ Grade Equivalent (Table E.6)	

Graphical Profile

0.1% 2.2% 13.6% 34.1% 34.1% 13.6% 2.2% 0.1%

-5SD -4SD -3SD -2SD -1SD Avg. +1SD +2SD +3SD +4SD

Standard Score   20 30 40 50 60 70 80 90 100 110 120 130 140 150 160

Percentile

NCE

Stanine

Description Extremely Low Score   Moderately Low Score   Low Average Score   High Average Score   Moderately High Score   Extremely High Score

Recommendations

Figure 4.2. John Smith's results from the Peabody Picture Vocabulary Test–Fourth Edition. (From Dunn, L.M., & Dunn, D.M. [2007]. *Peabody Picture Vocabulary Test* [4th ed.]. Minneapolis, MN: Pearson; reprinted by permission.)

it is within the confidence for her "true" score) even without intervention. So SEM scores, when they are available for a standardized test, help us to determine when a score changes, whether or not that score was likely to have happened without any intervention.

Standardization   In order for a test to be fair, everyone should take it under the same conditions. It would not be fair if some people taking a math test were allowed to use a calculator whereas others were not. That is why consistency in administration and scoring is necessary in a standardized test. The manual for administering the test should provide very specific instructions for administering and scoring the test, and clinicians need to follow these instructions in detail in order to ensure that test administrator or testing environment has minimal effect on the test taker's performance.

Validity   When a test accurately measures what it claims to measure, we say the test is valid. For example, a valid measure of your running speed could involve your running on a treadmill for a given length of time and then computing the distance run divided by the time you spent running. But having you run on a crowded street where you have to avoid running into people and have to stop at street corners to wait for the light to change would be a less valid measure of how fast you can run. Standardized tests have metrics that are used to measure their

validity; these metrics usually involve comparing them to other, well-established tests that are known to test the same thing. So if we create a new test to measure a child's understanding of vocabulary, we might give clients both our new test and an established test, such as the Peabody Picture Vocabulary Test–Fourth Edition (Dunn & Dunn, 2007), and compare the scores to show that our test is measuring the same thing as the more familiar Peabody. This comparison would serve as one measure of the test's validity. Validity is usually reported in test manuals as a correlation statistic that can range from 0.0 to 1.0. A correlation of 0.0 is very poor, indicating no reliability, whereas a correlation of 1.0 is considered perfect. Validity statistics can vary, but the higher the statistic, the more likely the test is to be a valid measure.

Reliability When a test score remains stable, or similar, regardless of who gives the test or when the client takes it, the test is considered reliable. Two commonly used measures of reliability are interrater and test–retest reliability. **Interrater reliability** is measured by having one tester give a client a test and score it and then having a second tester do the same and comparing the two scores. These two scores should be quite close together in order to show that the test has high interrater reliability. **Test–retest reliability** refers to a test's consistency over time. The same test is administered to the same person more than once; obtaining the same or similar results would indicate a test has good test–retest reliability. Test manuals report reliability data, like validity, as correlation coefficients. Reliability measures should be at least .90 for a test to be considered reliable. Norbury and Paul (2012) give more detail on these and other psychometric properties of standardized tests. Table 4.2 presents examples of standardized tests frequently used by SLPs.

It is also important to note whether individuals with communication disorders are included in the norming sample for a test. A norming sample that includes only typically developing clients will be helpful in showing whether a person is significantly different from the norm, though that may not be the question we want the test to answer. For example, we already know that John, our child with CP, has speech that is significantly impaired. We may want to compare him to others with CP, instead of typically developing individuals, in order to determine how severely he is affected. For this purpose, we may want to choose a test that includes individuals with a specific communication disorder in the norming sample. For example, the Stuttering Severity Instrument–Fourth Edition (SSI-4; Riley, 2009) includes preschool children, school-age children, and adults who stutter in the norming sample. Therefore, the SSI-4 allows the clinician to compare stuttering severity among individuals who have the same diagnosis.

Other Considerations Figure 4.2 illustrates some of the terms that were just introduced using the Peabody Picture Vocabulary Test–Fourth Edition (Dunn & Dunn, 2007), which is an example of a norm-referenced test commonly used in communication assessment.

Norm-referenced tests are excellent tools for determining whether a client is significantly different from the norming sample and for establishing eligibility for services. However, by their nature, such tests do not allow for variation or accommodations during test administration. In addition, the testing situation may not be natural or familiar to the person being tested and may therefore negatively

Table 4.2. Examples of tests for adults and children used to assess speech, language, and communication

Name	Age	Assessment area
Articulation and phonology		
Arizona Articulation Proficiency Scale–Third Revision (Arizona-3; Fudala, 2000)	1.5–18 years	Articulation
Goldman-Fristoe Test of Articulation–Second Edition (GFTA-2; Goldman & Fristoe, 2000)	2–21 years	Articulation
Hodson Assessment of Phonological Patterns–Third Edition (HAPP-3; Hodson, 2004)	3–8 years	Phonological processes
Khan-Lewis Phonological Analysis–Second Edition (KLPA-2; Khan & Lewis, 2002)	2–21 years	Phonological processes
Fluency		
Stuttering Severity Instrument for Children and Adults–Fourth Edition (SSI-4; Riley, 2009)	2 years–adult	Fluency
Test of Childhood Stuttering (TOCS; Gillam, Logan, Pearson, 2009)	4–12 years	Fluency
Language		
Child		
Clinical Evaluation of Language Fundamentals–Fifth Edition (CELF-5; Semel, Wiig, & Secord, 2013)	5–21 years	Language: receptive and expressive morphology, syntax, semantics; auditory memory
Comprehensive Assessment of Spoken Language (CASL; Carrow-Woolfolk, 1999)	3–21 years	Language: comprehension, expression, lexical and semantic retrieval, syntax, pragmatics, supralinguistic areas
Diagnostic Evaluation of Language Variation (DELV; Seymour, Roeper, & de Villiers, 2005)	4–9 years	Language: syntax, pragmatics, semantics, phonology
MacArthur-Bates Communicative Development Inventories –Second Edition (CDIs; Fenson et al., 2007)	8–37 months	Language: receptive and expressive vocabulary, gestures, syntax, morphology
Peabody Picture Vocabulary Test–Fourth Edition (PPVT-4; Dunn & Dunn, 2007)	2.5–90+ years	Language: receptive vocabulary
Preschool Language Scales–Fifth Edition (PLS-5; Zimmerman, Steiner, & Pond, 2011)	Birth–7 years	Language: receptive and expressive semantics, syntax, morphology, articulation
Test of Adolescent and Adult Language–Fourth Edition (TOAL-4; Hammill, Brown, Larsen, & Weiderholt, 2007)	12–24 years	Language: receptive and expressive semantics and syntax; reading, writing, auditory comprehension
Test for Auditory Comprehension of Language–Third Edition (TACL-3; Carrow-Woolfolk, 1998)	3–9 years	Language: auditory comprehension of semantics, syntax, morphology
Adult		
Boston Diagnostic Aphasia Examination–Third Edition (BDAE-3; Goodglass, Kaplan, & Barresi, 2001)	Adult	Language (aphasia): auditory and written language comprehension, oral expression, writing
Boston Naming Test–Second Edition (BNT; Kaplan, Goodglass, & Weintraub, 2000)	Adult	Language (aphasia): word retrieval
Communication Activities of Daily Living–Second Edition (CADL-2; Holland, Frattali, & Fromm, 1999)	Adult	Language (aphasia/brain damage): semantics, pragmatics, reading, writing
Western Aphasia Battery–Revised (WAB-R; Kertesz, 2006)	Adolescent to adult	Language (aphasia): auditory comprehension, verbal fluency, naming, information content
Cognition		
Assessment of Language-Related Functional Activities (ALFA; Baines, Heeringa, & Martin, 1999)	16–95 years	Language-related functional activities

(continued)

Table 4.2.　*(continued)*

Name	Age	Assessment area
Behavior Inattention Test (BIT; Wilson, Cockburn, & Halligan, 1987)	19–83 years	Functional skills relevant to visual neglect
Cognitive Linguistic Quick Test (CLQT; Helm-Estabrooks, 2001)	18–89 years	Attention, memory, executive functions, language, visuospatial skills
Detroit Tests of Learning Aptitude–Fourth Edition (DTLA-4; Hammill, 1998)	6–17 years	Cognition
Reading Comprehension Battery for Aphasia–Second Edition (RCBA-2; LaPointe & Horner, 1998)	Adolescents and adults	Reading comprehension
Ross Information Processing Assessment–Second Edition (RIPA-2; Ross-Swain, 1996)	15–90 years	Memory, temporal orientation, spatial orientation, problem solving, abstract reasoning, auditory processing and retention
Scales of Cognitive Ability for Traumatic Brain Injury (SCATBI; Adamovich & Henderson, 1992)	Adolescents and adults	Perception/discrimination, orientation, organization, recall, reasoning

influence that individual's performance. For example, a client like Alexa, who stutters, may be particularly uncomfortable in a testing environment with an unfamiliar examiner and may therefore exhibit more dysfluencies during testing than she would during a typical conversation. A further consideration is that norm-referenced tests are appropriate for individuals who are represented in the norming population. It is important that clinicians be careful about choosing tests with norming populations that represent the client's characteristics in terms of age, ethnic and socioeconomic status, and language experience. Therefore, all tests are not appropriate for all clients, especially those who come from backgrounds that are culturally and linguistically different from the mainstream. Chapter 10 discusses these issues in more detail.

Criterion-Referenced Procedures

Unlike norm-referenced tests, **criterion-referenced tests** do not compare an individual's performance to others. Instead, criterion-referenced measures compare skills to certain predetermined expectations. An example of a criterion-referenced assessment is the Rossetti Infant–Toddler Language Scale (Rossetti, 2006), shown in Figure 4.3, which we might use to assess our toddler Sam's language level. The scoresheet shows that there are certain skills that are expected to be present in the 21–24 month age range, such as these: *follows a two-step related command* and *uses new words regularly*. Criterion-referenced assessments may or may not be standardized; some outline specific procedures to elicit responses to items, other instruments do not. The strengths of criterion-referenced assessments are that they can be administered in a naturalistic environment and modifications can be made to observe or elicit certain behaviors. Their main disadvantage is that a standard score is not obtained, which many times is required to document the need or the continuation of therapy in certain settings such as public schools. But if eligibility has already been established with a standardized test, criterion-referenced assessment can be very helpful to determine what

21–24 months

| page 35 | Interaction–*attachment* | *Notes* |

No items at this age level

| page 49 | Pragmatics |

No items at this age level

| page 58 | Gesture |

O E R

16. Gestures to request action
17. Gestures to indicate toileting needs
18. Pretends to pour from a container
19. Pushes a stroller or shopping cart
20. Flies a toy airplane

| page 78 | Play |

O E R

33. Puts away toys on request
34. Attempts to repair broken toys
35. Stacks and assembles toys and objects

| page 111 | Language comprehension |

O E R

57. Chooses one object from a group of five upon verbal request
58. Follows novel commands
59. Follows a two-step related command
60. Understands new words rapidly

| page 153 | Language expression |

O E R

63. Uses two-word phrases frequently
64. Uses 50 different words
65. Uses new words regularly
66. Relates personal experiences
67. Uses three-word phrases occasionally
68. Refers to self by name
69. Uses early pronouns occasionally
70. Uses a mean length of 1.25–1.50 morphemes per utterance

Figure 4.3. Skills tested in children 21–24 months of age on the Rossetti Infant–Toddler Language Scale. (From Rossetti, L. [2006]. *The Rossetti Infant–Toddler Language Scale*. East Moline, IL: LinguiSystems; reprinted by permission.) The Rossetti Infant-Toddler Language Scale is divided into six areas of development (i.e., interaction, pragmatics, gesture, play, language comprehension, and language expression). For each area (e.g., language expressive) for each age range, (e.g., 21–24 months) there are certain skills that are tested. Each skill can be observed (O), elicited (E), or reported (R). The skills that are observed, elicited, or reported are considered to be mastered and therefore an age equivalent estimating the child's functioning can be obtained.

communicative functions a client can and cannot perform, and such assessment can guide the development of the intervention plan.

Informal Tools

Interviews   When clients are very young or are impaired due to stroke or injury, they may not be able to accurately report their history or describe their current strengths and needs, so clinicians often turn to family members to gain this information. There are a variety of instruments designed to assist in collecting this history and current function information from individuals of all ages. Table 4.3 provides a few examples. In addition to using these structured tools for gathering client information, clinicians may also use **interviewing,** more open-ended conversations about the client's history, concerns, and perceptions about his or her communication skills, to understand why evaluation is being sought. Interviewing also allows the SLP to understand the concerns and perceptions of family members. A detailed discussion of interviewing and case history gathering can be found in Chapter 7.

Behavioral Observation   Tests and criterion-referenced measures compare a client's performance to a standard; behavioral observations describe behavior in a systematic way, without reference to predetermined criteria. Behavioral observations are conducted in settings where the client typically communicates (e.g., home, child care, school, work, social situations), in order to describe communication strengths and weaknesses in real-world contexts. Behavioral observation checklists such as the Functional Communication Profile–Revised (FCP-R; Kleinman, 2003) can be used to note clients' communication and interaction

Table 4.3.   Examples of checklists and interview instruments for assessing communication

Measure	Age range	Areas of communication
Communication and Symbolic Behavior Development Profile Infant–Toddler Checklist (CSBS DP–ITC; Wetherby & Prizant, 2003)	6–24 months	Emotion and gaze Communication Gestures Sounds Words Understanding
Language Use Inventory (LUI; O'Neill, 2007)	18 months–4 years	Pragmatics Communicative functions Sentences and stories
Children's Communication Checklist–2 (CCC–2; Bishop, 2003)	4–16 years	Speech Syntax Semantics Coherence Pragmatics
Vineland Adaptive Behavior Scales–II (Vineland–II; Sparrow, Cicchetti, & Balla, 2005)	Birth–80 years	Communication Socialization Daily living skills Motor skills Maladaptive behavior
Social Communication Questionnaire (SCQ; Rutter, Bailey, & Lord, 2003)	4 years–adult	Communication skills Social function
Aphasia Needs Assessment (Garrett & Beukelman, 2006)	Adult	Functional communication

skills. In addition, SLPs can use structured sampling events (McLaughlin & Cascella, 2008) to observe a particular communication behavior that seems to be causing trouble. We might observe Sally, for example, in her English class, where it is reported she is getting into trouble by interrupting and calling out. We might keep track of what triggers these behaviors, how others react, and what rules the other students follow to get a turn to talk. This observation could be discussed with Sally and used to develop an intervention plan. Recording samples of connected speech and analyzing the properties of the words, sounds, and sentences used is also a rich source of information about clients' communicative competence. Speech and language sampling is covered in more detail in Chapter 5.

Dynamic Assessment   Tasks in most assessment procedures are presented to clients without any support from the clinician. We might, for example, ask Eddie, our recovered stroke client, to tell a story from a picture, or explain how to cook spaghetti, in order to get a look at how he is able to organize his language output and note where he shows difficulties when producing extended talk on his own. Dynamic assessment (Haywood & Lidz, 2007), though, allows the clinician to determine how clients respond to different support strategies. One of the goals of dynamic assessment is to determine what approaches or intervention techniques will promote change in the client. For example, when evaluating Alexa's dysfluency, the SLP can teach different strategies (e.g., easy onset, reduced rate of speech) and observe which help Alexa most. Dynamic assessment procedures can aid in determining which therapeutic techniques may be beneficial.

AREAS OF ASSESSMENT

The next sections of this chapter discuss areas of assessment, including language, speech, voice, fluency, hearing, alternative and augmentative communication (AAC), and sensorimotor assessment, in clients ranging in age from infancy through adulthood. Each area of assessment is divided into age categories: 0 to 5 years: infants, toddlers, and preschoolers; 6 to 17 years: elementary school age and adolescents; and 18+ years: adults.

Language

Thorough language assessment will include each of the domains of language: semantics, phonology, syntax, morphology, and pragmatics. For each component, both receptive (understanding) and expressive (productive) aspects should be assessed. For all ages, receptive language may be somewhat challenging to assess because when we understand language, that understanding happens inside our mind and may not produce any obvious behavior. We typically make inferences about an individual's language comprehension by asking clients to demonstrate understanding through indicating pictures or objects or answering questions, so receptive language tasks typically involve pointing to objects or pictures (e.g., "Point to the cat") or following instructions (e.g., "Pick up the keys"). If an individual does not successfully complete the task, it may be difficult to determine whether he or she did not understand the instructions (*point to*) or the target word (*cat*), did not possess the fine motor skills necessary to achieve this act (e.g., an

individual with limited physical skills), or was simply noncompliant (not cooperative, interested, or attentive). For this reason, it is often helpful to supplement
receptive testing with methods other than formal testing such as interviewing
caregivers, using dynamic assessment, and engaging in behavioral observation.

Assessment of language production involves eliciting speech samples from
clients to evaluate semantic, phonological, morphological, syntactic, and pragmatic aspects of language. Tasks used to assess these areas include a variety of discourse types such as naming pictures, repeating sentences, describing pictures or
picture scenes, completing sentences, telling stories, and providing spontaneous
language sampling. These are discussed in more detail in Chapter 5.

An additional aspect of language that may be assessed is reading readiness,
for young children, and other literacy-related skills for older students. Individuals
with a history of language delay are at risk for reading, writing, and literacy difficulties (e.g., Schuele & Boudreau, 2008). Audiologists and SLPs should be aware
of the need to assess this area in children who experience these risks. Cognitive
status, which can also have an impact on language function, is another important
element in the assessment of clients with communicative disorders. Usually this
aspect of the assessment is accomplished through collaboration or referral to a
psychologist.

Infants, Toddlers, and Preschoolers   Assessment of language comprehension
in young children involves such tasks as pointing to objects, pictures of objects,
body parts, and clothing items, and following directions and routines. This can
be achieved using formal procedures (e.g., Preschool Language Scale–Fifth Edition, PLS-5; Zimmerman, Steiner, & Pond, 2011) or such informal procedures as
play routines and observation. Depending on the age of the client, parent report
of these skills may be more valuable than direct observation. For example, our
toddler Sam's parents may report that he can point to six body parts during bath
time, but when asked during the evaluation he does not respond to this direction.
There could be several reasons why Sam does not comply, apart from the fact that
his parents are mistaken about his ability: He may unfamiliar with being asked to
"perform" in this way; or his temperament may be very shy, so interacting with
an unfamiliar adult is uncomfortable for him. The assessment process involves
the clinical judgment to make sense of apparent contradictions like these and to
devise strategies for resolving them.

Language production can be elicited by engaging in play routines to name
objects or pictures of objects, respond to questions, or describe pictures. Parent report may be valuable as well when assessing early language production
because a young child may not respond to language probes during an evaluation. There are parent-report checklists such as the MacArthur-Bates Communicative Development Inventories–Second Edition (CDIs; Fenson et al., 2007),
which examines receptive vocabulary, expressive vocabulary, morphology, and
syntax in young children (<30 months). The parent interview can yield information about how a child communicates in different settings and with different
people (e.g., at home versus child care; with parents, grandparents, siblings, and
peers). Another useful tool among children age birth to 3 years is the Receptive-
Expressive Emergent Language Scale–Third Edition (REEL-3; Bzoch, League, &
Brown, 2003).

The use of communication to accomplish intentions is also an important part of the assessment for young children, particularly for those with very limited speech. Skills that should be noted include using eye contact, taking turns, and initiating and responding to communication with adults, family, and peers. Sometimes this assessment approach includes structured sampling tasks, where, for example, the clinician deliberately "tempts" a child to communicate by placing an attractive toy in a tightly closed jar the child needs help to open.

Because literacy is so important for success in our society and because speech, language, and hearing disorders put children at risk for reading disorders, preliteracy may be part of the assessment for young children. Practitioners involved in this aspect of assessment may use formal tests (e.g., Test of Preschool Early Literacy [TOPEL]; Lonigan, Wagner, & Torgesen, 2007); criterion-referenced methods, such as having children produce rhymes or name letters; or behavioral observation to observe how toddlers hold books, turn pages, and so forth.

Elementary School and Adolescents   Children in the school-age years need language not only to communicate but also to learn the academic curriculum. Therefore, in addition to assessing understanding and production of semantics, syntax, morphology, phonology, and pragmatic forms, it is necessary to assess their ability to meet the demands of the classroom. Understanding of classroom discourse rules (when students are allowed to talk, for example), decontextualized language (talk about objects and events removed from the immediate setting), and metalinguistic skills (using language to talk about language, such as knowing what a *word* or *sentence* is) should be assessed (Paul & Norbury, 2012). There are many standardized tests available to assess the core aspects of language (e.g., CELF-5; Semel, Wiig, & Secord, 2013). Classroom observation, teacher interviews, and collaboration enable the SLP to assess the influence of a child's oral language skills on his or her functioning in the classroom. In addition, literacy skills should be assessed in each school-age and adolescent child. This task can be accomplished using standardized tests and criterion-referenced procedures in collaboration with the reading specialist. A language assessment for John, our child with CP, for example, might include whether he can not only understand spoken sentences but also demonstrate phonological awareness by indicating how many sounds are in the word *hot* (3: /h/, /a/, /t/) or selecting a picture of a word that rhymes with *cat*.

Adults   Language assessment in adults is typically completed in a medical or rehabilitative setting. **Aphasia** is a loss of language that may result from a stroke, degenerative disease, tumor, or traumatic brain injury, among others. There are a number formal tests for aphasia (see Table 4.2), with the Boston Diagnostic Aphasia Examination–Third Edition (BDAE-3; Goodglass, Kaplan, & Barresi, 2001) and the Western Aphasia Battery–Revised (WAB-R; Kertesz, 2006) the most commonly used. The areas usually considered for assessment of aphasia are naming, fluency, repetition, and comprehension. Assessing these areas allows the clinician to determine a diagnosis of the major type of aphasia. As part of an aphasia assessment, cognition is also screened; this screening is done in collaboration with a psychologist.

Naming and Word Retrieval   A common characteristic of all types of aphasia is anomia, or word-finding problems. The components of word retrieval that are assessed include confrontation naming (e.g., verbal naming of pictures, objects, actions), defining referents (e.g., "What does bed mean?"), category naming (e.g., "Tell me all the animals you can think of"; "A rose, tulip, and carnation are all _____"), and automatic closure naming (e.g., completing an open-ended sentence or phrase such as "You sit on a _____"). Although it is important to assess naming because of its functional role in communication, naming is not a characteristic that allows one to determine the specific type of aphasia because virtually all aphasia involves word-finding difficulty.

People with aphasia produce paraphasic errors, unintended word or sound substitutions such as saying *book* for *magazine*, or they produce nonwords (also called pseudowords), such as *scrat* when they mean *rug*.

Verbal Fluency   In aphasia and language assessment, the degree of fluency is determined by the number of words produced in connected, grammatical utterances. Fluent speech is defined as eight or more grammatically connected words; nonfluent speech is defined as fewer than five connected words (Goodglass & Kaplan, 1972). Determining fluency involves not just counting words but also determining whether the words are ordered grammatically. (It is important to be aware that *fluency* refers to verbal connected discourse when discussing aphasia, rather than the smoothness of speech, as it is when discussing stuttering.)

Repetition   Repetition is assessed by presenting words that range from single syllables (*dog*) to multisyllabic (*doggedly*), and from phonemically simple (e.g., *man*) to complex (e.g., *sphinx*). Sentences used for repetition assessment range from highly probable (e.g., "I heard him speak on the radio last night") to highly improbable sentences (e.g., "The spy fled to Greece"). Repetition is assessed because performance on these tasks helps in determining the type of aphasia present.

Comprehension   Comprehension is tested at multiple levels. At the single-word level, the patient points to a picture from a choice of pictures (e.g., "Show me the shoe"). At the sentence level, the patient follows simple commands (e.g., "Point to the ceiling and then to the floor") and complex commands (e.g., "Keeping your eyes shut, tap each shoulder twice with two fingers"). At the paragraph level, the patient listens to paragraphs read by the clinician and then answers comprehension questions (Goodglass et al., 2001). Performance on these kinds of tasks also helps the examiner determine the type of aphasia.

Cognitive Screening   Cognition can be screened by a psychologist using a formal measure such at the Mini–Mental State Examination (MMSE; Folstein & Folstein, 2010), or it can be screened informally, in order to determine the need for referral to a psychologist. Thus, SLPs can screen orientation by asking the client, "What is your name?" "Where are you?" "What year it is?" "What is the month?" and "What is the day?" Attention may be screened by asking the client to spell the word *world* backward. Sequencing, organization, and planning may be screened by having the client describe five steps to an activity, such as *how to make a cup of coffee* or *how to make spaghetti.*

Speech

Speech production requires articulation, or the motor processes involved in the planning and execution of movement of the articulators (tongue, lips, jaw) in order to achieve overlapping gestures that result in speech. Speech intelligibility refers to how well a speaker is understood by clinicians and familiar and unfamiliar listeners. The SLP should consider both speech perception and production when examining articulation and speech intelligibility. Speech perception testing involves listening to pairs of sounds (in syllables or words) and indicating whether they are the same or different. It is also important to assess the oral mechanism to examine the structure and function of the articulators in a nonspeech context. Oral mechanism assessment will be discussed below.

Speech production assessment typically involves examining an individual's ability to produce speech sounds in isolation (e.g., *k*), in syllables (e.g., *ka*), in words (e.g., *cat*), and in running speech (I have a *cat* named Tiger). Speech production testing is often accomplished by asking an individual to name pictures, read words or sentences, tell a story, or engage in conversation while the SLP analyzes incorrect patterns. Speech intelligibility testing involves judging how well an individual is understood by his or her listeners. This testing can be accomplished by collecting a spontaneous speech sample and analyzing the percentage of words understood by familiar and unfamiliar listeners. The SLP also performs speech stimulability testing to observe the client's ability to imitate correct production of sounds the client is currently producing in error. Stimulability is usually tested in sounds in isolation first and then in syllables and words.

Infants, Toddlers, and Preschoolers   Children typically master the production of most of the sounds of their native language by the time they are 3 or 4 years old, and they refine production of a few residual errors on sounds such as /r/, /s/, /ʃ/, /z/, and /th/ between the ages of 3 and 7 (Fudala, 2000). Typical levels of intelligibility (Paul & Norbury, 2012) are

- 50% at 2 years

- 75% at 3 years

- 100% (with some errors persisting, but still understandable) at 4 years

In evaluating young children's articulation, then, it is important to understand the range of normal variation in this development.

In addition, clinicians should be aware of the close connection between speech and language development. Children who use few words may not produce enough speech sounds to determine their articulation or intelligibility (Bauman-Waengler, 2012), let alone to assess the characteristics of childhood apraxia of speech (CAS), which include inconsistency of speech sound errors and errors in vowel production and intonation. Differential diagnosis for the underlying cause of delayed speech can be difficult to determine, and it may be premature to diagnose apraxia or articulation disorder before the child is using connected speech. In this case, it may make sense to provide intervention for word production and monitor the development of articulation as words are acquired. An additional consideration in this age group is that speech perception may be difficult to assess because the child may not understand the linguistic concepts required to indicate whether two words are the same or different.

Elementary School and Adolescents Motor speech and articulation skills are usually mastered in children by the mental age of 7 (Fudala, 2000). Children at this developmental level should be able to complete speech perception and speech production testing; a combination of standardized articulation testing and criterion-referenced procedures involving oral motor assessment, stimulability, and spontaneous speech sampling should provide a comprehensive picture of articulation and intelligibility. It will be important to consider children's speech production skills at the phoneme, word, and sentence level and the influence of word length (one syllable, two syllables, three syllables) on overall intelligibility. In addition, SLPs assess the impact of speech production on interactions in a variety of settings (e.g., home versus school) and with different communication partners (teachers versus peers versus family). This can be accomplished through behavioral observation or interviewing the client, caregivers, teachers, and so forth.

Adults Adult acquired speech disorders can arise secondary to a variety of medical diagnoses, including stroke, degenerative diseases, tumors, and traumatic brain injury, among others. Acquired **apraxia of speech** and acquired **dysarthria of speech** are referred to as motor speech disorders (Duffy, 2005). Apraxia of speech is defined as impaired capacity to plan or program sensorimotor commands necessary for directing movements that result in phonetically and prosodically normal speech. Dysarthria of speech is a collective name for a group of neurologic speech disorders resulting from abnormalities in strength, speed, range, steadiness, tone, or accuracy of movements required for the control of the respiratory, phonatory, resonatory, articulatory, and prosodic aspects of speech production. Based on clinical presentation and the assessment, apraxia of speech and/or one or more of the different types of dysarthrias are diagnosed by the SLP. The reader is referred to differential diagnosis of dysarthria in Duffy (2005) for an in-depth description of this process.

The assessment of speech in an adult with an acquired speech disorder involves perceptual (e.g., Speech Oral Motor Examination; see later in this chapter), and instrumental (e.g., acoustic assessment via instrumentation) methods, as well as speech intelligibility assessment. The Assessment of Intelligibility of Dysarthric Speech (Yorkston & Beukelman, 1982) is a structured intelligibility measure that allows the calculation of percent speech intelligibility for single words and sentences. Perceptual, instrumental, and speech intelligibility assessments combine to inform the clinician regarding the specific type of motor speech disorder.

Voice

Voice assessment is completed to evaluate strengths and weaknesses of vocal function, including the identification of impairments, associated activity, and limitations in participation in communication interactions (Gallena, 2007). Patients with voice disorders are often first evaluated by a physician, usually an otolaryngologist (an ear, nose, and throat physician), prior to a voice evaluation by an SLP.

Basic voice evaluation equipment includes a tape recorder, a microphone, a pitch pipe, a stop watch, and a flashlight, as well as a mirror, tongue depressors, and gloves. In addition, laryngeal visualization and imaging via stroboscopy allow for a direct assessment of vocal fold structure and function. In general, for all ages the overall clinical voice assessment involves obtaining a speech sample, pitch range, dynamic range, the *s/z* ratio (completed by having the client produce *s* for as long as possible, and *z* for as long as possible), ratings regarding vocal abuse, and observation of muscular tension.

Toddlers and Preschool Children   A speech sample is obtained through play interactions or reciting familiar texts like nursery rhymes or the *ABC*s. Clinicians can provide activities to elicit pitch range, such as having a toy climb up and down a play structure while modeling high pitch on the way up, and low pitch on the way down. To elicit dynamic range for loud versus quiet speech, the SLP can use a puppet that can open its mouth wide and loud or small and soft. Props to help obtain the *s/z* ratio include use of a snake for the *s* and a bumble bee for the *z*. To elicit the child's production of the /s/ the clinician can model a hissing sound such as /s/ in play and then play a game with two snakes, one for the child and one for the clinician. The goal is to have the child's snake "beat" the clinician's snake in making a longer /s/ sound, prompting the child to prolong the /s/ as long as possible. A similar game format can be employed for production of the /z/ with the child and the clinician playing a bumble bee and producing /z/. A stopwatch is used to time the prolongation of /s/ and /z/; then the longest /z/ is divided into the longest /s/. The purpose of the *s/z* ratio is to indirectly determine whether there is glottal closure during phonation and a ratio of 1:1.4 is within normal limits. Any *s/z* higher than 1.4 indicates air leakage through the glottis on the /z/ (Boone, McFarlane, Von Berg, & Zraik, 2010).

Elementary School Children, Adolescents, and Adults   Variations of the above described techniques may be used with younger elementary school children, whereas older elementary school children and adolescents are likely to be assessed similarly to the way adults are assessed. Specific measures of voice are obtained from older children by

- Asking the client to show respiratory support for speech by taking a breath and saying /a/ for as long as he or she can

- Asking the client to demonstrate pitch range by modeling "singing" from the client's lowest pitch to his or her highest pitch

- Asking the client to speak as loudly and softly as possible to assess dynamic range

- Explaining and modeling prolonged /s/ and /z/ production to assess the *s/z* ratio

In addition to these measures, rating scales that allow clinicians to record observations of vocal performance, such as the Voice Handicap Index (VHI; Jacobson et al., 1997), are often used with older children and adults.

All these evaluation techniques can be considered a part of a perceptual voice assessment. In addition to perceptual measures, instrumentation is also used to assess vocal function. The Computerized Speech Lab (CSL, by KayPENTAX) assesses vocal parameters such as pitch (in hertz) and loudness (in decibels) from speech directed into a microphone connected to the computer. The CSL can be used with children and adults to obtain quantitative measures of several aspects of vocal function.

Fluency

Stuttering has been described as a fluency disorder involving affective, behavioral, and cognitive components (Cooper & Cooper, 1993). The affective component is the emotional aspect of the disorder, whereas the behavioral component is the type and frequency of specific dysfluent elements (i.e., repetitions, blocks, prolongations). The cognitive component of stuttering refers to what the speaker thinks about his or her actual dysfluencies. One person who stutters may have speech disruption on 5% of words and think he or she stutters severely. Another person with the same percentage may think he or she stutters mildly.

A novice clinician often video- or audiotapes a fluency assessment in order to ensure accuracy of the dysfluency count, but with experience, clinicians are usually able to calculate percentage of speech dysfluencies as the person is speaking. Along with the behavioral assessment or dysfluency counting, much of the information in the assessment and diagnosis of stuttering comes from the case history and the assessment of feelings and attitudes. Before we get to these areas, let us consider the behavioral component of stuttering or the actual percentage of dysfluencies that the speech-language pathologist computes during the assessment.

Regardless of the client's age, a central aspect of the assessment of stuttering concerns documenting the frequency and type of dysfluencies produced. Dysfluencies are generally counted in three speaking contexts: no structure, no pressure; structure, no pressure; structure and pressure (Shapiro, 2010); as well as when reading if the client is school age or older. In each of these speaking situations, the percentage of dysfluent syllables is determined by counting the number of times a core behavior of stuttering occurs during three 100-syllable samples of speech. Core behaviors of stuttering (Guitar, 2014; Van Riper, 1971) include "blocks," such as a tense pause before the word *book*; "part-word repetitions," such as *ta-ta-table*; and "prolongations," such as *mmmmmmmmooon* (see Table 4.4). In addition to determining the percentage of stuttered syllables in each speaking situation, the evaluator observes and records the frequency and type of secondary behaviors (e.g., eye blinks, head nods, arm movements, postponing behaviors, instances of avoiding a word or avoiding a speaking situation). This information contributes to the assessment of severity of stuttering behavior. Table 4.5 provides examples of activities that can be used to elicit speech in various contexts.

Table 4.4.   Core behaviors of stuttering

Core behaviors of stuttering	Example in speech
Block	"__book" (hard tense pause with physical tension in initial place of articulation precedes production)
Initial phoneme repetition	"b,b,b, book"
Initial phoneme prolongation	"sssssand"

Table 4.5.   Activities used to elicit speech in three speaking contexts

Speaking situation context	Toddlers and preschoolers	School-age children and younger adolescents	Older adolescents and adults
No structure, no pressure	Free play with props: farm and animals; house and people; dolls and clothing, bottle, and so forth	Description of an ideal birthday party, free play with Legos, open-ended questions about hobbies or activities	Open-ended questions about school, work, history of speech and stuttering
Structure, no pressure	Direct questions regarding free play props, story retell using picture book	Direct questions regarding no structure activities, story retell using book or movie retell	Direct questions, story or movie retell, procedural discourse such as steps to brush teeth
Structure, pressure	Structured activities with clinician interruptions and clinician rapid rate	Structured activities with clinician interruptions and clinician rapid rate	Structured activities with clinician interruptions and clinician rapid rate

Table 4.6.   Other behaviors related to making stuttering diagnosis

Likely to be true stuttering	Unlikely to be true stuttering
Language delayed	Language skills advanced for age
Mean length of utterance (MLU) less than expected for age	Mean length of utterance (MLU) greater than expected for age
Phoneme or part-word repetitions	Whole-word repetitions or phrase repetitions
Syllabic repetitions with tension	Easy syllabic repetitions with no tension
Blocks with visible tension	Pauses without tension
Physical concomitants and avoidance behaviors	No obvious physical concomitants or avoidances
Family history of stuttering as an adult	No family history of adult stuttering
Disfluencies present for more than 1 year	Disfluencies present less than 1 year

The Stuttering Severity Instrument–Fourth Edition for Children and Adults (SSI-4; Riley, 2009) is an assessment tool that relies on speech samples to estimate stuttering severity (primary and secondary behaviors). There are norms for preschool-age children, school-age children, adolescents, and adults.

In addition to the above-described measures used for counting dysfluencies and determining severity for all age groups, specific assessment procedures and methods are used for each specific age group as well. These are described below under each designated age level.

Toddlers and Preschoolers   As for any client, case history information is helpful in understanding the disorders of preschoolers with dysfluency. Specific case history questions for the parent include these: "When did your child first start stuttering?" "How did it sound when stuttering first was noticed?" "Has the stuttering changed since it was first noted?" "Does anyone else in the immediate family stutter?" "Do any relatives stutter?" and "How does the child react to the stuttering?"

The first question a clinician needs to answer about a young child with dysfluency concerns whether the child is presenting with developmental dysfluencies that are likely to resolve without turning into true stuttering. Table 4.6 is included as a guideline to help the clinician decide whether specific behaviors that likely suggest a diagnosis of stuttering are present. In general, the more "high risk" the behaviors, the greater the chance that true stuttering will develop.

School-Age Children and Younger Adolescents Older children may be evaluated for the first time in the school setting. Additional case history questions at the school-age level include these: "Has the child ever been evaluated or treated for stuttering?" "How does the stuttering affect the child in the school setting?" and "How does the stuttering affect the child's relationship with peers?"

Formal assessment measures include the Test of Childhood Stuttering (TOCS; Gillam, Logan, & Pearson, 2009) and the Overall Assessment of the Speaker's Experience of Stuttering (OASES; Yaruss & Quesal, 2010). The TOCS assesses speech fluency skills and stuttering-related behaviors in school-age children. The OASES addresses the effect of stuttering on a person's life. This assessment presents the client with specific scenarios, and the client rates each one based on his or her perceived degree of dysfluency and his or her emotional reaction to speech in the situation.

A sample of reading is typically obtained for school-age children and adults. In the reading sample, the percentage of dysfluencies is computed and compared to the percentage of dysfluencies in an average of the three speaking contexts.

Older Adolescents and Adults Additional case history questions for adults include these: "How does stuttering affect your ability to participate in work activities?" "How does the stuttering affect your ability to participate in social activities?" An acquired stuttering disorder in an adult (cf. neurogenic stuttering) is not considered here. Neurogenic stuttering poststroke is rare and has similarities and differences from developmental stuttering that has advanced from childhood to adulthood.

Assessment for dysfluency, in summary, involves the computation of the frequency and types of stuttering behaviors as well as a more comprehensive examination of the effects of the dysfluency on the client's communicative competence. As with any communication disorder, dysfluency occurs not in isolation but in the context of the client's family, friends, and other social settings. A thorough assessment includes a consideration of the effects of these contexts on the communication problem.

Sensorimotor Speech Examination

The sensorimotor speech examination is an assessment of the structure and function of the oral motor mechanism that supports speech and swallowing. This examination is a necessary aspect of all speech-language evaluations. Assessing the speech-motor system consists of examining facial symmetry; dentition; the structure and function of the lips; tongue, jaw, and velopharynx; and respiratory, phonatory, and resonance functions as they are used for speech. Paul and Norbury (2012) and Shipley and McAfee (2008) provide some guidance in conducting and interpreting the oral-facial examination. McCauley and Strand (2008) provide a review of standardized measures for assessing oral-motor functions. It is essential to use universal precautions to protect both the clinician and the client from infection. These precautions include cleaning all surfaces and instruments with disinfectant before use and washing the clinician's hands with antibacterial soap before and after putting on gloves, which should be worn throughout the examination. Figure 4.4 provides a form that can be used to record the observations from this assessment.

Name: _____   Date: _____

1. Lips

    a. Structure

        Touch when teeth are in occlusion: yes _____ no _____

        Upper lip length: normal _____   short _____   long _____
        (describe)

        Evidence of cleft lip or other structural impairment: yes _____ no _____

    b. Function

        Can retract unilaterally

            Left: yes _____   no _____

            Right: yes _____   no _____

        Equal retraction bilaterally: yes _____   no _____

        Number of times can produce /pʌ/ in 5 seconds:

            trial 1 _____   trial 2 _____   trial 3 _____

        Does stabilizing the jaw facilitate the activity?   yes _____ no _____

    c. Adequacy for speech: 1 _____ 2 _____ 3 _____ 4 _____

2. Teeth

    a. Structure

        Occlusion: normal   _____   neutroclusion _____

                            distoclusion _____   mesioclusion _____

        Anteroposterior relationship of incisors: normal _____

        Mixed (some in labioversion, some in linguoversion) but all upper and lower teeth con-
        tact; all upper incisors lingual to lower incisors but in contact _____ not in contact _____

        Vertical relationship of incisors: normal _____   openbite _____   closebite _____

        Continuity of cutting edge of incisors: normal _____   rotated _____   jumbled _____

                                    missing teeth _____   supernumerary teeth _____

        If lack of continuity, identify teeth involved and describe nature of deviation.

Figure 4.4. Oral mechanism evaluation form. (Republished by permission of Delmar Learning, from Tomblin, J.B., Morris, H.L., & Spriestersbach, D.C. [2000]. *Diagnosis in speech-language pathology* [2nd ed., pp. 95–97]. Clifton Park, NY: Delmar Learning; permission conveyed through Copyright Clearance Center, Inc.)   _____

(continued)

b. Dental appliance or prosthesis: yes _____ (describe)   no _____

c. Adequacy for speech: 1 ____   2 ____   3 ____   4 ____

3. Tongue

a. Structure

Size in relation to dental arches: too large _____   appropriate _____   too small _____

symmetrical _____   asymmetrical _____

b. Function

Can curl tongue up and back: yes _____   no _____

Number of times can touch anterior alveolar ridge with tongue tip without sound in 5 seconds:

trial 1 _____   trial 2 _____   trial 3 _____

above average _____   average _____   below average _____

Number of time can touch the corners of mouth with tongue tip in 5 seconds:

trial 1 _____   trial 2 _____   trial 3 _____

above average _____   average _____   below average _____

Number of times can produce /tʌ/ in 5 seconds:

trial 1 _____   trial 2 _____   trial 3 _____

above average _____   average _____   below average _____

Number of times can produce /kʌ/ in 5 seconds:

trial 1 _____   trial 2 _____   trial 3 _____

above average _____   average _____   below average _____

Restrictiveness of lingual frenum:

not restrictive _____   somewhat restrictive _____   markedly restrictive _____

c. Adequacy for speech: 1 ____   2 ____   3 ____   4 ____

4. Hard palate

a. Structure

Intactness: normal _____   cleft, repaired _____   cleft, unrepaired _____

Figure 4.4.   *(continued)*

Palatal fistula: yes _____ (describe)   no _____

Alveolar cleft: yes _____ (describe)   no _____

Palatal contour:

   normal configuration _____ flat contour _____ deep and narrow contour _____

b. Adequacy for speech: 1 _____   2 _____   3 _____   4 _____

5. Palatopharyngeal mechanism

  a. Structure

  Soft palate

  Intactness: normal _____ cleft, repaired _____ cleft, unrepaired _____

              symmetrical _____   asymmetrical _____

  Length: satisfactory _____   short _____   very short _____

  Uvula

      normal _____   bifid _____   deviated from midline to right _____

      to left _____   absent _____

  Oropharynx

      Depth: shallow _____ normal _____   deep _____

      Width: narrow _____   normal _____   wide _____

  b. Function

  Soft palate

      Movement during prolonged phonation of /ɑ/:

          none _____   some _____   marked _____

      Movement during short, repeated phonations of /ɑ/:

          none _____   some _____   marked _____

      Movement during gag reflex:

          none _____   some _____   marked _____

      If some movement, then amount:

          same for both halves _____ more for right half _____ more for left half _____

(continued)

Oropharynx

   Mesial movement of lateral pharyngeal walls during phonation of /a/:

      none _____   some _____   marked _____

   Mesial movement of lateral pharyngeal walls during gag reflex:

      none _____   some _____   marked _____

Audible nasal emission while blowing out a match:
   yes _____ (describe) no _____

Inconsistency in nasal emission during speech or blowing tasks:
   yes _____ (describe) no _____

Patient stimulable to oral productions of pressure consonants:
   yes _____ (describe) no _____

Nares construction during speech or blowing tasks:
   yes _____ (describe) no _____

Oral manometer ratio (instrument _____)

      trial 1: nostrils open_____   nostrils closed_____   ratio_____

      trial 2: nostrils open_____   nostrils closed_____   ratio_____

      trial 3: nostrils open_____   nostrils closed_____   ratio_____

   c. Adequacy for speech: 1 _____   2 _____   3 _____   4 _____

6. Fauces

   a. Structure

      Tonsils: normal _____   enlarged _____   atrophied_____   absent _____

      Pillars: normal _____   scarred _____   inflamed _____   absent _____

      Area of faucial isthmus: above average _____   average _____   below average_____

   b. Function

      Posterior movement during phonation of /a/:none_____   some_____   marked_____

      Mesial movement during phonation of /a/:   none_____   some_____   marked_____

      Restriction of velar activity by pillars: none_____   some_____   marked_____

   c. Adequacy for speech: 1 _____   2 _____   3 _____   4 _____

Figure 4.4. *(continued)*

There are standard protocols for this assessment, including the Clinical Assessment of Oropharyngeal Motor Development in Young Children (Robbins & Klee, 1987), Frenchay Dysarthria Assessment–Second Edition (FDA-2; Enderby & Palmer, 2008), Mayo Clinic Motor Speech Examination (Darley, Aronson, & Brown, 1969), and Verbal Motor Production Assessment for Children (VMPAC; Hayden & Squire, 1999). The sensorimotor speech assessment begins with the examination of the external visible structures (including the face) and progresses to structures within the oral cavity. Swallowing is screened during the assessment by the dry swallow and by swallowing liquids as well as solids of various consistencies. The gag reflex may also be observed. Materials used in the sensorimotor speech examination include a pen light, a stopwatch, a mirror, tongue depressors, gauze pads, and gloves.

Infants, Toddlers, and Preschoolers   For toddlers and preschoolers, it is important to speak to the child in age-appropriate language and to speak at the child's level. Use of props such as bubbles for blowing to assess lip rounding or making playful requests ("Open your mouth really wide so I can see if there are any elephants in there!") may be helpful in young children. Allowing the child to "examine" the clinician's mouth first and letting the child handle the pen light and stopwatch and put on gloves may enlist the youngster's cooperation.

Elementary School Children and Adolescents   By elementary school age, most children are able to follow directions adequately so that much of the examination can be done as it would be with an adult. Most elementary school children and adolescents can perform the repetitions necessary for diadochokinetic tasks (Fletcher, 1978), which assess the ability to produce rapid sequences of nonsense syllables (e.g., "papapapapa, pataka"), although younger students may need some initial coaching to accomplish these tasks. It may be helpful to provide the elementary school child with the same props the examiner uses, allowing the child to "evaluate" the clinician as well.

Adults   In adults with acquired brain damage, the oral-motor examination is obtained with special attention to the impaired cranial nerves. See Table 4.7, which describes the types (sensory or motor), innervations, symptoms, and functions of cranial nerves related to speech, swallowing, and hearing. The SLP notes the presence or absence of cranial nerve impairment during the oral-motor assessment.

Hearing

The interaction between hearing and speech and language skills has been well established; therefore, early identification and management of hearing loss will result in the best outcomes for speech and language skills. To ensure hearing health as early as possible, the majority of states in the United States have established universal hearing screening laws, where all newborn babies receive a hearing screening shortly after birth. Hearing can change over time and should be revaluated throughout the life span. Because SLPs may conduct hearing screenings, they can screen clients for hearing loss; middle ear pathology (ASHA, 2007) and all speech and language evaluations should include a hearing screening.

Table 4.7.   Summary of physical examination results and patient complaints for cranial nerves V, VII, X, and XII

Cranial nerve	Function	Technique of examination	Patient complaints	Changes in structure
V—Trigeminal	Motor—masticatory muscles	Opening the mouth, clenching the teeth for palpation of the masseter and temporalis muscles	Motor—chewing difficulty, drooling, jaw difficult to close;	Jaw may hang open
	Sensory—face and mucosal surfaces of the eyes, tongue, and parts of the nasopharyngeal space		Sensory—decreased sensation in face, cheek, tongue, teeth, or palate	
VII—Facial	Muscles of expression	Furrowing the brow, screwing up the eyes, sniffling, whistling, pursing the lips	Drooling, biting the cheek or lip when chewing or speaking, difficulty keeping food in the mouth	Affected side sags at rest; nasolabial fold is often flattened
X—Vagus (recurrent branch only)		Vocal characteristics; laryngoscopic examination		
XII—Hypoglossal	Innervation of tongue muscles	Tongue protrusion	Problem with oral articulation and chewing; difficulty handling saliva; tongue feels "thick"	Atrophy on the weak side
X—Vagus (above the pharyngeal branch)	Motor and sensory— innervation of the muscles of the soft palate, pharynx, and larynx	Gag reflex symmetry; vocal characteristics; laryngoscopic examination	Changes in voice and resonance; nasal regurgitation during swallowing	Soft palate hangs lower on the side of the lesion
X—Vagus (superior branch only)		Vocal characteristics; laryngoscopic examination	Voice changes	

Source: This table was published in *Motor Speech Disorders: Substrates, Differential Diagnosis and Management,* by J.R. Duffy. Copyright Mosby 1995.

Audiologists are the professionals who are responsible for the prevention, identification, assessment, and rehabilitation of hearing, auditory function, and balance systems (ASHA, 2003). If a client fails a hearing screening or if there are concerns about hearing, auditory, or balance function, it is appropriate to refer the client to an audiologist.

Infants, Toddlers, and Preschoolers   In order to test the hearing of young children, audiologists employ specialized methods that rely on automatic responses or behaviors. **Otoacoustic emissions** (OAEs) and **auditory brainstem**

responses (ABRs) are automatic physiological responses that can be detected in individuals of all ages and can be measured without requiring a behavioral response. Actually, OAEs and ABRs can be obtained when an individual is sleeping, thus making such tests an ideal method to evaluate hearing in newborns and infants. Conditioning procedures, such as **visual reinforcement audiometry** (VRA) and **play audiometry,** are used with toddlers and preschoolers to obtain hearing information. When gathering medical history information, it is important to note the presence or history of ear infections because otitis media with effusion (OME) may be associated with early speech and language delay (Gravel et al., 2006).

Elementary School Children and Adolescents It is typical for all elementary school children to receive a hearing screening yearly, or at least as they enter kindergarten. For children who are receiving speech and language intervention, it is important for hearing to be tested annually, especially if they are diagnosed with a condition in which hearing can be affected (e.g., Down syndrome, craniofacial anomalies, Wardenberg syndrome). Another aspect of hearing ability that should be noted is classroom acoustics because children with speech and language disorders (as well as typically developing children) may have difficulty perceiving speech in noisy classrooms (Moeller, Tomblin, Yoshinaga-Itano, Connor, & Jerger, 2007).

Adults As with children, adults' hearing should be screened as a part of a comprehensive evaluation process. Audiologists should be involved if any concerns about hearing arise. When gathering a medical history, it is important to note whether the client has a condition that is associated with hearing loss (e.g., noise exposure, use of ototoxic drugs, head trauma). In addition, many adults experience presbycusis, or gradual hearing loss due to the typical aging process. Presbycusis initially affects the high-frequency sounds and is typically observed bilaterally, or in both ears. Hearing loss could have a negative influence on speech perception and speech production skills; therefore, it is important to understand the nature of each client's hearing status, including the degree, slope, and type of hearing loss, when developing a therapy plan.

Alternative and Augmentative Communication

Alternative and augmentative communication (AAC) systems can be used by any client to supplement restrictions in speech and language production and/ or comprehension (ASHA, 2004). For some individuals, AAC systems serve as the primary means of communication; whereas for others, AAC systems are a supplementary mode of communication and may include vocalization, gestures, and body language. Information about assessment of AAC systems applies to clients of all ages; therefore this section will not be separated into the different age groups.

Alternative augmentative systems can be simple (e.g., gestures, two pictures pasted on a piece of paper) or complex (e.g., electronic devices with voice output). Most often, AAC systems are used by clients who have severe cognitive or physical disabilities. When clinicians assess an individual for candidacy for communication intervention, unmet communication needs should be the primary consideration (Beukelman & Mirenda, 2013). This communication needs model (Beukelman & Mirenda, 2013) of assessment should include the following:

1. Documentation of the communication needs of an individual

2. Identification of needs met through current communication techniques

3. Development of a plan to meet the unmet communication needs through AAC interventions

There is no standard battery of tests that comprise an AAC evaluation (ASHA, 2004); therefore, nonstandardized procedures, behavioral observation, and interviews with the client's caregivers and family as well as interviews with other professionals (e.g., physical therapist, occupational therapist, teachers) are used to determine the AAC needs for each client. An AAC evaluation determines the goodness of fit between the client and the equipment and contexts in which the client communicates. Dynamic assessment procedures are helpful in determining whether a client can benefit from an AAC system and which system may work best. For example, the SLP might present a client like John, with CP, with a variety of AAC systems (e.g., low-technology picture boards, high-technology electronic devices) and provide support for the client to try each for a variety of communication purposes (e.g., requesting a response, initiating communication) and with a variety of communication partners.

As clients age or gain new communication skills, their communication needs change; thus AAC assessment of a client of any age should consider three general phases (Beukelman & Mirenda, 2013):

Table 4.8.   Phases of alternative and augmentative communication assessment

Phase	Characteristics
I: Initial assessment for today	Assess current communication needs Assess physical, cognitive, sensory capabilities Goal: to develop a basic communication system to facilitate interactions with family, friends, and individuals familiar with the client
II: Detailed assessment for tomorrow	Assess communication needs in client's expected settings and communication partners (e.g., in school, at work) Goal: to develop a communication system to support use in environments beyond familiar ones
III: Follow-up assessment	Periodically examining communication equipment Assessing needs of the abilities of communication partners, reassessing an individual's capabilities as he or she changes Goal: to maintain a comprehensive alternative and augmentative communication system that meets the changing needs and lifestyles of the individual

Source: Beukelman and Mirenda (2013).

1. Initial assessment for today

2. Detailed assessment for tomorrow

3. Follow-up assessment to document change and response to intervention

Table 4.8 presents the information that should be included in each phase. Other aspects to consider when assessing the AAC needs of a client include participation patterns and needs, in addition to opportunity barriers (Beukelman & Mirenda, 2013). Chapter 11 considers these issues in more detail.

CONCLUSIONS

When we consider the range of clients assessed by communication disorders professionals—from toddlers like Sam to elderly folks like Mary; from people like Eddie and Sally with mild, subtle disabilities, to those like John and Molly with more obvious impairments—we gain some appreciation of the wide scope of our professions. For each client, the purpose of assessment is to identify the core problem so that optimal services can be put in place, establish baseline function, identify appropriate goals for intervention, and explore the methods of intervention that will be most effective. And the job of evaluation does not end there: Ongoing assessment will be necessary to document progress and ensure that the client's time and money are being effectively spent.

STUDY QUESTIONS

1. To determine test–retest reliability:
   a. The same test would be administered to the same person more than one time.
   b. A different test would be administered to the same person a day after the first test was administered.
   c. The results of the first half of a test are compared o the results of the second half of the test.
   d. The results of the odd-numbered questions on a test are compared to the results of the even-numbered questions on a test.
2. Norm referencing refers to which of the following?
   a. The process of measuring overall performance of a group of individuals on two tests that are compared
   b. The process of measuring the performance of a group of individuals on a given subset of items on a test
   c. The process of measuring performance of each test item on a group of individuals so the average performance of that group can be determined
   d. The process of measuring performance of different individuals on each test item on a test to look at different levels of performance

3. Which is not true about criterion-referenced tests?
    a. They may be standardized.
    b. An individual's performance is compared to others.
    c. They are administered in a naturalistic environment.
    d. All of the above.
4. Acquired apraxia of speech is defined as which of the following?
    a. Impaired language abilities
    b. Impaired capacity to plan or program sensorimotor commands
    c. Impaired ability to control respiration
    d. A phonatory disorder
5. True stuttering or developmental dysfluency is a question asked at what point?
    a. At birth
    b. During adolescence
    c. In adulthood
    d. During the preschool years
6. What are the aspects of language that should be included in an assessment?
    a. Comprehension
    b. Cognition
    c. Reading, writing, and literacy
    d. All of the above

FURTHER READING

Dollaghan, C.A. (2007). *The handbook for evidenced-based practice in communication disorders.* Baltimore, MD: Paul H. Brookes Publishing Co.
Shipley, K.G., & McAfee, J.G. (2009). *Assessment in speech-language pathology: A resource manual* (4th ed.). Clifton Park, NY: Cengage Learning.

REFERENCES

Adamovich, B.B., & Henderson, J. (1992). *Scales of cognitive ability for traumatic brain injury.* Austin, TX: PRO-ED.

American Speech-Language-Hearing Association. (2003). *Scope of practice in audiology.* Retrieved from http://www.asha.org/policy/SP2004-00192

American Speech-Language-Hearing Association (2004). *Roles and responsibilities of speech-language pathologists with respect to augmentative and alternative communication: technical report.* Retrieved from http://www.asha.org/policy/TR2004-00262

American Speech-Language-Hearing Association. (2005). *Evidence-based practice in communication disorders.* Retrieved from http://www.asha.org/policy/PS2005-00221

American Speech-Language Hearing Association. (2007). Scope of practice in speech-language-pathology. Retrieved from http://www.asha.org/policy/SP2007-00283

Baines, K.A., Heeringa, H.M., & Martin, A.W. (1999). *Assessment of language-related functional activities.* Austin, TX: PRO-ED.

Bankson, N.W., & Bernthal, J.E. (1990). *Bankson-Bernthal Test of Phonology.* Austin, TX: PRO-ED.

Bauman-Waengler, J. (2012). *Articulatory and phonological impairments a clinical focus* (3rd ed.). Boston, MA: Pearson.

Beukelman, D.R., & Mirenda, P. (2013). *Augmentative and alternative communication: Supporting children and adults with complex communication needs* (4th ed.). Baltimore, MD: Paul H. Brookes Publishing Co.

Bishop, D. (2003). *Children's Communication Checklist–2*. San Antonio, TX: Pearson.

Blakely, R.W. (2000). *Screening Test for Developmental Apraxia of Speech* (2nd ed.). Austin, TX: PRO-ED.

Boone, D.R. (1993). *The Boone Voice Program for Children* (2nd ed.). Austin, TX: PRO-ED.

Boone, D.R., McFarlane, S.C., Von Berg, S.L., & Zraick, R.I. (2010). *The voice and voice therapy* (8th ed.). New York, NY: Allyn & Bacon.

Bzoch, K.R., League, R., & Brown, V.L. (2003). *Receptive-Expressive Emergent Language Test—Third Edition*. San Antonio, TX: Pearson.

Carrow-Woolfolk, E. (1998). *Test for Auditory Comprehension of Language* (3rd ed.). Austin, TX: PRO-ED.

Carrow-Woolfolk, E. (1999). *Comprehensive Assessment of Spoken Language*. San Antonio, TX: Pearson.

Cooper, E.B., & Cooper, C.S. (1993). Fluency disorders. In D.E. Battle (Ed.), *Communication disorders in multicultural organizations* (pp. 189–211). Boston, MA: Andover Medical Publishers.

Coplan, J. (1993). *Early Language Milestones Scale*. Austin, TX: PRO-ED.

Darley, F.L., Aronson, A.E., and Brown, J.R. (1969). Differential diagnostic patterns of dysarthria, *Journal of Speech and Hearing Research, 12*, 246–269.

Dollaghan, C.A. (2007). *The handbook for evidenced-based practice in communication disorders*. Baltimore, MD: Paul H. Brookes Publishing Co.

Duffy, J.R. (1995). *Motor speech disorders: Substrates, differential diagnosis and management*. St. Louis, MO: Mosby.

Dunn, L.M., & Dunn, D.M. (2007). *Peabody Picture Vocabulary Test* (4th ed.). Minneapolis, MN: Pearson.

Enderby, P., & Palmer, R. (2008). *Frenchay Dysarthria Assessment* (2nd ed.). Austin TX: Pro-Ed.

Fenson, L., Marchman, V.A., Thal, D.J., Dale, P.S., Reznick, J.S., & Bates, E. (2007). *MacArthur-Bates Communicative Development Inventories (CDI) words and gestures* (2nd ed.). Baltimore, MD: Paul H. Brookes Publishing Co.

Fletcher, S. (1978). *Diagnosing speech disorders from cleft palate*. New York, NY: Grune & Stratton.

Fluharty, N.B. (2000). *Fluharty Preschool Speech and Language Screening Test* (2nd ed.). Austin, TX: PRO-ED.

Folstein, M.F., & Folstein, S.E. (2010). *Mini–Mental State Examination–Second Edition* (MMSE-2). Lutz, FL: Psychological Assessment Resources.

Fudala, J.B. (2000). *Arizona Articulation Proficiency Scale–Third Revision*. Torrance, CA: Western Psychological Services.

Gallena, S.K. (2007). *Voice and laryngeal disorders*. St. Louis, MO: Mosby.

Garrett, K., & Beukelman, D. (2006). *Aphasia assessment materials*. Retrieved from http://aac.unl.edu/screen/screen.html

Gauthier, S.V., & Madison, C.L. (1998). *Kindergarten Language Screening Test* (2nd ed.). Austin, TX: PRO-ED.

Gillam, R.B., Logan, K.J., & Pearson, N.A. (2009). *Test of Childhood Stuttering*. Austin, TX: PRO-ED.

Goldman, R., & Fristoe, M. (2000). *Goldman-Fristoe Test of Articulation* (2nd ed.). San Antonio, TX: Pearson.

Goodglass, H., & Kaplan, H. (1972). *The assessment of aphasia and related disorders*. Philadelphia, PA: Lea & Febiger.

Goodglass, H., Kaplan, H., & Barresi, B. (2001). *Boston Diagnostic Aphasia Examination* (3rd ed.). Philadelphia, PA: Lea & Febiger.

Gravel, J.S., Roberts, J.E., Roush, J., Grose, J., Besing, J., Burchinal, M., ... Zeisel, S. (2006). Early otitis media with effusion, hearing loss, and auditory processes at school age. *Ear and Hearing, 27*(4), 353–368.

Guitar, B. (2014). *Stuttering: An integrated approach to its nature and treatment* (4th ed.). Baltimore, MD: Lippincott Williams & Wilkins.

Hammill, D.D. (1998). *Detroit tests of learning aptitude* (4th ed.). Austin, TX: PRO-ED.

Hammill, D.D., Brown, V.L., Larsen, S.C., & Wiederholt, J.L. (2007). *Test of Adolescent and Adult Language* (4th ed.). San Antonio, TX: Pearson.

Hayden, D., & Squire, P. (1999). *Verbal Motor Production Assessment for Children* (VMPAC). San Antonio, TX: Pearson.

Haywood, H.C., & Lidz, C.S. (2007). *Dynamic assessment in practice: Clinical and educational applications*. New York, NY: Cambridge University Press.

Helm-Estabrooks, N. (2001). *Cognitive Linguistic Quick Test*. San Antonio, TX: Pearson.

Helm-Estabrooks, N., & Hotz, G. (1991). *Brief Test of Head Injury*. Austin, TX: PRO-ED.

Hodson, B.W. (2004). *Hodson Assessment of Phonological Patterns* (3rd ed.). Torrance, CA: Western Psychological Services.

Holland, A.L., Frattali, C.M., & Fromm, D. (1999). *Communication Activities of Daily Living* (2nd ed.). Austin, TX: PRO-ED.

Jacobson, B.H., Johnson, A., Grywalski, C., Silbergleit, A., Jacobson, G., Benninger, M.S., & Newman, C.W. (1997). Voice Handicap Index. *American Journal of Speech-Language Pathology, 6*, 66–70.

Kaplan, E., Goodglass, H., & Weintraub, S. (2000). *Boston Naming Test* (2nd ed.). Austin, TX: PRO-ED.

Kertesz, A. (2006). *Western Aphasia Battery* (Rev. ed.). San Antonio, TX: Pearson.

Khan, L., & Lewis, N. (2002). *Khan-Lewis Phonological Analysis* (2nd ed.). San Antonio, TX: Pearson.

Kleinman, L.I. (2003). *Functional Communication Profile–Revised* (FCP-R). East Moline, IL: LinguiSystems.

LaPointe, L., & Horner, J. (1998). *Reading Comprehension Battery for Aphasia* (2nd ed.). Austin, TX: PRO-ED.

Lonigan, C.J., Wagner, R.K., & Torgesen, J.K. (2007). *Test of Preschool Early Literacy*. Austin, TX: PRO-ED.

Mardell, C., & Goldenberg, D.S. (2011). *Developmental indicators for the assessment of learning* (4th ed.). Minneapolis, MN: Pearson.

McCauley, R.J., & Strand, E.A. (2008). A review of standardized tests of nonverbal oral and speech motor performance in children. *American Journal of Speech-Language Pathology, 17*, 81–91.

McLaughlin, K., & Cascella, P.W. (2008). Eliciting a distal gesture via dynamic assessment among students with moderate to severe intellectual disability. *Communication Disorders Quarterly, 29*(2), 75–81.

Moeller, M.P., Tomblin, J.B., Yoshinaga-Itano, C., Connor, C.M., & Jerger, S. (2007). Current state of knowledge: Language and literacy of children with hearing impairment. *Ear & Hearing, 28*, 740–753.

Morgan, D.L., & Guilford, A.M. (1984). *Adolescent Language Screening Test*. Austin, TX: PRO-ED.

O'Neill, D. (2007). *Language use inventory*. Waterloo, Canada: Knowledge in Development.

Paul, R., & Norbury, C. (2012). *Language disorders from infancy through adolescence* (4th ed.). St. Louis, MO: Elsevier.

Riley, G.D. (2009). *Stuttering Severity Instrument for Children and Adults* (4th ed.). Austin, TX: PRO-ED.

Robbins, J., & Klee, T. (1987). Clinical assessment of oropharyngeal motor development in young children. *Journal of Speech and Hearing Disorders, 52*, 271–277.

Rossetti, L. (2006). *The Rossetti Infant–Toddler Language Scale*. East Moline, IL: LinguiSystems.

Ross-Swain, D. (1996). *Ross Information Processing Assessment* (2nd ed.). Austin, TX: PRO-ED.

Rutter, M., Bailey, A., & Lord, C. (2003). *Social Communication Questionnaire*. Torrance, CA: Western Psychological Services.

Schuele, C.M., & Boudreau, D. (2008). Phonological awareness intervention: Beyond the basics. *Language, Speech, and Hearing Services in Schools, 39*, 3–20.

Semel, E.M., Wiig, E.H., & Secord, W. (2013). *Clinical evaluation of language fundamentals* (5th ed.). San Antonio, TX: Pearson.

Seymour, H.N., Roeper, T.W., & de Villiers, J. (2005). *Diagnostic evaluation of language variation*. San Antonio, TX: Pearson.

Shapiro, D.A. (2010). *Stuttering intervention*. Austin, TX: PRO-ED.

Shipley, K.G., & McAfee, J.G. (2009). *Assessment in speech-language pathology: A resource manual* (4th ed.). Clifton Park, NY: Cengage Learning.

Sparrow, S., Cicchetti, D., & Balla, D. (2005). *Vineland Adaptive Behavior Scales–II*. San Antonio, TX: Pearson.

St. Louis, K.O., & Ruscello, D.M. (2000). *Oral Speech Mechanism Screening Examination* (3rd ed.). Austin, TX: PRO-ED.

Tomblin, J.B., Morris, H.L., & Spriestersbach, D.C. (2000). *Diagnosis in speech-language pathology* (2nd ed.). Clifton Park, NY: Delmar Learning.

VanRiper, C. (1971). *The nature of stuttering*. Englewood Cliffs, NJ: Prentice-Hall.

Vanryckeghem, M., & Brutten, G.J. (2010). *Communication Attitude Test for Preschool and Kindergarten Children Who Stutter*. San Diego, CA: Plural Publishing.

West, J., Sands, E., & Ross-Swain, D. (1998). *Bedside Evaluation Screening Test* (2nd ed.). Austin, TX: PRO-ED.

Wetherby, A., & Prizant, B. (2003). *Communication and Symbolic Behavior Scales Developmental Profile Infant–Toddler Checklist and easy-score user's guide.* Baltimore, MD: Paul H. Brookes Publishing Co.

Wilson, B.A., Cockburn, J., & Halligan, P.W. (1987). *Behavioral Inattention Test.* San Antonio, TX: Pearson.

Yaruss, J.S., & Quesal, R.W. (2010). *Overall assessment of the speaker's experience of stuttering.* Minneapolis, MN: Pearson.

Yorkston, K.M., & Beukelman, D.R. (1982). *Assessment of intelligibility of dysarthric speech.* Austin, TX: PRO-ED.

Zimmerman, I.L., Steiner, V.G., & Pond, R.E. (2011). *Preschool language scales* (5th ed.). San Antonio, TX: Pearson.

CHAPTER **5**

Communication Sampling Procedures

Patrick R. Walden, Monica Gordon-Pershey, and Rhea Paul

CHAPTER OBJECTIVES

After reading this chapter, students will be able to

- Describe the importance, purpose and aims of communication sampling.
- Provide strategies for sampling nonverbal communication, language, and speech.
- Provide tools for analyzing communication samples.
- Provide introductory information for interpreting language sample analysis results.

One of the earliest means of studying children's language was the diary study. Parents who were deeply interested in language development—Charles Darwin among them—kept detailed recordings of their children's early speech productions (Bar-Adon & Leopold, 1971). This method not only yielded a great deal of quantitative information about what children say at various points in development, it also introduced the idea of carefully observing, recording, and analyzing natural behavior as a means to understand language use. These early studies were focused on a small number of children, on a small range of questions concerning single-word use and the beginning of two-word combinations, on a narrow age range, on production only, and on typical development only. Nonetheless, the studies set the stage for the development of a broader use of language sampling procedures to address a range of issues in clinical work with people with communication disorders.

The use of communication sample analysis in the evaluation of children's speech-language abilities has seen much recent attention in the literature and has become recommended practice in clinical contexts, especially for culturally diverse populations, such as speakers of nonmainstream dialects and English-language learners (Horton-Ikard, 2010; Rojas & Iglesias, 2009, 2010). This may be in part due to the nature of standardized tests of language abilities. Despite their widespread use in schools, standardized tests of language abilities may be insufficient to differentiate children with disorders and those who are typically developing, depending on the assessment used (Plante & Vance, 1994). Further, standardized evaluations of language abilities often fail to provide the diagnostic information necessary to plan treatment goals and objectives (Price, Hendricks,

& Cook, 2010). Costanza-Smith (2010) reported four benefits of language sample analysis in clinical evaluation of language abilities: 1) increased sensitivity for diagnosis of language disorder, 2) increased ecological validity, 3) improved compliance for children who are difficult to test, and 4) ability to use assessment results to guide treatment planning.

Botting (2002) reported that use of narrative analysis to describe children's language production abilities should be a routine part of language assessment protocols, due to the large amount of normative data available, the predictive ability of narrative competence for later literacy skills, and the utility of narrative analysis in differentiating children with primarily linguistic deficits from those with primarily pragmatic deficits. Narrative retell tasks have been shown to sufficiently elicit complex syntactic structures for both typically developing and language-impaired children (Gummersall & Strong, 1999; Merritt & Liles, 1989) in an authentic manner (Udvari & Thousand, 1995).

Another justification for sampling communication behavior comes from changes made since 2001 in systems for classifying disorders, most notably the International Classification of Functioning, Disability and Health (ICFDH; World Health Organization, 2001). This classification system views disorders from the point of view of their effect on everyday life, that is, whether disorders can result in limitations to aspects of an individual's well-being, beyond the use of speech. For example, a person with a voice disorder may have limitations on career choice because of an inability to project the voice sufficiently to be heard by a group of people. This limitation on functioning may affect the person's vocational goals and decisions, if, for example, a teaching career is being considered. In traditional clinical evaluations, this issue may be overlooked because the person might be able to communicate adequately in a clinical setting. Thus, use of communication sampling contributes to the ability to perform functional assessment. **Functional assessments** of communication add to the understanding of the impact of communication disorders on a person's functioning in a variety of real-world settings. In these days of increased accountability for the costs of speech-language pathology services, speech-language pathologists (SLPs) need to be able to demonstrate that treatments make real, functional differences in clients' lives. Using communication sampling as a form of functional assessment meets this requirement.

An important consideration in communication sampling is to establish that samples bear a strong resemblance to the kinds of interactions in which clients really engage. This consideration is known as the **representativeness** of the sample. Although clinicians try to attain a representative sample, the communication SLPs observe during sampling may not be quite like the client's communication in everyday settings. A sample that is not representative may not show what a client is really able to do. This difference may occur because SLPs meet clients in clinical settings that are unfamiliar to them, or because clients are participating in an interaction with an unfamiliar partner (i.e., the clinician, whom the client may not know well), or because the client and clinician may be members of different cultural or linguistic communities. It is part of the SLP's job to ensure that the sample is as representative as possible. Methods for maximizing representativeness of the sample are addressed throughout this chapter, but keep in mind that for every client, the clinician must be attentive to the relevance of the sampling procedures and to **cultural sensitivity** regarding members of culturally and/or linguistically different (CLD) populations. Cultural sensitivity means realizing that the rules for talking and interacting differ among various communities. To get a valid sample of a client's language, clinicians need to attend to the cultural rules that govern conversation for that person. For instance, in some communities, it may not be acceptable for children to talk to strangers; in others, it may be rude to ask a question to which the answer is obvious (e.g., "What color is that shirt you are wearing?").

A clinician may or may not be familiar with the cultural and/or linguistic characteristics of some clients. Several sources can help a clinician gain information on CLD clientele (see, e.g., American Speech-Language-Hearing Association [ASHA], n.d., 2010, 2011; Anderson, 2009; Griffer & Cheng, 2009; Chapter 10). To monitor the representativeness of a speech-language sample collected from CLD clients, SLPs will want to learn something about conversational practices in the client's community. Other than by reading about the client's cultural and/or linguistic group, the clinician can interview community members to learn about cultural and linguistic characteristics. In addition, the clinician may want to sample the client in several conversational situations and then select the most representative and functional sample to use as the basis for a speech-language sample analysis. It also is a good idea to ask a client's family member whether the sample to be analyzed sounds like the way the client usually talks. Stockman (1996) offers other considerations for analyzing samples produced by children from specific CLD groups. Stockman suggests that a sample should attempt to reveal at least the child's minimum competency. Second, sampling should allow the clinician to differentiate the child's behaviors from performance that is considered normal or typical in the child's community. The sample will ideally reveal that the child shows behaviors or weaknesses that typical children from that community do not demonstrate.

With clients for whom English is not the dominant or preferred language, clinicians may sample while the client interacts in his or her dominant or preferred language with a family member or other fluent speaker of that language. The audio or video recording of the sample can be transcribed by an interpreter, but the interpreter must comply with the clinician's request to have the transcription accurately represent the client's production. If the interpreter *normalizes* the speech and/or language (i.e., correcting the client's errors to produce a corrected transcription), an important source of information about the client's speech and linguistic capabilities is removed.

In summary, it is important to remember that language is always embedded in culture. The way people talk differs not only on the basis of their abilities and disabilities but also on the basis of their own community's conversational rules, which may be different from those of the clinician's culture or community (see Chapter 10 for more considerations).

Communication sampling can be used with clients of all ages to investigate a broad range of speech and language problems. Clinicians may use samples of communication to examine the understanding and use of words (**semantics**) and sentences (**syntax**) in conversations, narratives, and explanations; explore the appropriateness of communication in context (**pragmatics**); analyze the client's sound system and its **intelligibility (phonology)**; observe speech **fluency;** evaluate the use of **paralinguistics** (such as **prosody**) in speech; and observe the quality and **resonance** of the speaking voice. Sampling and analysis techniques are applicable in three broad categories:

- *Nonverbal communication:* sampling that documents all communicative intentions expressed nonverbally; accounts for the amount, rate, or frequency of communication (i.e., nonverbal participation in conversational turns); and evidences the means by which the client's communications are produced, be that with gestures, vocalizations, body movements, facial expressions, or other nonword means

- *Language:* sampling that documents semantics, syntax, and pragmatics

- *Speech:* sampling that documents phonology, prosody, fluency, and voice

In this chapter's discussion of communication sampling, sampling procedures for nonverbal communication are discussed first. Second, sampling language across a range of developmental levels is explored. Third, sampling for aspects of speech production is discussed.

NONVERBAL COMMUNICATION

Some clients are *nonverbal,* meaning that they do not use any spoken language. Other clients are *minimally verbal,* meaning that they use very limited speech. Still, many of these clients actually do communicate quite well without producing words. Some may produce a great number of nonword communications. Nonverbal clients include children who are at *preverbal* levels of development, meaning that they have not yet acquired symbolic language. Other nonverbal or minimally verbal clients include older children, adolescents, or adults with developmental disabilities whose long-standing levels of functioning have precluded symbolic language learning. Third, some nonverbal clients had previously been typical language users but lost their skills due to injury or illness.

Collecting a representative sample from nonverbal clients is particularly challenging. Often these individuals are difficult to engage. Very young children may be unwilling to interact with an unfamiliar examiner. Clients with lifelong developmental disabilities who have had a lesser level of functioning throughout their life spans may be exceedingly passive or withdrawn after years of inability to communicate. If clients have lost communicative ability after, for instance, a stroke or an accident, they may be deeply frustrated with the mismatch between the intents they have to express and the means available to them for expression.

The purpose of communication sampling for nonverbal individuals varies according to developmental level. For young children who are not talking, clinicians sample current level of functioning in order to determine whether to set goals for oral speech and/or for some other form of symbolic communication, such as the manual signs used in **American Sign Language** (ASL; see Figure 5.1) or the iconic symbols used in **Blissymbols** (see Figure 5.2). Clinicians look for the potential to use **augmentative and/or alternative communication devices** (AAC), which could include low-technology picture boards or high-technology electronic communicators with a synthesized speech output. SLPs plan the interventions that would be appropriate based on clinical judgment of the extent and effectiveness of the child's current means and rate of communication.

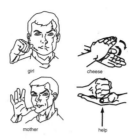

Figure 5.1. Examples of signs from American Sign Language. (© 2004 http://www.Lifeprint.com. Used by permission.)

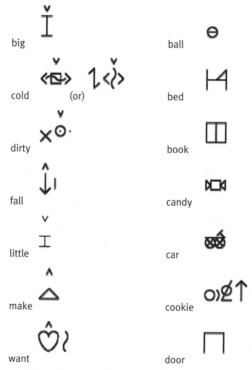

Figure 5.2. Examples of Blissymbols. (Blissymbols used herein copyright Blissymbols Communication International, Göteborg, Sweden, http://www.blissymbolics.org. Exclusive licensee since 1982.)

In working with preverbal children, clinicians have yet another purpose of communication sampling, namely, to assist in differential diagnosis. For example, clinicians expect children with developmental disorders such as intellectual disability, specific language impairment, or hearing impairment to show fairly typical skills in nonverbal communication, even when verbal language is absent. However, for children with more pervasive and complex developmental communication disorders, such as autism spectrum disorders, both language and nonverbal communication are affected. Communication sampling may assist the diagnostic team in determining the child's primary and secondary disorders.

For older clients who have developmental delays, clinicians may consider a more sophisticated form of the AAC system, which may relate to the use of a personal computer, iPad, iPhone, or some similar device. Clinicians need to determine what kinds of ideas the client is attempting to communicate in order to match the assistive system to the client's needs. Assistive systems can allow clients to make choices and express their wishes. When working with clients who have acquired losses, SLPs may need to determine what kinds of communication skills have been spared and then identify the best intervention strategies for making use of the communicative functioning that the client still has; clinicians also need to consider whether the client demonstrates the skills needed to use assistive technologies. Previously typical adults may have retained some of their reading and writing abilities, which can afford them many more options.

For all nonverbal clients, communication sampling is used to answer the following diagnostic questions:

- What can the client respond to during a linguistic interaction; that is, what are the client's functional comprehension skills like?

- What types of communicative intentions can the client express? Is a range of intentions available, or is the range very limited?

- How frequently does the client attempt to communicate? Can the client initiate communication as well as respond?

- By what means does the client attempt to get messages across? Does he or she use gestures, gaze, vocalizations, words, behaviors, or some combination of these? Does the client have any ability to associate pictures, printed symbols, or written language with his or her communicative intents?

- Does the client show the cognitive-linguistic correlates of communication, such as attentiveness to the communications going on around him or her; visual scanning of pictures, computer screens, or other media; behaviors that reveal the client's recall of past events; choice making; manual sequencing of steps to complete a task; and simple cause-and-effect behaviors?

Collecting the Sample

Collecting a representative sample from a nonspeaking client necessitates using a sampling context that is as similar as possible to the client's typical interactive contexts. For very young clients, this task will usually mean a play session with developmentally appropriate toys and a familiar interlocutor, such as a parent. For children with motor impairments, clinicians need to be especially careful to provide opportunities for the child to express wants, needs, and intents. Many children with fewer motor skills get used to having the people around them anticipate their desires; these children may become passive communicators (Calculator, 1997). When sampling older clients with severe developmental communication disorders and adult clients with acquired disorders, it is important to choose developmentally appropriate materials and arrange for a sampling context where communication is a large part of the activity that goes on in that context. This may mean observing the client in a daily living setting and noting various daily behaviors, such as choosing food items from a menu or completing vocational activities that involve interaction. It is important to ask individuals who know the client well to judge whether the interaction observed is typical of the client's current communication. The sample should be long enough to enable the client to exhibit a broad range of communicative behaviors. Generally, clinicians want to continue collecting data until the sample includes at least 20 purposeful acts of communication from the client. For active communicators, 15–20 minutes is usually a long enough time period for a reasonable sample. For clients who take communication turns less frequently, SLPs may need to spend a longer amount of time collecting a sample.

Recording the Sample

It is generally necessary to video record nonverbal clients. It is likely that the bulk of their communicative interactions will be visually observable and that audio recording will not capture a representative sampling of their communicative performance. Video recording the communication sample lets the clinician analyze the sample after the sampling session ends. Video recording allows the clinician to watch the interaction several times and to score one aspect of communication during each viewing. This makes it possible to use only one sample of communication to answer all the diagnostic questions that were posed prior to the assessment. Video recording has become much easier in recent years due to the availability of video recorders built into laptops, smartphones, and iPads.

Analyzing the Sample

When analyzing the sample of an individual who is nonverbal, clinicians try to answer the first diagnostic question posed earlier in this chapter: What can the client respond to during a linguistic interaction; that is, what are the client's functional comprehension skills like? Communication sampling allows clinicians to determine whether the client comprehends the communicative behaviors of the other individuals in the sampling setting. Clinicians may be able to make some inferences about how the language spoken to the client in a natural setting influences the client's behavior. The analysis documents the degree to which the nonverbal client's behavior suggests an understanding of language. This information provides an important adjunct to formal testing of language comprehension. Client behaviors in the sampling context show whether the client uses what Chapman (1978) called "comprehension strategies." The use of comprehension strategies allows a client to act in context as if language comprehension has occurred, even though linguistic knowledge of specific words and grammatical forms may be lacking. These strategies operate in typically developing children. For example, when a mother looks at a ball, points to it, and says, "See the ball?" to her 12-month-old child, the baby does not have to understand the word *ball* in order to appear to understand; he or she has only to look at what the mother is pointing to in order to make a contextual response. This looking behavior gives the impression that the child knows the word, even though the child might not be able to identify *ball* in an array of several objects without the mother's gaze and point cues. If the client seems to comprehend

Context	Client response		
	Responds appropriately	Responds inappropriately (describe)	Does not respond
Partner gives verbal instruction.			
Partner asks question.			
Partner offers choice verbally.			
Partner suggests joint activity.			
Partner remarks on object or event.			

Figure 5.3.   Assessing comprehension in natural contexts.

better in these natural interactions than during standardized testing of language comprehension, the sample has gathered an important piece of information: the client takes advantage of interactive cues in the environment. SLPs can learn about many of the client's skills, such as receptive vocabulary, ability to follow directions, and comprehension of contextual behavioral routines. Clinicians can compare adequate performance in an interactive context with how well the client performs on standardized testing. Some clients do well on both natural-istic tasks and testing, some do well on one task or the other, and other clients perform poorly on formal receptive testing and do not use comprehension strategies in natural situations.

Figure 5.3 presents an observation form that may be used to examine a non-verbal client's receptive behaviors during naturalistic communication sampling. The form records the frequency and context of behaviors that appear to suggest language comprehension. (Keep in mind that an assessment like this can be help-ful for clinicians working with young children who have a hearing impairment, in order to assess the degree to which residual hearing is used to support natural communication.)

The other diagnostic questions posed earlier relate to a nonverbal client's means of communication, range of intents, and frequency of communications expressed. Again, using a video-recorded sample of representative communica-tion, clinicians can assess how often, in what form, and for what purpose the client communicates. In assessing the communications of nonspeakers, it is important that clinicians be conservative about attributing intention to the client's actions. It may be inaccurate to regard the client's every act as an act of communication. In order for the client's action to count as a communicative act, the action should meet more than one of the following criteria:

1. It should be directed by means of gaze, body orientation, or gesture toward the interlocutor.

2. It should have an effect on the interlocutor.

3. It should convey a recognizable message that could be translated into words.

4. It should be persistent; if the act does not immediately gain its objective, it should be repeated or revised.

Communicative function	Form				
	Gaze	Body movement	Gesture	Vocalization	Word approximation
Request object or action					
Protest					
Comment (joint attention)					
Greeting or social interaction					
Request information					
Give new information					
Acknowledge partner's remark					

Figure 5.4. Assessment of nonverbal communication behaviors.

An observation form like the one in Figure 5.4 can be used to summarize the actions that represent communicative functions. In some cases, the behaviors observed during sampling sessions can be analyzed by applying formal procedures for assessment of preverbal communication in children in the early stages of communicative development. One sample instrument is the Communication and Symbolic Behavior Scales (CSBS; Wetherby & Prizant, 2002), an assessment procedure with known reliability and validity (Wetherby, Allen, Cleary, Kublin, & Goldstein, 2002). The CSBS procedure involves a structured play session, a parent-report checklist, and a caregiver follow-up questionnaire. In addition, clinicians can consult the comprehensive suggestions offered by Crais (2011) for recommended practices in screening, evaluation, and assessment of infants and toddlers.

When assessing nonverbal communication in adolescent and adult clients who have not developed spoken language or who have lost speech and language, the same diagnostic questions apply. Clinicians use methods that are designed to provide opportunities for communicative responses and then examine the communication that is present. Ogletree, Fischer, and Turowski (1996) describe assessment protocols for use with older nonverbal clients with developmental disabilities. In some cases, the clinician offers *communicative temptations* in order to stimulate the production of client behaviors. McLaughlin and Cascella (2008), for example, describe a communicative temptations procedure for eliciting gestural responses during a choice-making activity. During the assessment of a nonverbal or minimally verbal client, the clinician generally investigates trial usage of manual communication systems and/or AAC devices. He or she explores all means of communication that the client could use to increase the client's communicative capacity. Although AAC assessment is beyond the scope of this chapter, readers will find many useful resources in Fishman (2011), Proctor and Oswalt (2008), and Beukelman and Mirenda (2013). Regarding the assessment of previously typical individuals who have lost communication abilities, Threats (2009) describes how the ICFDH guidelines provide some parameters for assessment. Lasker (2009) and Buzolich (2006) provide assessment protocols that implement trial usage of AAC strategies.

LANGUAGE SAMPLING

Clinicians sample client language in order to observe the meanings expressed (semantics), the forms used for expression (syntax), and the appropriateness of communication in a social context (pragmatics). Because language changes and develops over the life span, clinicians use somewhat different methods at each level of development. Language sampling covers broad developmental periods: the preschool level (1–5 years), the school-age level (6–16 years), and the adult level (older than 16 years).

Sampling Language in Preschoolers

Children between 1 and 5 years of age are typically acquiring basic words and sentence structures. Communication sampling often focuses on establishing that children produce the syntactic structures and morphological markers that are significant indicators of language growth during this developmental phase, but clinicians assess semantics (vocabulary, word knowledge, and word usage) and pragmatics (interactional capabilities) as well.

Collecting the Sample   Clinicians usually collect language samples from preschoolers during play interactions. Owens (2004) reports that the choice of play materials has the potential to make a difference in the content and quality of the samples obtained. Play interactions that include familiar people, activities, materials, and topics tend to elicit the most representative sample. Manipulable materials (i.e., items that require using one's hands and that children can play with in many ways) stimulate opportunities for producing language that is more complex. Often the best toys represent familiar domestic objects and actions. These toys stimulate the everyday vocabulary that accompanies the use of these items. Pretend play to enact routine domestic interactions, such as bathing, dressing, food preparation, housekeeping, and running errands, is appropriate for small children of both genders. Play items include toy kitchenware and foods; shopping toys, such as baskets, carts, and play money; dress-up items; dollhouses with toy people and furniture; and toy community settings, such as a gas station, playground, farm, or zoo. Creative materials also stimulate language, such as Play-Doh and cookie cutters or multistep craft activities that the child and clinician complete together. Children respond well to container play with "sand box" materials that are safer than sand: substances like uncooked macaroni noodles, grains of rice, or rolled oats (i.e., old-fashioned raw oatmeal). "Sand box" play elicits talk about digging, pouring, dumping, rolling, and other play actions. Blocks and other construction toys can elicit language about directionality (e.g., building up, falling down). In summary, children tend to talk more about familiar, mundane items than about items with which they have had little or no experience. Toy objects that are too novel or unfamiliar tend to elicit quiet exploratory play. Toy vehicles and action figures that are too exciting may stimulate more vocalization (e.g., "Vroom! Vroom!") than verbalization (O'Brien & Nagle, 1987). Electric toys are useful if they require manipulations, not just flipping a switch and then watching the toy.

Even the most appropriate materials will not necessarily get a preschooler to talk, however. Miller (1981) suggests some strategies to help establish rapport and elicit talk from young children. Initially, for the first few minutes, the clinician is to say very little except "Hi" and general words of welcome. The clinician presents the child with toys and waits for the child to speak. Some children may not understand that they need not remain quiet in this quiet setting. If the child does not initiate conversation, the clinician may begin to *parallel play* with the child and offer intermittent comments about ongoing actions (e.g., "You're stacking the blocks; I'll stack mine, too!"). As the play progresses, the clinician can initiate some interactive play, though it is best for the clinician to maintain a lower frequency of conversational turns for the first few minutes. The adult must not overwhelm the child with instructions or lead the child to expect to simply answer adult questions. When the child appears comfortable with the clinician and is speaking, the clinician may begin trying to elicit verbal responses from the child that expand upon the child's previous utterances. If the child says, "I'm stacking blocks," the clinician may say something that leads the child to respond but that does not supply the child with an actual modeled utterance, for example, "I think this looks like something," and perhaps add, "Can you guess what it looks like?" The clinician needs to refrain from talking too much after the child has become comfortable. Even though the clinician may have "broken the ice," the child must be able to speak freely, at length, and without interruption. The clinician should not contaminate the sample by offering labels for items or other semantic or syntactic cues. The idea is to allow the child to express a sample of the semantics and syntax that he or she has already acquired. The clinician should not influence what the child has to say.

The clinician's own use of language pragmatics is critical for obtaining a representative language sample. In a study of the effects of parental questions versus topic continuations, Yoder and Davies (1990) found that adult *topic continuations* elicited children's responses. Multiword replies from children were most likely to occur after explicit prompts that continued the child's topic (e.g., Child: "Baby cry." Examiner: "Oh! That's sad! What can we do?"). Open-ended or loosely structured questions can be used effectively to "break the ice" early in the session and to determine the child's interest in a specific topic, but it is unwise to ask many yes-no or **closed questions** (e.g., "What is that?" "Where is the dog?" "Who is this?") because these typically elicit one-word responses. When this happens, the length of utterance that the child produces may be quite short, and the child may appear to have less verbal fluency than he or she actually has. The sample would not be representative of the child's true skills. On the other hand, the technique of *parallel talk*, by which the clinician describes what the child is doing, is often more effective for eliciting language. Clinicians describe the child's present actions ("I see that you are building something") and then lead into an **open-ended question** or comment (e.g., "Tell me about that").

Repetition of a child's utterance, perhaps with a change of inflection, can be used effectively to increase the child's output. People tend to say more if what they have just said is validated. If the child says, "A tower," and the clinician repeats the utterance with a tone of interest and enthusiasm, the child may then elaborate. Some clinicians repeat the child's utterances with a rising intonation that signals a question and that invites the child to say more. Further, it is useful for the clinician to repeat a child's utterance when the child has reduced intelligibility. This allows the child to confirm or disconfirm that the clinician has heard correctly. Repeating the child's utterance is a precaution that makes audio or video recordings more accurate. Many clinicians are surprised to find that although they understood what a client was saying during the sampling interaction, it is much more difficult to understand the client when listening to the recording after the session is over. Clinicians may make written notes as they collect the sample to remind them of what was happening and what was said.

Another effective technique is to offer a one-word response followed by silence. An example is "Really?" because it shows interest and implies wanting to know more. Playful statements that are obviously false can be useful in eliciting more elaborated forms (e.g., Examiner: "My doggy is green!" Child: "No it not!").

How long should a language sample from a preschooler be? Most authorities (Miller, 1981; Nelson, 1998) suggest 50–100 utterances. If it is possible to collect two 50-utterance samples in two different settings, this is ideal. For children functioning at the 1–5-year level, a sample of this length can generally be collected during a 15-minute interaction. If the child's language or general development is delayed, a somewhat longer sample of 20–30 minutes may be needed to obtain enough spoken language to analyze.

Recording the Sample   It may not be necessary to video record a communication sample with a preschool-age child. Because clinicians are interested in the spoken language, audio recording will usually be sufficient for sampling purposes. Exceptions include children who communicate by using a visual communication system such as ASL or who are so unintelligible that the clinician will need the nonverbal context to help decipher what they are saying. However, because devices such as personal computers, iPhones, and iPads offer audio- and video-recording options, the choice to video record may be just as easy as the choice to audio record, and video allows for a complete record of verbal and nonverbal interactions. When planning to analyze a sample from an audio or video recording, the clinician must bear in mind that it is important that the sampling setting be conducive to quiet recording. This means that background noise should be minimal and that the recording instrument and microphone should be carefully chosen and situated in the room. Although many devices have high-quality internal microphones, an external, unidirectional microphone that can be placed fairly close to the child is generally recommended. It is wise to consult the user manual accompanying the device or the device manufacturer's web site to determine whether a peripheral microphone is a better choice than an internal microphone. It is critical that a clinician test the functioning of the recording device and microphone before the session begins. There is nothing more frustrating than spending 15–20 minutes of time obtaining a speech and language sample only to find that the recorder failed to work or had not been turned on!

Transcribing the Sample   Transcribing a spoken language sample yields a tangible document that clinicians can examine in a variety of ways. Transcription retains all the errors that the child produces. Clinicians examine language sample transcripts to discover the errors or error patterns that they will address in intervention.

A challenging aspect of transcribing a sample involves how to separate the child's speech stream into utterances. *Utterance boundaries* are important because clinicians calculate the average number of particular structures per utterance.

Table 5.1.   Sample transcription format

Adult	Child	Context
1. What have you got there?		Child plays with toy dog and bone.
2. Is it a doggy?	1. Uh-huh.	
3. I have a dog at home.		
4. Tell me about who's at your house.	2. We have kitty.	Child leaves toy and looks up at examiner.
5. Oh, cool!		
6. I like cats.		
7. Tell me about yours.	3. Black.	
	4. It have white foots.	
8. I'll bet it's pretty!		Child returns to playing with toy dog.

Source: Retherford (2000).

Generally, clinicians make decisions regarding utterance separation by observing syntactic, intonational, contextual, and pausing features. For preschoolers, Leadholm and Miller (1992) suggest using either a falling or rising intonational contour or a pause of more than 2 seconds to indicate the end of one utterance and the start of another. Lund and Duchan (1993) present rules for using intonational, syntactic, and contextual information to identify utterance separations.

There are various formats for transcribing language samples. A sample transcript using the three-column format suggested by Retherford (2000) appears in Table 5.1. The column labeled "Context" describes exactly what the child is doing as each utterance is produced. The context may describe the antecedent event that caused the child to produce language, for example, Context: The child drops the doll. Child: 1. "Oops." Adult actions are transcribed when they affect the child's communication, for example, Context: Mother points to a ball. Child: 1. "Ball." In this case, the mother's pointing is the antecedent that caused the child to speak.

Analyzing the Sample   When clinicians look closely at language samples to discover patterns of error and areas of strength, they cannot truly separate *form* (syntax and morphology), *content* (meaning or semantics), and *use* (pragmatics). Analyses often artificially divide these aspects of language, but it is wise to remember that in real communication, these aspects are integrated. Clinicians can employ procedures to analyze each of these areas of language but should remember that, in fact, they all work together to express the client's intents. In analyzing the sample, the clinician's main job is to determine the area(s) of relative strength and the area(s) of relative weakness and to observe how well the areas work together. Sometimes a stronger area can compensate for some weaknesses. Other times, a weak area makes it difficult for stronger areas to be used to their full potential.

Semantics and Syntax   Analyzing language samples is one of the most time-consuming aspects of clinical practice. For this reason, it is important that clinicians use language sampling judiciously. Sampling and standardized testing (see Chapter 3) work together to establish a clear picture of a client's language skills. For some clients, it is more efficient to administer standardized tests first; if an expressive language deficit is found, then sampling can be carried out to shed light on how this deficit affects functional communication. In other cases, testing is inconclusive, so sampling is carried out to gain more information. Other clients are not candidates for standardized tests, or suitable tests for this type of client are not available, so sampling is used as the primary diagnostic method. A sample may be compared to the language milestones that are summarized on developmental checklists. In this way, the child's development is compared to that of his or her peers.

The clinician's goal in language sampling is not to obtain a score but to answer questions about the client's communication ability and to identify appropriate intervention goals. When completing a language sample analysis, some questions to ask include these:

- How does the language sample compare to other aspects of the client's receptive and expressive language performance? (Performance indicators can be test scores, information derived from checklists, environmental performance observations, or reports from family members, teachers, and others.)

- Is the child consistently using the language structures that are expected at a particular developmental level or stage? (In other words, can the child's semantic, syntactic, and pragmatic levels of functioning be ascertained?)

- Is there variety in the types of utterances that the client uses, or does he or she use the same utterance constructions over and over?

- Are there consistent error patterns, or are errors inconsistent and erratic? Are the errors consistent with language maturation and therefore expected at the child's age level, or are the errors apparently not consistent with the refinement of language that usually takes place during the developmental period?

Usually, when clinicians collect a language sample, in addition to thinking about general questions like these, they employ formalized analyses that help understand the sample more fully. There are two basic methods of analyzing language samples: manual methods and computer-assisted procedures.

Manual Methods   Various paper-and-pencil methods have been developed to examine language during the preschool period. In particular, manual methods of language analysis allow clinicians to carefully consider syntactic development. Some examples of procedures for exploring the development of syntactic form are given in Table 5.2. Perhaps the most widely used of all language sample analysis procedures is the computation of the mean length of utterance (MLU) in morphemes. Roger Brown (1973), in his pioneering research on the stages of acquisition of morphology and syntax, first used MLU to index morphological and syntactic development in young children. A **morpheme** is a minimal meaningful unit of language. Computing the MLU involves counting the total number of morphemes in a language sample and dividing by the total number of utterances. A client's MLU can be compared to normative values reported by Leadholm and Miller (1992), Owens (2004), or Paul and Norbury (2012) to decide if the client's performance represents a delay. The MLU can be a useful tool to measure a child's syntactic growth. Clinicians who compute an MLU as part of an initial assessment battery establish the child's baseline; the clinician can then compare the child's subsequent MLUs at reassessment.

Table 5.2.   Examples of language sampling procedures

Procedure	Reference
Mean length of utterance (MLU)	Brown (1973)
Language Assessment, Remediation, and Screening Procedure (LARSP)	Crystal, Fletcher, and Garman (1991)
Assigning of Structural Stage Procedure (ASSP)	Miller (1981)
Developmental sentence scoring (DSS)	Lee (1974)
Language Sampling, Analysis, & Training (LSAT)	Tyack and Gottsleben (1974)
Index of Productive Syntax (IPSyn)	Scarborough (1990)

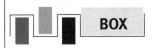 **BOX** | # Rules for Counting Morphemes and Computing Mean Length of Utterance

Counting Morphemes

1. Use only completely intelligible utterances.

2. Count the morphemes in the first 50 consecutive utterances.

3. Repetitions or false starts within an utterance are assigned morphemes only in the most complete form (e.g., in "My my mom is pretty," count only "My mom is pretty"). If the repetition is for emphasis, count each word (e.g., in "My dad is big BIG," count all words, including the repetition for emphasis).

4. Fillers (e.g., *um*, *well*, *oh*) are not counted. *Hi*, *no*, and *yeah* are counted.

5. Compound words (e.g., *birthday*, *somebody*), proper names (e.g., *Mickey Mouse*), and ritualized reduplications (e.g., *choo-choo*, *night-night*) are counted as one morpheme.

6. Diminutive forms (e.g., *doggie*, *daddy*, *toesie*) are counted as one morpheme.

7. Auxiliary verbs are counted as one morpheme, even if they are contracted (e.g., "He is running" has three morphemes; "He's running" has three morphemes).

8. Catenatives (e.g., *gonna*, *wanna*, *gotta*, *hafta*) count as just one morpheme.

9. All inflections (e.g., possessive *s*, plural *s*, regular past *-ed*) are counted as two morphemes (e.g., *shoes* has two morphemes; *baby's* has two morphemes).

10. Negative contractions (e.g., *can't*, *don't*, *won't*) are assigned two morphemes only if there is evidence elsewhere in the transcript that the child uses each part of the contraction separately.

Computing Mean Length of Utterance

1. Count the total number of morphemes produced by the speaker.

2. Divide by the number of utterances counted (usually 50).

Source: Brown (1973).

In addition to computing an MLU, clinicians use other analyses that can give more in-depth information about a child's syntactic and semantic development. Using the framework of Brown's stages of morphological and syntactic development (1973), the Assigning of Structural Stage Procedure (ASSP; Miller, 1981) counts the occurrences of the 14 grammatical morphemes originally studied by Brown (1973) and deVilliers and deVilliers (1973). The ASSP allows the clinician to chart the child's use of various simple sentence constructions that correspond to Brown's stages and identifies the child's stage of development of noun and verb phrase elaborations, negations, questions, and complex sentences. Assigning stages shows where a child may have strengths and weaknesses in the development of syntax and morphology. The process requires a detailed knowledge of the sequence of normal syntactic acquisition. Justice and Ezell (2008), Miller (1981), Owens (2004), Paul and Norbury (2012), and Retherford (2000) provided information on syntactic development that clinicians are obliged to know.

The ASSP is qualitative in nature and allows clinicians to look at patterns in the child's use of language. Figure 5.5 presents a worksheet that might be used to record and summarize information about syntactic development using the ASSP.

Scarborough (1990) presented an extension of Miller's procedure (1981). Scarborough's Index of Productive Syntax (IPSyn) includes structures from the ASSP as well as additional syntactic forms that Scarborough found to be

Brown's stage	Grammatical morphemes	Noun phrase	Verb phrase	Negation	Yes–No Qs	Wh- Qs	Complex sentences
I							
II	-ing 100% in 100% plural 100%		‖‖‖				
III	on 100% Possessive 100%	‖‖‖ ‖‖‖ ‖‖‖	‖‖‖ ‖‖‖	‖‖‖ ‖	‖‖	‖	
IV		‖‖‖ ‖‖‖	‖‖‖ ‖	‖			‖
V	Copula *be* 33% Regular past 45% Irregular past 50% Regular third-person singular 25%						
V+	Auxilliary *be* 33% Irregular third person singular						
V++							

Figure 5.5. Sample Assigning of Structural Stage Procedure worksheet. Key: Qs, questions. (*Source:* Miller, 1981.)

diagnostic. Use of the IPSyn involves counting the first two correct occurrences of each of these structures to determine whether each is part of the child's repertoire. The IPSyn provides both norm-referenced and criterion-referenced information that can be useful in selecting treatment goals and in measuring progress in language usage.

Another language sample analysis procedure is Lee's Developmental Sentence Analysis (DSA; 1974). This procedure has two components: developmental sentence types (DST) and developmental sentence scoring (DSS). The DST component is a criterion-referenced analysis for young children whose language is at the one-word and two-word utterance level. This procedure analyzes five utterance categories to determine 1) which categories are frequent in the child's speech, 2) which categories should be used as a basis for developing longer utterances, and 3) which categories are infrequent and should be elicited first in one- to two-word utterance forms. The DSS component, which is for use with children who use subject-verb sentences consistently, is rather widely used by clinicians and provides both norm-referenced and criterion-referenced information. This component analyzes eight syntactic categories that appear in the language of young children and that have certain developmental characteristics. The DSS scores are standardized for ages 2-0 (2 years, 0 months) to 6-6 (6 years, 6 months). Scores below the 10th percentile indicate a language deficit. But as with the ASSP and IPSyn, it is the qualitative information obtained from a DSS analysis that provides the most useful information for characterizing a child's language and for determining treatment goals and measuring intervention progress.

Computer-Assisted Procedures   There are several computer programs for language sample analysis. Miller, Freiberg, Rolland, and Reeves (1992) described the benefits of computer technology for language sampling in the areas of transcription, analysis, accuracy, and interpretation. The ability to perform multiple analyses on the same transcript is perhaps the biggest advantage in using a computer program. Larson and McKinley (2003) cautioned that it is still up to the clinician to obtain a reliable and representative language sample and to transcribe it accurately.

The widely used Systematic Analysis of Language Transcripts (SALT) was developed by Miller and Chapman (2000, 2012). The software manages the processes of eliciting, transcribing, and analyzing language samples. The software includes a transcription editor, report generator, and reference databases for age-matched comparisons. (The software package includes narrative elicitation materials to use with speakers who are old enough to produce narratives.) Analyses include MLU and several kinds of word counts: 1) *type–token ratio* (TTR), a semantic measure of the number of different words used in the sample divided by the total number of words; 2) *number of different words* (NDW), a measure of semantic maturity and diversity (Long et al., 2005); and 3) *total number of words* (TNW), a measure of general language proficiency that reflects talkativeness (Long, McKinley, Thormann, Jones, & Nockerts, 2005). Miller and colleagues (1992) showed that both MLU and NDW are sensitive to language development and delay during the preschool and school-age periods. Frequency counts of errors in syntax, morphology, and semantics are also calculated. These error types may be particularly helpful in differentiating language differences from an actual disorder in clients who are learning English as a second language or who speak a nonmainstream dialect of English. The SALT program has features that allow users to design their own analyses.

The SALT program provides a reference database that acknowledges linguistic diversity and incorporates several different language groups. This allows a client's performance to be compared to that of children from a culturally relevant reference sample. The SALT 2012 program can be purchased in clinical, research, instructional, and student versions (see http://www.saltsoftware.com).

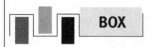 **BOX**   **Computer-Assisted Language Analysis Procedures**

The Child Language Data Exchange System (CHILDES; MacWhinney, 2012a) is an online system for sharing transcripts and studying child language. The CLAN (Computerized Language ANalysis) software program (MacWhinney, 1996, 2000, 2012b) is designed to analyze transcripts that are formatted for the CHILDES system. The CLAN program provides a host of analyses, including MLU, DSS, TTR, word frequency counts, and morphosyntactic analyses.

Computerized Profiling (Long, Fey, & Channell, 2000; Long, 2008) is available online. Among its many features are utterance count, number of different sentence types, number of complete and intelligible sentences, semantic analyses, and early vocabulary analysis of single-word and early multiword productions. In addition, the program features the Language Assessment, Remediation, and Screening Procedure (LARSP; Crystal, Fletcher, & Garman, 1989)—a system for profiling children's syntax—as well as the IPSyn, the DSS and an adapted DSS for speakers of African American Vernacular English, phonology analyses, prosody analysis, the Conversational Acts Profile (CAP; Fey, 1986), and narrative analysis. The software allows users to compare two samples or two analyses, which facilitates clinical progress monitoring (see http://childes.psy.cmu.edu).

Pragmatic Language   *Pragmatics* is defined as the study of how language is used in the context of communication. Evaluating a child's pragmatic skills is a natural extension of evaluating a language sample because pragmatics must be assessed in a communicative context. The goal of assessment in this area is to compare a child's pragmatic skills with his or her skills in the areas of syntax, semantics, and phonology to help determine the communicative basis the client has for learning language.

Several organizational schemes can be used to evaluate pragmatic skills as observed during a language sample. One that is widely used is Prutting and Kirchner's Pragmatic Protocol (1983). This method allows a clinician to look at pragmatic behaviors as they occur within the context of a language sample and then make an overall judgment as to whether the behaviors are generally appropriate or inappropriate. An adaptation of this coding scheme appears in Figure 5.6. Owens

Communicative act	Appropriate	Inappropriate	No opportunity to observe
Utterance acts			
A. Verbal/paralinguistic			
1. Voice quality			
2. Vocal intensity			
3. Prosody			
4. Fluency			
B. Nonverbal			
1. Proximity			
2. Posture			
3. Gestures			
4. Gaze			
5. Facial expression			
Expression of meaning			
A. Word use			
1. Specificity			
2. Accuracy			
B. Relations between words			
1. Word order			
2. Given/new information			
C. Register variation			
1. To adults			
2. To peers			
Communicative functions			
A. Speech acts			
1. Remarks relevant to conversation			
2. Uses a broad range of communicative functions[a]			
B. Topics			
1. Selection			
2. Introduction			
3. Maintenance			
4. Change			
C. Turn taking			
1. Initiation			
2. Response			
3. Repair or revision			
4. Pause time			
5. Interrupts			
6. Gives feedback			
7. Quantity and conciseness			

Figure 5.6. A form for recording pragmatic behaviors in communication samples. (From Prutting, C.A., & Kirchner, D. [1983]. Applied pragmatics. In T.M. Gallagher & C.A. Prutting [Eds.], *Pragmatic assessment and intervention issues in language* [pp. 29–64]. San Diego, CA: College-Hill Press.)

[a]Some examples of communicative functions are requests information, follows narrations, provides explanations, gives predictions, pretends, reasons, gives new information, plans conversations, and comments on the conversation.

(2004), Paul and Norbury (2012), and Roth and Spekman (1984a, 1984b) provided additional guidelines for analyzing communication intention and discourse organization during conversational language interaction between a preschool-age child and an adult.

Language Sampling in School-Age Children and Adolescents

In the school-age developmental period, basic sentence structures, vocabulary, and conversational rules have been learned. Analysis focuses on the refinement and elaboration of communication skill.

Collecting the Sample In collecting a spontaneous speech and language sample from a school-age child, Evans and Craig (1992) found that the use of an interview format elicited more representative language behaviors than did free play with toys and games. They suggested using the following three open-ended questions to elicit 15 minutes of speech and language from children in the 7- to 12-year age range:

1. Tell me about your family.

2. Tell me about your school.

3. What do you do when you are not in school?

For school-age children or teens, it may be especially useful to have at least part of the language sample collected during the client's interaction with a peer. Peer conversation tends to contain more complex language than does conversation with adults. School-age children or teens may tend to take a relatively passive role in interacting with authority figures but may communicate more assertively with others of their own age. If a peer interaction can be arranged, this sample can be analyzed in conjunction with the interview sample. Suggested topics for a peer conversation could include shared interests (e.g., games, sports) or popular entertainments (e.g., music, TV, movies); or the clinician can ask the client to explain a game or activity to a peer. The peers might engage in a game or activity that involves verbalizations. The clinician may be able to remain an observer and thus obtain a more naturalistic and representative sample of the child's or teen's communication.

Recording and Transcribing the Sample In general, as mentioned in the section on recording preschoolers' language, although audio recording of school-age children or teens is sufficient, the availability of video recording devices on laptops, smartphones, and iPads makes it very easy to capture the sample on video.

There are some different procedures needed for transcribing school-age children's language samples that have to do with how utterances are segmented. Hunt (1965) developed an utterance segmentation system called the **T-unit,** or terminal unit, which is used to segment lengthier utterances into units for analysis. Hunt observed that school-age children sometimes produced run-on sentences, something like this:

> Well, last weekend I went skiing with my buddies from school and it was gonna be a long trip so I packed a sandwich and a bottle of pop and I put them on my seat on the bus so I would have them for later and I wouldn't get too hungry before we stopped at McDonald's and had some dinner on the way home from the trip but then I got hungry and ate half the sandwich before we got to the mountain.

Hunt (1965) reasoned that to count such a long utterance as just one sentence was not representative of the complexity of the child's language. He devised the

T-unit to compensate for these run-on sentences. A T-unit is defined as one main clause with all the subordinate clauses and nonclausal phrases attached to it. The preceding sample sentence is divided into T-units as follows:

1. Well, last weekend I went skiing with my buddies from school

2. and it was gonna be a long trip

3. and I packed a sandwich and a bottle of pop

4. and I put them on my seat on the bus so I would have them for later

5. and I wouldn't get too hungry before we stopped at McDonald's to have some dinner on the way home from the trip

6. but then I got hungry and ate half the sandwich before we got to the mountain.

Once the sample is segmented into the T-units, various analyses can be completed, including MLU per T-unit. Computer-assisted language analysis programs analyze T-units in a variety of ways. Owens (2004) reports an increase in words per T-unit from an average of about seven in Grades 3–4 to about eleven in Grades 10–11.

Analyzing the Sample   At this developmental period, language sample analysis focuses less on missing forms and more on the degree to which communication is complex and flexible. The computer-assisted methods of analysis that SLPs use with preschool-age samples can be used with school-age children and adolescents.

Semantics and Syntax   There are fewer procedures developed to analyze the expressive language of children and teens in the school-age period. Most clients at this developmental level have mastered the basic syntax, morphology, semantics, pragmatics, and phonology of communication. The difficulties they have tend to be in contexts that demand more specific, complex language skills related to literacy and school success. Some of the analyses discussed for preschoolers can be used with younger school-age clients. The DSS can be used up to age 7, which usually corresponds to second grade. The SALT reference database contains information on MLU, NDW, and TNW, as well as use of **bound morphemes,** personal pronouns, questions words, negative markers, **conjunctions,** and **modal verbs** (i.e., *can, will, shall, may, could, would, should, must, might*) for children from 3 through 13 years of age as long as the SALT protocols for language sampling are followed.

Another analysis that provides important information about school-age clients and teens has been adapted from the analyses used for preschoolers. Craig and Washington (2002) and Paul and Norbury (2012) argued that a school-age client's less skillful use of **complex sentences** can reveal language delay because complex sentences reflect the speaker's ability to combine ideas within a sentence. Moreover, combined sentences are an important aspect of the literate language used in written text. An example of a complex combined sentence that could be found in literate text is "The hillside village was an assembly of small wooden cabins and stone huts that crouched below the large, solid church of stone, bricks, and mortar that stood tall near the top of the hill." A school-age child might paraphrase this literate sentence using complex spoken sentences in this way: "In the village there were small wooden cabins and stone huts on the hillside and a large church near the top of the hill that was made of stone, bricks, and mortar." A school-age child whose language is atypical might need to reduce the sentence complexity and recite a series of simple sentences thus: "There was a village. There were cabins. There was a church."

Paul and Norbury (2012) recommend reviewing a transcript for its complex sentences and analyzing the transcript in three areas:

1. The proportion of complex sentences to total sentences in the sample

2. The types of complex forms used (e.g., infinitive clauses, relative clauses)

3. The number and type of conjunctions (e.g., *and, if, because, when, so*)

An analysis of sentence complexity reveals whether a student is not using appropriately complex language and suggests which aspects of complex language ought to be addressed in an intervention program. A sample worksheet for this analysis appears in Figure 5.7.

In addition, Paul and Norbury (2012) and Scott and Stokes (1995) suggested looking at other measures of advanced language use, such as the presence of noun and verb phrase components, adverbs, and morphological features such as prefixes and suffixes. Clinicians may want to look for the usage of other aspects of language form that are frequently problematic for students with language disabilities, as noted by Miller and colleagues (1992):

- Utterance formulation difficulties, including false starts, repetitions, and reformulations

- Word-finding problems as evidenced by single-word reformulations and/or circumlocutions

- Semantic deficits as evidenced by limited vocabulary and use of general words as opposed to specific names (e.g., *thingy, stuff, whatchamacallit*)

Pragmatics Larson and McKinley (2003) developed the Adolescent Conversational Analysis, a tool to analyze a school-age student's role as both a listener and a speaker. Larson and McKinley recommend analyzing a sample of the student speaking with each of several partners, including the clinician (i.e., an unfamiliar adult) and a peer. As in Prutting and Kirchner's procedure (1983) for analyzing the pragmatic language of younger children, the Adolescent Conversational Analysis evaluates the student's conversational behaviors as *appropriate*, *inappropriate*, or *not observed* in 10-minute samples of conversation. As a listener, the client's ability to understand the vocabulary and main ideas of the speaker is evaluated, in addition to how the client responds to nonverbal feedback. As a speaker, the client is evaluated for specific language and paralinguistic features (e.g., rate of speech, tone of voice, use of pauses and fillers), as well as for the use of communication functions and conversational rules. A sample worksheet for this analysis appears in Figure 5.8.

Brinton and Fujiki (2004) found that the clinician's use of probes during the sampling interaction increases the efficiency of the sampling session and can

Student name: _A. J. Nevarow_   Data of birth: _11/20/01_

Teacher: _R. Paul_   Grade: _6_

Clinician: _E. Reuler_   Date of examination: _10/10/13_

School: _Ruttles Middle School_   Samplingcontext: _Interview_

Number of T-units in sample: _50_

Number of complex sentences in sample: _22_

Percentage of complex sentences in sample: _44%_

Complex sentence type	T-unit	Conjunction used
Sentence-conjunction-sentence	5. He plays soccer, and I play baseball. 9. I like ice cream, but I don't want yours.	and but
Simple infinitive	14. I need to go home right after school. 34. He wants to beat me at that game.	
Adverbial clause	16. After I get home, I watch TV. 46. If my mom isn't home, I get a snack	after if
Propositional clause	27. I wish that I had the new Star Wars DVD.	that
Wh- clause	3. Mom knows where I am. 41. I don't know who that is.	where who
Sentences with three or more verbal phrases	18. I want to go see it, but my mom won't take me. 23. After we go to the circus, we like to stop for ice crease	but after
Relative clause	25. That's the kind I like. 30. They're the kids that I play ball with.	that that
Infinitive clause with different subject	15. He wants me to go with him. 20. My teacher wants you to teach me.	
Infinitive with wh-	19. I know how to do that. 28. Did you tell me when to stop?	how when
Passive infinitive	7. He doesn't want to get hit by the truck. 10. Do you want to be picked by the teacher?	
Gerund clause	26. Snowboarding is fun 49. My favorite thing is playing computer games.	

Figure 5.7. Sample worksheet for complex sentence analysis (with sample utterances).

target whether the client can produce various pragmatic behaviors. Some probes that they found to be effective are these:

- Initiating new topics in the midst of conversation (e.g., "By the way, I went skiing last weekend") to look for client responsiveness, maintenance of the new topic, and the relevance of the client's response to the comment

Communicative skill	Appropriate	Inappropriate	No opportunity to observe
Listening skills			
1. Understands partner's vocabulary and syntax			
2. Follows conversational topics introduced by others			
3. Indicates understanding or misunderstanding with verbal feedback			
Speaking skills			
A. Linguistic features			
1. Produces a variety of forms			
2. Uses some figurative language, slang			
3. Uses precise vocabulary			
4. Produces few mazes or false starts			
B. Paralinguistic features			
1. Inflection			
2. Pausing			
3. Rate			
4. Fluency			
5. Intelligibility			
C. Communicative functions			
1. Gives information			
2. Requests information			
3. Describes objects and events			
4. Expresses beliefs, intentions, or feelings			
5. Persuades listener to do, believe, or feel			
6. Solves problems with language			
D. Discourse management			
1. Initiates conversation			
2. Chooses topic			
3. Maintains topics			
4. Shifts topics			
5. Repairs or revises when necessary			
6. Yields floor			
7. Interrupts			
E. Conversational rules			
1. Manages quantity (does not talk too much or too little)			
2. Makes sincere comments			
3. Makes relevant comments			
4. Expresses thoughts clearly and concisely			
5. Uses tact, politeness			
F. Nonverbal behaviors			
1. Makes gestures and facial expressions			
2. Makes eye contact and holds gaze			
3. Maintains proximity			

Figure 5.8. A worksheet for adolescent conversational analysis. (*Source:* Larsen & McKinley, 2003.)

- Requesting repairs in the context of ongoing conversation (e.g., "What kind of music was it?") to look for responsiveness, adjustment to listener needs, and appropriateness of repair strategies

- Inserting sources of communication breakdown (e.g., "Can you get me the scissors?" when no scissors are available) to look for assertiveness, ability to monitor the interaction, and requests for clarification

Narrative and Expository Language   Farmer (2000) proposed that as communication skills mature, speakers move from simply participating in conversation to using narration and exposition. Narration and exposition require strong receptive and expressive language skills and increasingly take written form over verbal as the child progresses through his or her education.

Narration involves recounting an event or an experience. A true-life event may be recounted or a fictionalized story may be told. More complex narration describes a series of events, which may take the form of a plot. In narration, the narrator plays a role in the story itself (*Narration*, n.d.). The narrator may speak (or write) as a participant, that is, as if from within the story, or as an observer of the story. Consider how children's storybooks describe events. There is a main character who is part of the story or who has seen the events of the story occur. Consider, also, how certain subject matter is taught to children in school. Narration is used to make the material accessible to children and easier to understand. In a history class, for example, the story of the *Mayflower* may be told from the perspective of a girl who was on board. A science experiment is recorded in student diaries and then students talk about what they observed and learned. Mastery of oral and written narrative forms is critical to school success.

Expository language is used to deliver and explain information. The speaker (or writer) must describe, illustrate, and interpret information so that a listener (or reader) can comprehend the information. In complex exposition, the speaker or writer provides an orderly, sequential, factual report, which might be quite lengthy.

Informal written language might be as simple as an e-mail, text, tweet, chat, instant message, or Facebook update. A narration might read, "I forgot my sunscreen and got burned at the pool today. Ouch!" (Given the code of conduct for social media, though, many variants in spelling are likely. Written conversation is yet to be fully explored in the language literature since the advent of the Internet and texting. This area may be particularly difficult for older children with language disorders—and for older adults as well!—given the "shorthand" versions of written conversation often seen in electronic communications.)

An exposition might read, "The White Sox have taken first place from the Indians!" Gillam (1999) and Larson and McKinley (2003) suggested that for older students, clinicians should sample oral and written narrative and expository language because these forms are critical to successful communication in and out of school. These more demanding, literate uses of language may reveal weaknesses not seen in ordinary conversation (Scott & Windsor, 2000; Westby, 2005). In fact, face-to-face conversation may not be the most important communication medium for adolescents. Today's youth rely on virtual reality in order to participate socially and academically (Bauerlein, 2009; Berg, 2011; Lenhart,

2012; Tuttle, 2010). Given that written narration and exposition are the sum and substance of online social networking, adolescents need to master these forms of expression in order to enjoy social success. Because so much subject matter is accessed online and has interactive features, teachers expect students to be able to use online communication tools to participate in academic assignments.

A variety of methods are available for analyzing narratives and determining whether clients' narrative skills are age-appropriate. High-point analysis explores how well speakers organize their narratives into episodes (Labov & Waletzky, 1967). Applebee (1978) proposed that children develop the ability to structure their narratives as they advance through six successive phases where the logical and temporal nature of story structure becomes refined. Story grammar analysis (Stein & Glenn, 1979) examines whether a speaker uses traditional elements of narration, such as characters, plot, and setting. Other methods are found in Bliss, McCabe, and Miranda (1998); Gillam and Pearson (2004); Hedberg and Westby (1993); Hughes, McGillivray, and Schmidek (1997); Larson and McKinley (2003); McCabe and Peterson (1991); McCabe and Rollins (1994); Nelson and Van Meter (2007); and Strong (1998).

Larson and McKinley (2003) recommended that clinicians obtain two narrative samples: a reformulation task, in which the client retells a story; and a formulated task, in which the client relates a personal experience. If clients' narratives are less mature than would be expected for grade level, intervention can be aimed at advancing both the understanding and production of narrative.

Guidance on collecting and analyzing expository oral and written language samples can be found in Paul and Norbury (2012), Scott (2005), Scott and Stokes (1995), and Westby (2005). Clinicians may also use the rubrics and scoring instruments that are available to teachers. Although these are not diagnostic tools, they provide a point of reference for what is expected for grade level. These tools can be obtained from English and language arts teachers, from district or state offices on student assessment, or online from many commercial and noncommercial sources.

Language Sampling in Adults with Acquired Language Disorders

Adults who acquire a language disorder through certain injuries or illnesses are said to have aphasia. Forms of aphasia, which most frequently arise due to a stroke, can affect the ability to understand words and sentences, to retrieve words, and to formulate sentences. Some forms of aphasia can even hamper the ability to imitate the language spoken by another person. Clinicians also treat adults with **cognitive-communication disorders** that occur due to traumatic brain injuries, strokes, or illnesses. In a cognitive-communicative disorder, individuals have difficulty using thought to regulate their use of language. They may have difficulty communicating because of confusion, memory disturbances, disorganized thinking, poor reasoning, or other difficulties. Clinicians sample language produced by adults with aphasia and cognitive-communicative deficits for the same reasons that they sample child language: to examine the functional use of language in real communicative situations and to supplement standardized evaluation procedures with information from more naturalistic assessments. Clinicians ascertain a baseline level of functioning so that they can then note progress toward recovery.

Acquired language disorders often present with concomitant disruption of speech production. These disruptions may make assessment of language more difficult. Motor speech disorders commonly found alongside aphasia are discussed later in this chapter.

 **BOX**   **Collecting the Sample**

Shadden (1998) and Doyle et al. (2000) suggested several contexts for eliciting language samples from adults:

- Engaging in interactive conversation about a familiar topic.
- Describing a picture of a common scene, such as people watching television in a living room; of a well-known picture, such as a Norman Rockwell painting; or of a commonly used clinical stimulus, such as the "cookie theft" picture from the Boston Diagnostic Aphasia Test (Goodglass & Kaplan, 1983), or "Broken Window," a series of four pictures depicting a storyline in which a boy breaks a window with a ball. Here, the patient is instructed to tell the story starting with the first picture and proceeding through the last picture.
- Retelling a story heard verbally.
- Generating a story from a set of pictures, often based on familiar stories such as "Cinderella." In this protocol, the patient is asked to look through a short picture book about Cinderella. The clinician then removes the book and asks the patient to tell the story.
- Listing procedures involved in a familiar event in daily living, such as shopping in a grocery store or making a peanut butter and jelly sandwich.

Shadden (1998) and Liles and Coelho (1998) emphasized the importance of collecting samples that involve different sorts of communication tasks and/or that involve more than one context or setting. Sampling a client more than once using different conversational probes can reveal the client's ability to deal with differing levels of difficulty in discourse situations. Just as when sampling child language, clinicians want to be sure that adult samples are valid representations of communicative ability.

Recording and Transcribing the Sample   Most of the recording and transcription conventions used for younger clients are appropriate for transcribing adult language as well. T-unit segmentation is often used for the same reasons that it is used with younger populations. Likewise, the same computer-assisted procedures, such as the SALT, CLAN, and Computerized Profiling programs, can be used to analyze adult discourse, but the developmental normative comparisons are disregarded. The AphasiaBank database established in CHILDES provides transcription conventions and some standard analyses appropriate for discourse samples of adults with acquired language disorders (MacWhinney, 2012a). It is a great resource for sampling discourse in aphasia and related disorders.

Analyzing the Sample In analyzing language samples produced by adults with aphasia, clinicians look for disruptions in well-learned language processes, such as naming items and formulating sentences. Clinicians also note situations when frustration occurs due to the client's inability to find the words or forms to express the intentions that he or she has in mind.

Phonological errors include unintended nonword responses that share some of the phonemes composing the target word and would be understood by a naïve listener as a substitution for the target word, with phonemic errors not arising from articulatory deficits secondary to **apraxia of speech** or **dysarthria of speech.**

Syntax According to Shadden (1998), adult language analysis includes 1) sentence length; 2) syntactic complexity, diversity, and completeness; and 3) use of morphological forms. In analyzing adult language, SLPs can apply some of the same procedures of analysis that were discussed for school-age children and teens, including MLU per T-unit and percentage of complex sentences. Shadden (1998) suggested some additional analyses that can be helpful for adults:

- Words/clause: total number of words divided by total number of clauses

- Clauses/T-unit: total number of clauses (both independent and subordinate) divided by total number of T-units

- Percentage of 1-, 2-, and 3+-clause sentences

All these analyses can be used as baseline measures for monitoring progress during the course of a therapy program designed to increase syntactic complexity.

As an index of syntactic accuracy and completeness, Shadden (1998) suggested assigning each T-unit a plus (+) if it is fully grammatical and a minus (−) if it contains errors. Errors could include

- Verb-marking errors (e.g., errors in use of bound morphemes or suffixes, or omission of bound morphemes or suffixes)

- Obligatory word omissions

- Additions of extra elements (e.g., repetitions or circumlocutions)

- Incomplete forms (e.g., partial sentences or partial words)

- Morphological errors

- Pronoun errors

- Word order errors

A clinician can then calculate the percentage of syntactically accurate and complete T-units and compare this percentage across discourse tasks. Repeated sampling can be used during a course of intervention to track the client's production of these types of errors.

Semantics A similar plus-or-minus procedure can be used to assess semantic accuracy and completeness, with minus scores given for such errors as these:

- Empty or vague word use

- Given/new information errors

- Neologisms or paraphasias

- Inaccurate information

- Ambiguous or low-content information

- Inappropriate word use

- Incompleteness

- Lack of semantic diversity and accuracy

- Real words used incorrectly, in contexts where the target word shares an association or feature with the error word

Semantic analysis for adult clients concerns the amount, efficiency, conciseness, accuracy, and completeness of the information that the client can convey. A semantic analysis involves determining how well a client uses words meaningfully and readily.

Semantics is an important component of successful discourse. Shadden (1998) suggested that many adults with acquired language and cognitive-communicative disorders have specific difficulty with the **informativeness** of their discourse; that is, they have difficulty using words to convey the appropriate amount of information. They may struggle to convey information of sufficient quality without producing irrelevancies, redundancies, off-topic interjections, or overly personalized content. Efficiency and conciseness may be problematic for these clients, who may produce discourse that is unfocused and prone to delay, errors, excessive detail, and effortful production. Several approaches have been developed to provide clinical analysis of these kinds of discourse problems.

Content unit analysis or *correct information unit analysis* (Capilouto, Wright, & Wagovich, 2005; Doyle, Tsironas, & Goda, 1996) involves developing a list of content units (relevant and expected words) that would apply to a particular stimulus, such as a picture of a scene from daily living. The clinician compares a client's response to that stimulus to a list of responses generated by the clinician or a panel of typical controls. The purpose is to determine whether the client produces content that would be considered typical and relevant. The clinician can document if the client does not generate information that would be considered relevant, correct, and meaningful. Content units can be derived for a variety of discourse tasks, including procedural descriptions such as "going shopping" or "eating in a restaurant." The number of content units included within a client's response can be tabulated along with the number of units (words) that are irrelevant, redundant, or inaccurate.

An example of a content unit analysis that might be developed for a picture description task (The Birthday Party picture; Nicholas & Brookshire, 1993) is provided. The Birthday Party picture appears in Figure 5.9. Figure 5.10 presents an analysis for the Birthday Party picture that represents a client's productions at two points in time. Capilouto et al. (2005) and Nicholas and Brookshire (1995) reported that a content unit analysis allows a clinician to look for increases in quantity of appropriate information and decreases in inappropriate utterances as indices of progress in therapy.

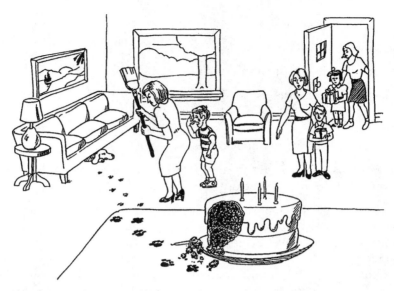

Figure 5.9. Sample picture used in content unit analysis. (From Nicholas, L., & Brookshire, R. [1993]. A system for quantifying the informativeness and efficiency of the connected speech of adults with aphasia. *Journal of Speech and Hearing Research, 36,* 346. © American Speech-Language-Hearing Association; reprinted by permission.)

Content units	Time 1	Time 2	Interpretive units	Time 1	Time 2
Woman	X	X	Mother	X	X
Standing with broom	X	X	Angry		X
Looking at dog	X	X	For stealing cake	X	X
Little boy	X	X	Birthday child		
Crying	X	X	Upset		X
Standing beside	X	X	About cake	X	X
Women and children	X	X	Guests and mothers		
Coming into living room	X	X	Surprised		X
With boxes	X	X	With birthday gifts		X
Dog	X	X	Afraid to come out	X	X
Under sofa	X	X	After eating cake		X
Left footprints	X	X	Ruined party		
TOTALS	12/12	12/12		4/12	9/12
Irrelevant/i ncorrect/ inaccurate units	3	1			

Figure 5.10. Content unit analysis for the birthday party picture. (*Sources:* Myers, 1979; Nicholas & Brookshire, 1993, 1995; Shadden, 1998; Ulatowska, Doyle, Freedman-Stern, Macaluso-Haynes, & North, 1983.)

BOX   **Content Unit Analysis Example**

Nicholas and Brookshire's Birthday Party Picture (1993), shown in Figure 5.9, would be analyzed in this way:

woman	little	women coming	dog
mother*	boy	in with children	under couch/sofa
standing (with broom)	crying	to living room	hiding*
	sad*	mothers*	afraid to come
looking (at dog)	standing beside	guests*	out*
angry*	mother*	carrying boxes	left footprints
for stealing cake	upset about	birthday gifts*	after eating cake*
	cake*	surprised*	ruined party*

Sources: Capilouto, Wright, and Wagovich (2005); Myers (1979); Nicholas and Brookshire (1993, 1995); and Shadden (1998).

*interpretative units

Informational content analysis is used to assess the efficiency of communication. Here, the ratio of meaningful to nonmeaningful units of information can be tracked across several discourse contexts as well as over time. Cheney and Canter (1993) provided data on normal ranges for this analysis. Figure 5.11 provides a sample worksheet for an information content analysis that can be used to examine production across several discourse tasks. **Verbosity,** or excessive talking, is often seen in acquired aphasias. Gold, Andres, Arbuckle, and Schwartzman (1988) suggested distinguishing two kinds of verbosity: *off-target verbosity* or irrelevant speech, where clients speak about topics not relevant to the current topic; and *digressive speech*, where clients remain on topic but say too much about it. Verbosity can be measured in a variety of ways; these involve the following:

- Calculating the number of information units per minute (Yorkston & Beukelman, 1980)

- Calculating number of words per story or discourse unit (Gleason et al., 1980)

- Calculating the number of content units in the first 50 words in a discourse task (Arbuckle, Gold, Frank, & Motard, 1989)

Pragmatic Analysis   As in the assessment of older children and teens, clinicians assess the pragmatic aspects of adults' conversation and narrative. In some cases, particularly for adults who would like to return to work, clinicians will assess the client's pragmatic skills during exposition. To analyze conversation, formats used for younger clients, such as Prutting and Kirchner's Pragmatic Protocol (1983) and Larson and McKinley's Conversational Analysis (2003), can be used. Halper, Cherney, Burns, and Mogil (1996) developed a rating scale specifically for assessing adult communication skills. An adaptation of this form appears in Figure 5.12.

Student name: _____ Date of birth: _____

Teacher: _____ Grade: _____

Clinician: _____ Date of examination: _____

School: _____ Sampling context: _____

Task/sample date	Meaningful units		Nonmeaningful units				Efficiency (number of meaningful/nonmeaningful)
	Essential	Elaborations	Irrelevant	Redundant	Inacurate	Off-topic	
Cookie theft picture description Date:							
How to make scrambled eggs procedure description Date:							
Story retelling Date:							
Conversion Date:							
Normal range (from Cheney & Canter, 1993)	40%–78%	10%–33%	7%–38%	0%–6%	0%–1%	0%	4%–14%

Figure 5.11. Sample worksheet for information content analysis. (*Source:* Shadden, 1998.)

	1 Markedly abnormal	2 Limited or inconsistent	3 Appropriate most of the time	4 Consistently appropriate
Nonverbal communication				
Intonation				
Facial expression				
Eye contact				
Gestures				
Proxemics				
Verbal communication				
Conversational initiation				
Turn-taking				
Topic maintenance				
Referencing				
Response length				
Repair and revision				
Quantity of information				

Figure 5.12.   A rating scale for adult conversational skills. (*Source:* Halper, Cherney, Burns, & Mogil, 1996.)

For narrative and expository analyses, many of the tools used to assess older children and teens can be used with adult clients (Biddle, McCabe, & Bliss, 1996; Coelho & Flewellen, 2003). Assessments may include story retelling or story generation, with or without picture supports. In a pragmatics assessment, clinicians are less focused on the content of the story (as during a semantic analysis) and more concerned with the pragmatic elements of storytelling, that is, how well the speaker communicates a purposeful, logical, coherent, and contextually appropriate message. Doyle and colleagues (2000) showed that a wide variety of productive language variables, including measures of language form, content, and use, can be reliably measured using a story-retelling procedure with adult clients. Hughes and colleagues (1997) outlined several narrative assessments designed for school-age clients that can be used effectively with adults.

One analysis that can help clinicians assess adult pragmatics during conversation, narration, and exposition is the analysis of **cohesive ties,** that is, how the client uses words to mark the structural connections among the parts of a text (Halliday & Hasan, 1976). Liles and Coelho (1998) identified a set of linguistic markers of cohesion, which includes examples of words that link one sentence to the next. For example, if a client says, "I ate breakfast *but* I did not like *it*," *but* is the cohesive conjunction that provides the link between the two ideas in this sentence, and *it* is a cohesive pronoun that is substituted for the noun *breakfast*. Figure 5.13 presents a summary of the cohesive ties identified by Liles and Coelho (1998).

Cohesive market type	Examples	Cohesive element in client discourse (word)	Found in T-unit number;	Cohesive adequacy		
				Complete	Incomplete	Error
Reference						
Personal	He, she, mine, it					
Demonstrative	This, that, these, those					
Conjunction						
Casual	Because, to that end, otherwise					
Adversative	Yet, although instead, but					
Temporal	Then, afterward, subsequently					
Additive	Likewise, furthermore, incidently					
Lexical						
Reiteration						
• repetition	I have a house on the beach. It is a tiny house.					
• synonym	He's a good boy. One of the finest lads...					
• superordinate	You can have the carrot. I don't like vegetables.					
• general word	I gave john the money. The doofus lost it					
Collacation	I'll get the doctor. You look sick.					
Ellipsis						
Nominal	What do you want to drink? Coke					
Verbal	Who's coming to the store? We are.					
Clausal	Has he done it all? He has.					
Substitution						
Nominal	I need a coat. Would you get me one?					
Verbal	I don't know how to fix this, and I don't think you do either.					
clausal	They won, didn't they? Unfortunately not.					

Figure 5.13.   A worksheet for assessing cohesive adequacy. (*Source:* Liles & Coelho, 1998.)

Table 5.3.   Ratings of coherence in narrative

Rating	Global coherence[a]	Local coherence[b]
1	Unrelated	No relation to content of previous utterance
2	Utterance contains more than one clause; one clause relates to the general topic, but the other clause does not	Utterance contains more than one clause; one clause relates to the previous utterance, but the other clause does not
3	Utterance possibly relates to the general topic, but the topic must be inferred; topic is evaluated without substantive information	Utterance relates to the previous utterance, but has a shift in focus or is vague or ambiguous to the point that the relation to the previous utterance must be inferred
4	Utterance contains more than one clause; one clause relates directly to the general topic, but the other clause relates indirectly	Utterance contains more than one clause; one clause relates directly to the previous utterance, but the other clause may not
5	Utterance provides substantive information that relates to the general topic	The topic of the previous utterance is continued by elaboration, sequencing, examples, or maintaining characters, events, or focus

Source: Coelho and Flewellen (2003).

[a]Relationship of content or meaning of the utterance to overall content of the story.
[b]Relationship of content or meaning of the utterance to previous utterance.

Clinicians can use this form to assess the cohesive adequacy of adult discourse samples.

To provide even more detail, cohesive markers within discourse samples can be rated as complete, incomplete, or erroneous, as shown here:

Complete: Information referred to by the tie is easily found and defined without ambiguity.

Example: Alice was hungry. She ate some cake.

Incomplete: Information referred to by the tie is not provided in the text.

Example: James walked home from school. He saw them at the bus stop.

Erroneous: The tie guides a listener to ambiguous information.

Example: Tom and Dick were at the video arcade. He had lots of quarters.

A second pragmatic analysis that can be used with adult conversation, narration, and exposition involves scoring the sample for **coherence.** Coherence relates to how well a discourse event hangs together. Discourse that coheres flows logically and smoothly. *Local coherence* shows that one sentence follows the next in a reasonable order. *Global coherence* describes how each utterance contributes to the overall point of a discourse. Coelho and Flewellen (2003) developed a rating system, summarized in Table 5.3, which can be used to examine coherence in oral or written language. LaPointe (2004) and Spreen and Risser (2003) discussed additional communication sampling techniques for adults with acquired language disorders.

SPEECH SAMPLING

Very often, the same sampling protocols for eliciting language can be used to elicit speech samples. Further, many language samples can also be analyzed with speech production as the clinician's analysis goal. When analyzing a sample for speech production, clinicians attend to the following areas: articulation, intelligibility, fluency, prosody, voice quality, and resonance. The examination of speech sampling here follows the same three developmental periods (preschool, school-age, and adult) used earlier, in the language sampling portion of this chapter.

Preschool Speech Sampling

Speech sampling with the preschool child often focuses on achieving seven goals: 1) determining the number of articulation errors as well as any patterns in these errors; 2) providing a description of the child's sound inventory; 3) determining **intelligibility,** or the total number of correctly articulated sounds or words in a sample; 4) determining the child's **stimulability** for speech sound productions or the child's ability to more closely approximate correct production of error sound(s); 5) determining screening voice, fluency, and resonance; 6) determining baseline speech performance in a naturalistic context for later comparison during and after treatment; and 7) planning treatment that focuses on the child's identified strengths and weaknesses in a variety of communicative contexts.

Collecting the Sample   Approximately 30% of children who experience a delay in the development of speech sound production also experience impairment in one or more language domains (Shriberg, Tomblin, & McSweeney, 1999). Communication sampling is a means to use the same sample to assess both speech and language domains. Therefore, there may not be any need to collect separate samples for language analysis versus speech analysis. Although the focus here is on assessment of articulation and phonology, it is important to be aware that preschool-age children may also present with aberrant voice quality, dysfluent speech behaviors, and/or inappropriate nasal resonance. These latter three areas are discussed further in the school-age and adult speech communication sampling sections later in this chapter. Communication sampling procedures are similar for voice, fluency, and resonance no matter the client's age.

Recording and Transcribing the Sample   One aspect to recording and transcribing a speech sample versus a language sample is that many aspects of the speech signal require high-quality recording equipment. Most of the time, this high-quality recording equipment is not necessary for communication sampling in the articulation and phonology realm. Whatever sampling context the clinician may choose (narrative retell, conversation, or picture description), he or she should audio record the child's sample so that it can be analyzed at a later time.

For articulation and phonology assessment in the preschool child, perceptual evaluation, rather than instrumental or computer-assisted acoustic analysis, will suffice for a valid and reliable assessment. The perceptual skills to identify sound error types do require that the new preservice clinician practice listening to speech sound errors and be able to explain these errors so that other professionals and family members will understand the child's speech production difficulties. The accepted way to do this is through use of the International Phonetic Alphabet (IPA). Because phonetic transcription may be more time consuming for the new clinician than orthographic transcription, it has been suggested that a 100-word portion of the speech sample be chosen to phonetically transcribe using the IPA and diacritical markers (Grunwell, 1985). Frequently used diacritical markers can be found in Table 5.4.

Table 5.4.   Commonly used diacritical markers

Symbol	Description	Example
[ˌ]	Syllabic consonant	[r ɪ ʔ n̩] for "written"
[ʔ]	Glottal stop	[r ɪ ʔ n̩] for "written"
[w]	An /r/ production that is similar to /w/	[wɛd] for "red"
[ʰ]	Aspirated release of stop	[pʰ æ t⁼] for "pat"
[⁼]	Unaspirated release of stop	[pʰ æ t⁼] for "pat"
[˜]	Nasalized (this is sometimes due to coarticulation, especially for vowels)	[m ĩ n] for "mean"
[˜]	Denasalized	[n˜ɪ r] for "near" (may occur in Korean-accented English and is perceived as a stop to English ears
[˜]	Audible nasal emission	[s̃ ɪ s t ɚ] for "sister"
[·]	Short prolongation	[mer· bɪ] for "maybe"
[:]	Longer prolongation	[aʊːtʃ] for "ouch"
[ˌ]	Partial voicing	[sɪk] for "sick"
[₀]	Partial devoicing	[bɔɪz̥] for "boys"
[ ]	Dentalization	[s̪ ɪ s̪ t ɚ] for "sister"
[ ]	Lateralization	[s̴ e ɪ] for "say"

For very young children, speech intelligibility, especially for an unfamiliar listener, is often reduced. It is extremely difficult to assess speech production when the clinician does not understand what the child is intending to say. Activities that include talk about objects known to the clinician, such as toys in the environment or a sequence of familiar events (e.g., getting dressed) may aid the clinician in ascertaining the child's intended target word(s).

Analyzing the Sample   For the purpose of *identifying error patterns*, there are a variety of published methods that can be used to structure the coding and analysis of phonological errors. Some examples of formal articulation and phonology tests are listed in Table 5.5. Typically, these published methods are extensions of the basic phonemic contrasts of *place of articulation, manner of articulation,* and *voicing.* In addition, children, particularly those with phonological disorders, will still use methods of simplifying adultlike speech. These simplifications, called *phonological processes,* are a normal part of development and begin at a very early age. Yet, at the preschool age, children should be using very few, if any, phonological processes to simplify the motor act of producing running speech. Roberts, Burchinal, and Footo (1990) outlined the frequency of use of both common and uncommon phonological processes in a group of normally developing children ages 2½ to 8. These authors concluded that use of phonological processes after the age of 4 is rare for the typically developing child. Further, use of "uncommon phonological processes" after the age of 2½ may be a sign of phonological delay or impairment. Table 5.6 lists both common and uncommon phonological processes, provides an example of each, and lists the age at which Roberts et al. reported use of the phonological process less than 20% of the time in a normally developing sample.

Table 5.5. Examples of procedures for assessing sound errors and patterns

Test	Ages
Assessment of Phonological Processes–Revised (APP-R; Hodson, 2004)	3-0 to 12-0 years
Arizona Articulation Proficiency Scale–Third Edition (Arizona–3; Fudala, 2001)	1-6 to 18 years
Bankson-Bernthal Test of Phonology (BBTOP; Bankson & Bernthal, 1990)	3 to 9 years
Contextual Test of Articulation (CTA; Aase et al., 2000)	4-0 to 9-11 years
Goldman-Fristoe Test of Articulation–Second Edition (GFTA-2; Goldman & Fristoe, 2000)	2-0 to 21-0 years
Khan-Lewis Phonological Analysis, Second Edition (KLPA-2; Khan & Lewis, 2002)	2-0 to 5-11 years
Natural Process Analysis (NPA; Shriberg & Kwiatkowski, 1980)	2 years to adult
Photo Articulation Test–Third Edition (PAT–3; Lippke, Dickey, Selmer, & Soder, 1997)	5 to 10 years

[a]Ages are expressed in years and months with a hyphen dividing the two (e.g., 3-0 means 3 years, 0 months old).

In order to *assess the content of a child's sound inventory*, or the overall number of consonants a child can say (a measure of phonological maturity), the clinician can collect a **phonetic inventory**, a list of all the sounds the child produces in a sample of speech. Smit, Hand, Freilinger, Bernthal, and Bird (1990) reported norms for acquisition of consonants from 997 children between 3 and 9 years of age. The results of their research are presented as a clinical worksheet in Table 5.7. Clinicians may use this worksheet to build a consonant inventory by circling each consonant the child correctly produces. At the same time, the clinician may judge whether the child is following a typical pattern of speech sound acquisition by referring to the ages listed in the worksheet. Although the ages listed provide an idea of where the preschool child may be expected to be in terms of speech sound acquisition, the ages presented are not inflexible categories. Instead, they guide

Table 5.6. Common and uncommon phonological processes

Common process	Example	Age of cessation[a]	Uncommon process	Example	Age of cessation
Cluster reduction	[tap] for "stop"	4 years	Deletion of initial consonant	[ɔg] for "dog"	2.5 years
Deletion of final consonant	[kæ] for "cat"	2.5 years	Deletion of medial consonant	[peɪ ɚ] for "paper"	2.5 years
Reduplication	[wawa] for "water"	2.5 years	Addition of a unit	[bak təl] for "bottle"	2.5 years
Syllable deletion	[ba] for "bottle"	2.5 years	Metathesis	[pə skɛ dɪ] for "spaghetti"	2.5 years
Liquid gliding	[jɛ joʊ] for "yellow"	3 years	Backing	[gɔg]ˈ for "dog"	2.5 years
Fronting	[tet] for "cake"	2.5 years	Deaffrication	[ʃɛr] for "chair"	2.5 years
Stopping	[teɪ] for "say"	2.5 years	Apicalization	[tɔɪ] for "boy"	2.5 years
Assimilation	[gɔg] for "dog"	2.5 years	Labialization	[bɔɪ] for "toy"	2.5 years

Source: Roberts, Burchinal, and Footo (1990).

Note: [a]"Age of cessation" refers to Roberts, Burchinal, and Footo's report of phonological process use less then 20% of the time.

[b]If the child does not otherwise produce the /d/.

Table 5.7. Worksheet depicting ages of phoneme acquisition at 90% accuracy reported by sex

Age range	Males	Females
3-0 to 3-11	/m/, /n/, /h/, /w-/, /p/, /b/, /t/, /d/,/k/, /f-/	/m/, /n/, /h/, /w/, /p/, /b/, /d/, /k/, /g/, /f-/
4-0 to 4-11	/g/	/j-/, /t/, /ð-/, /tw/, /kw/
5-0 to 5-11	/j-/, /-f/, /v/, /tw/, /kw/	/-f/, /v/, /l/, /pl/, /bl/, /kl/, /gl/, /fl/
6-0 to 6-11	/l/, /pl/, /bl/, /kl/, /gl/, /fl/	/θ/, /ʃ/, /tʃ/, /dʒ/, /-l/
7-0 to 7-11	/-ŋ/*, /ð-/, /s/*, /z/*, /ʃ/, /tʃ/, /dʒ/, /-l/, /sp/*, /st/*, /sk/*, /sm/*, /sn/*, /sw/*, /sl/*, /skw/*, /spl/*, /spr/*, /str/*, /skr/*	/-ŋ/*, /s/*, /z/*,/sp/*, /st/*, /sk/*, /sm/*, /sn/*, /sw/*, /sl/*, /skw/*, /spl/*, /spr/*, /str/*, /skr/*
8-0 to 9-0	/-ŋ/*, /θ/, /s/*, /z/*, /r/, /-ɚ/, /sp/*, /st/*, /sk/*, /sm/*, /sn/*, /sw/*, /sl/*, /pr/, /br/, /tr/, /dr/, /kr/, /gr/, /fr/, /ɚr/, /skw/*, /spl/*, /spr/*, /str/*, /skr/*	/-ŋ/*,/s/*, /z/*, /r/, /-ɚ/, /sp/*, /st/*, /sk/*, /sm/*, /sn/*, /sw/*, /sl/*, /pr/, /br/, /tr/, /dr/, /kr/, /gr/, /fr/, /ɚr/, /skw/*, /spl/*, /spr/*, /str/*, /skr/*

Source: Smit, Hand, Freilinger, Bernthal, and Bird (1990).

Note: Ages depicted in years and months. The asterisk indicates a lack of mastery of phonemes or consonant clusters at the 90% criterion. Therefore, those sounds and combinations were reported from age 7-0 to age 9-0. However, clinicians should not wait until 9-0 to consider these sounds underdeveloped.

the clinician's thinking about the child's speech sound development. For example, if a 5-year-old child is not producing a sound that Smit et al. (1990) found to be mastered by age 3, the clinician has grounds to believe that this is not normal development. But, if the child is age 4½ and is not producing a sound typically mastered by 4-year-olds, the clinician should take a wider view and consider the natural variability that exists in the human species. Not every person will fall square-and-center into the norms.

To assess **intelligibility,** it is necessary to look at the number of consonant errors in relation to the total number of consonants produced. Traditionally, clinicians have used subjective judgments (i.e., overall educated guesses) of intelligibility. There are, however, more objective measurements that lead to quantifiable results, some of which take no longer than the collection of the sample.

To assess overall intelligibility of a speech sample using the word as the unit of analysis, the clinician transcribes the sample of at least 100 words and uses an X for any word that is unintelligible. The clinician then divides the number of unintelligible words by 100 (or the number of words produced in the sample if there are more than 100 words) and then multiplies that number by 100 to get an overall intelligibility percentage for the sample at the word level. This procedure does not require phonetic or phonemic transcription and can be performed "online" during collection of the speech sample. This overall intelligibility percentage is a gross measure of intelligibility, which does not give the clinician information about the types of errors causing decreased intelligibility.

A more detailed analysis of intelligibility at the phoneme level, percent consonants correct (PCC), was described by Shriberg and Kwiatkowski (1980). To calculate PCC, the clinician phonemically transcribes a 100-word speech sample using the IPA. For each consonant the child produces, the clinician provides a **gloss,** or the child's intended phoneme. For example, the child may say "wed." The clinician then transcribes this production phonemically with the IPA (/wɛd/) and then provides the gloss ("red" /rɛd/). To calculate the PCC, the clinician counts the total number of consonants that agree with their gloss and divides this by the total number of consonants that were glossed in the sample. The resultant number is multiplied by 100 to produce the PCC. The same type of measurement can be made for the 17 vowels and diphthongs in American English by substituting vowels and diphthongs correctly produced and vowels and diphthongs attempted (or glossed) for consonants in the PCC formula. In other words,

$$\frac{Total\ number\ of\ correctly\ produced\ consonants}{Total\ number\ of\ consonants\ attempted} \times 100 = PCC$$

but

$$\frac{Total\ number\ of\ correctly\ produced\ \frac{vowels}{diphthongs}}{Total\ number\ of\ \frac{vowels}{diphthongs}\ attempted} \times 100 = PVC$$

By deriving intelligibility ratings using PCC, one is comparing how many consonants were correctly produced in relation to how many should have been produced correctly. Most clinicians will likely focus on consonants rather than vowels because vowels are rarely distorted, substituted, or omitted after the age of 2½ (Shriberg, Austin, Lewis, McSweeney, & Wilson, 1997). It is also important to note, however, that relying on a PCC score for a child who produces all the consonants correctly might be misleading if the child produces only a few consonants. Therefore, it is necessary to use the PCC (or PVC) score in conjunction with the phonetic inventory and published developmental guidelines for speech sound acquisition to make a better informed decision regarding the child's speech development.

In addition to assessing a child's phonetic inventory, speech sound error patterns, and overall intelligibility, a clinician may wish to test a child's **stimulability** for error sounds. Sounds that were noted as a distortion, substitution, or omission in the transcript should be presented to the child by the clinician. To present the sound, the clinician produces the sound in isolation and asks the child to pay attention to how the clinician produces the sound with the mouth. The child is then asked to produce the target sound. If the child succeeds, stimulability at the phoneme level is established. This process is then repeated at the word level. If the child does not succeed, the clinician may cue the child visually or in a tactile manner. If the child succeeds using this cueing, stimulability with cueing for the target phoneme is established. If the child does not succeed in production of the target, the child is characterized as not stimulable for the target. Stimulability is an important part of the assessment process because it will guide treatment planning. In general, a clinician will target those sounds for which the child is stimulable first in treatment.

Screening for voice, fluency, and resonance can be accomplished during the collection of the speech sample or during analysis of articulation and phonology at a later time. (The methods one may use to screen these speech parameters are described later in this chapter under the school-age and adult sections.) The initial speech sample collected may serve as a baseline for documenting treatment progress in a naturalistic communication context. Standardized (norm-referenced) tests are useful for comparing one child to a group of other children with similar characteristics. Thus, standardized testing is very useful in comparing children to other like children as well as for determining to what extent any delay may be present (though this is not necessarily true for clients from linguistically diverse backgrounds). Standardized testing is not helpful, however, to document progress in therapy. Instead, communication sampling is the ideal choice.

School-Age Speech Sampling

When sampling speech communication in the school-age child, clinicians generally have goals similar to those outlined for the preschool period. School-age children may have persistent errors in articulation and phonology that are sampled and analyzed using the same methods one would use for the preschool child. During the school-age years, however, other difficulties with speech communication may become the salient features of problematic speech behavior. Specifically, disruption of the smooth flow of speech, or **dysfluency,** may occur. Further, as school-age children's language skills develop toward maturity, their longer utterances may better lend themselves to being analyzed with regard to the prosody of the speech sample, or the variation of intonation in the utterance for linguistic purposes. Prosodic variation can also, however, be analyzed with very short utterances.

Fluency   Two disorder types generally fall under developmental disorders of fluency: **stuttering** and **cluttering.** Van Zaalen, Wijnen, and De Jonckere (2009) cited multiple authors as differentiating stuttering and cluttering behaviors. These authors explain stuttering as "a disorder characterized by a high frequency of involuntary interruptions of the forward flow of speech, regarded by the person who stutters (PWS) as 'stutters,' which are often accompanied by a feeling of loss of control" (Van Zaalen et al., 2009, p. 138). On the other hand, they described cluttering as being "characterized by three main features: (1) a rapid and/or irregular articulatory rate; (2) a higher than average frequency of disfluencies, dissimilar to those seen in stuttering; and (3) reduced intelligibility due to exaggerated coarticulation ... and indistinct articulation" (2009, p. 138).

While stuttering and cluttering are considered different disorders, one assesses them in similar ways. A speech sample taken in multiple contexts and sometimes over several days is usually recommended, given the variability of dysfluent behaviors depending on the communication context as well as other factors, such as level of fatigue.

Collecting the Sample   In general, collection of a speech sample for fluency analysis is similar to collecting a sample for articulation analysis. However, in this case collecting more than one speech sample in various contexts is especially important, because context influences fluency so highly. For the school-age child, a conversational speech sample with a familiar communication partner (e.g., school friend) as well as an educationally relevant sample (e.g., giving a presentation in front of a small group of peers) may suffice. No matter which contexts are chosen for the samples, the goal is to analyze any changes in fluency based on communication context. No ideal length for a speech sample is reported in the literature. Myers (1986) reported using a 10-minute mother–child interaction as a basis for assessment of child fluency, whereas Ambrose and Yairi (1999) advocated eliciting a 1,000-syllable sample. How talkative a child is may be the most important factor in whether the clinician chooses to time a sample or to attempt to elicit a specified number of syllables to analyze.

Recording and Transcribing the Sample   Recording of the speech sample may be best accomplished using video recording rather than audio recording. One of the hallmarks of stuttering behavior is the addition of **secondary dysfluency behaviors,** which may consist of extraneous movements of the face or other body parts in addition to other behaviors, such as avoidance of certain sounds or speaking situations (Guitar, 2005). The clinician who does not have access to a video camera can, alternatively, audio record the sample and take written notes on any secondary behaviors identified during elicitation of the sample.

Transcribing the speech sample for fluency analysis does not require the clinician to phonetically or phonemically transcribe the speech sample. Instead, English-language spelling (orthography) may be used and any repetitions spelled out using the orthographic spellings. For example, a part-word repetition with three repetitions of the initial consonant in *cat* would be recorded as *c-c-c-cat*. Similarly, prolongation of sounds may also be spelled out and a note in the transcript logged regarding length of the prolongation. For example, a 2-second prolongation of the vowel in a word may be transcribed as *booook* (2 s). When transcribing the sample, it is important to note any interjections (such as *um* or *uh*) or pauses (as well as the length of the pause) in the transcript. All speech behavior should be transcribed, including any type of false start or revision (i.e., **maze behavior**).

Analyzing the Sample   Analysis of the speech sample for fluency should include a calculation of the number of different dysfluencies and number of repetitions for each dysfluency, as well as provide some measure of the percent dysfluencies of each type. It should also include speech rate, note any articulation errors, and probe stimulability. Ambrose and Yairi (1999) outlined a method for classifying dysfluency type and severity for young children (ages 2–5). The Ambrose and Yairi classification of dysfluency type and severity was used to create Figure 5.14. Once the speech sample is transcribed, the clinician may use Figure 5.14 as a guide in counting dysfluencies of different types as well as calculating a weighted score to compare to Ambrose and Yairi's reported norms. To use the worksheet, the number of occurrences for each dysfluency type should be logged into the chart. For part-word and single-syllable word repetitions, the number of repetitions should be counted. For example, if a child said, "b-b-b-b-baby," four repetitions would be logged for one occurrence of a part-word repetition. Also, if more than one dysfluency type occurs in a single word, each is counted separately.

Initial counting of each dysfluency type should be done on another piece of paper and final calculations performed on a copy of Figure 5.14. Using the formulas on the worksheet, the total number of Stuttering-Like Dysfluencies per 100 syllables may be calculated. In addition, a weighted score for Stuttering-Like

Dysfluency type	Example	Number of occurrences	Number of repetitions
Stuttering-like dysfluencies (SLD)			
• Part-word repetitions	"t- t- t- to"		
• Single-syllable-word repetitions	"to to to"		
• Dysrhythmic phonation			
• Prolongations	"booook"		
• Blocks	"#cat"		
• Broken words	"a#bout"		
Other dysfluencies (OD)			
• Interjections	"um"		
• Revision, abandoned utterances	"She screamed/ yelled."		
• Multisyllabic or phrase repetitions	"She said she said hi."		

Figure 5.14. Worksheet to record dysfluency type and frequency using Ambrose and Yairi (1999) classification.

Dysfluencies can be calculated. A general guide to interpretation of the results is also given at the bottom of the worksheet. It should be noted, however, that the norms reported are only for children between 2 and 5 years of age. Yet, the same type of information derived from the worksheet will be helpful in describing the fluency of a client no matter the age. If the clinician is in doubt, a norm-referenced, formal assessment of fluency may be used (e.g., Stuttering Severity Instrument–3; Riley, 1994).

Percent Dysfluencies of Each Type To calculate the percentage of occurrence of each dysfluency type, the clinician should use the completed worksheet (Figure 5.14). The process requires the clinician to add the number of occurrences of each of the dysfluencies listed in the worksheet. This is the total number of dysfluencies in the sample. Then, for each dysfluency type, the clinician must divide the number of occurrences for the individual dysfluency type by the total number of dysfluencies in the sample. For example, if there were 30 total dysfluencies (of all types) noted in the transcript and 10 of those were prolongations, the clinician would perform the operation 10 ÷ 30, which equals 0.33 or 33%. So, the clinician would record that 33% of the client's dysfluencies were of the prolongation type. Ambrose and Yairi (1999) reported that the number of Stuttering-Like Dysfluencies (SLD) is typically 65% or higher of the total number of dysfluency occurrences for children who stutter while the proportion of Other Dysfluencies (OD) is usually less than 35%.

Speech Rate Calculation of speech rate is particularly important when analyzing the speech behaviors of people with dysfluent speech. Speech rate may also help the clinician differentiate cluttering from stuttering (although they can co-occur). The clinician may want to calculate a speech rate that excludes dysfluencies and/or the rate of speech including dysfluencies. To calculate speech rate with dysfluencies, the clinician should count the total number of syllables produced in the entire speech sample and then divide that by the number of seconds the client took to produce the whole sample. This calculation will yield the number of syllables produced per second, including dysfluencies.

Clinicians interested in calculating speech rate exclusive of dysfluencies can follow the procedure recommended by Van Zaalen and colleagues (2009) by calculating the mean articulatory rate (MAR). To calculate the MAR, a stopwatch is necessary. The clinician will determine the average of five speech rate measures from 10 consecutive fluent syllables produced in the transcript. For example, the clinician will locate five areas in the transcript where 10 consecutive syllables are fluently produced. Each of these areas is then timed with a stopwatch in terms of how many seconds it took for the client to produce these 10 syllables. Then, the next identified string of 10 syllables is timed in the same way. When all five of the 10-syllable strings have been timed, these values are added together and divided by 5. This calculation will yield an estimate of the client's speech rate (in syllables per second), excluding moments of dysfluency.

Articulation Errors Articulation errors are often noted in clients who clutter (St. Louis, Myers, Faragasso, Townsend, & Gallaher, 2004). Therefore, it is important to note any errors in articulation when analyzing the speech sample transcript. The worksheet provided in Table 5.7 in the articulation and phonology section of this chapter may be used to note any of these types of errors.

Stimulability Last, the clinician may wish to assess a dysfluent client's stimulability for fluent speech. To do so, the clinician often uses the same techniques one would use in the treatment of a fluency disorder, such as asking the client to produce prolonged speech, gentle onset or airflow, reduced speech rate, or reduced articulatory effort (Shipley & McAfee, 2009). The client's responses to each of these techniques is recorded to note the level of success the client has with fluency using the chosen technique. Information about the client's stimulability for fluent speech will help guide treatment planning as well as aid in making prognostic statements about the client's likelihood of speech behavior change.

Prosody *Segmental features* of speech usually refer to the production of individual phonemes and syllables in an utterance. However, *suprasegmental features* of speech refer to changes in pitch, loudness, and duration of syllabics to communicate other information about the intended message. Shriberg et al. (2001) characterized prosody as the changing of suprasegmental features for grammatical, pragmatic, and affective purposes. *Grammatical prosody* includes syllable stress for syntactic differentiation as well as rising or falling pitch at the end of utterances to differentiate questions and statements. For example, a child may say the one-word utterance "Milk." If the child uses rising pitch during production of the word, it is likely the child is asking a question, such as "Can I have some milk?" Alternatively, grammatical prosody serves to indicate whether a word is used as a noun or a verb. For example, if a client says *CONflict*, the word is a noun. Yet, if the client says *conFLICT*, the word is a verb. Grammatical prosody is usually a required element to speech so that the listener fully understands the grammatical functions of the uttered words.

Pragmatic prosody (emphatic stress) is somewhat different than grammatical prosody, although both are produced by changes in pitch, loudness, and duration. Pragmatic prosody serves to alert the listener to a desired portion of an utterance by giving that part of the utterance prominence compared to other portions. For example, if a child says, "*He* did it," the child is giving prominence to the pronoun *he* and possibly clarifying that another child completed an act. Alternatively, if the child says, "he *did* it," the child gives prominence to the verb and is possibly drawing attention to the fact that another child has already completed some action.

Affective prosody is a more global type of prosody in that it may be used to reflect the speaker's mood or reflect speech patterns with different listeners. For example, a school-age child may raise his or her pitch when speaking to a baby. On the other hand, a child may increase the loudness of speech to signal excitement or surprise.

Clinical populations in which a clinician may wish to analyze a client's prosodic variation include individuals with autism, neurological insults, or hearing impairment, as well as client populations who wish to undergo treatment for accent modification. These populations are made up of children and adults; yet, all procedures for collecting, recording, transcribing, and analyzing the speech sample will be the same no matter the client's age. Obviously, clients with severe disorders that minimize verbal output would not be likely candidates for analysis of prosodic variation.

Collecting the Sample   Communication sampling for prosodic analysis may be accomplished through conversation elicitation, narrative retell, or spontaneous narrative. For maximal opportunity to vary prosody across grammatical, pragmatic, and affective purposes, a conversational sample is more likely to provide the clinician with more information than narratives. Conversations are more likely to consist of various utterance types (declaratives, interrogatives, and imperatives) than a narrative.

Recording and Transcribing the Sample   When recording the speech sample for prosodic analysis, it is important to ascertain that the background noise is reduced as much as possible. Since small fluctuations in pitch, intensity, and duration will be the units of analysis, background noise can be troublesome. In terms of transcription, it is not necessary to phonetically transcribe a speech sample when prosody is the main concern. If, however, the clinician is interested in articulation and phonology analysis, the same phonetically transcribed sample can be used to describe the child's prosodic characteristics across the sample.

Analyzing the Sample   Analysis of a transcribed speech sample for prosody requires the use of *pitch contours*, or a line drawn on the speech sample transcript that depicts the rising and falling pitch at the syllable and/or word level. Analysis of grammatical prosody requires the use of pitch contours at the syllable level and analysis of pragmatic prosody at the word level. Further, rising and falling intonation at the utterance level may be depicted on the transcript after the utterance as [↗] for rising intonation (for instance, with questions) or [↘] for falling intonation. Longer vowel durations (also a sign of prosodic variation) may be transcribed by inserting [:] after the vowel that was prolonged. Finally, loudness may also indicate prosodic variation. However, the IPA does not provide a set of transcription

Utterance Type	Phonetic Transcription	Orthographic Transcription
Interrogative	[hu wəʒʃi]	Who was SHE?
Imperative	[gɪv mi ðæt˥]	GIVE me that!
Declarative	[aɪ noʊ ɪt˥ wəʒ hɪm]	I KNOW it was him.

Figure 5.15. Sample transcriptions in which pitch contours have been added.

aids for variation in loudness. These may be handwritten on the transcript if the clinician feels too much or lack of variation of loudness is contributing to a client's communication difficulty (as in cases of neurological impairment that may cause sudden increases in vocal loudness). Figure 5.15 depicts sample transcriptions in which pitch contours have been added.

There are no established norms for determining whether a client's prosodic variation is within typical limits. Instead, the clinician uses his or her trained ear and subjective judgment as to whether the client's prosody variation (or lack thereof) draws undue or negative attention to itself. Speech sample analysis for prosody will give the clinician data on the client's ability to produce prosodic variation for various linguistic reasons. Still, it tells the clinician nothing of a client's ability to interpret prosodic variation in others. For this purpose, the clinician may wish to administer a structured test of a client's reception of prosody like the PEPS-C (Peppé & McCann, 2003).

Speech Sampling in Adults

Typically, the clinician assessing an adult's communication will be working with a patient who has lost some level of communicative function rather than with a person who has yet to develop a certain level of communicative function. Most often, but not always, adult communication assessments will occur due to some type of neurological damage that causes impairment in the adult's communication abilities. In terms of speech behavior, the adult's communication difficulties will stem from problems with respiration, phonation, articulation, and/or resonance.

Motor Speech Disorders   Dysarthria of speech is a "speech production deficit that results from neuromotor damage to the peripheral or central nervous system" (Freed, 2012, p. 50). On the other hand, apraxia of speech is a disorder in which the affected person is unable to correctly sequence the string of motor commands necessary to correctly produce speech. Unlike dysarthria of speech, apraxia of speech is not characterized by muscle weakness; like dysarthria, however, it can affect all the speech subsystems (i.e., respiration, phonation, articulation, resonation). Apraxia of speech and dysarthria of speech can co-occur.

A complete assessment of an adult with a suspected speech disorder will include a formal oral-motor examination as well as communication sampling. (For detailed information about oral-motor examination, see Chapter 4.) Often, oral-motor assessments and formal articulation tests give the clinician a lot of information about the impairment of each speech subsystem; yet, they give the clinician no idea of how the client's communication function is affected by the presence of a disorder. To ascertain this functioning, communication sampling is necessary.

Collecting the Sample Collecting a speech sample from an adult is not extremely different from collecting communication samples from school-age children. The sample may be collected during conversation, narration, or oral reading. If an adult is literate and does not have a concomitant language disorder that negatively affects his or her reading ability, asking the adult to read a passage orally has several advantages. First, a reading passage can function as a constant in assessment that can be used to measure progress in any subsequent treatment. Also, a reading passage may take some of the social pressure off a client if he or she is not familiar enough with the clinician to participate at great length in a conversation sample. On the other hand, oral reading samples can be used as a comparison to natural conversation and/or formal tests of articulation in order to better understand the client's communication in different contexts. An example of a reading passage often used clinically is "The Rainbow Passage" (Fairbanks, 1960, p. 127).

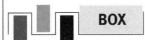 **BOX**   **The Rainbow Passage**

When the sunlight strikes raindrops in the air, they act like a prism and form a rainbow. The rainbow is a division of white light into many beautiful colors. These take the shape of a long round arch, with its path high above, and its two ends apparently beyond the horizon. There is, according to legend, a boiling pot of gold at one end. People look, but no one ever finds it. When a man looks for something beyond his reach, his friends say he is looking for the pot of gold at the end of the rainbow.

Throughout the centuries men have explained the rainbow in various ways. Some have accepted it as a miracle without physical explanation. To the Hebrews it was a token that there would be no more universal floods. The Greeks used to imagine that it was a sign from the gods to foretell war or heavy rain. The Norsemen considered the rainbow as a bridge over which the gods passed from earth to their home in the sky. Other men have tried to explain the phenomenon physically. Aristotle thought that the rainbow was caused by reflections of the sun's rays by the rain. Since then physicists have found that it is not reflection but refraction by the raindrops that causes the rainbow. Many complicated ideas about the rainbow have been formed. The difference in the rainbow depends considerably upon the size of the water drops, and the width of the colored band increases as the size of the drops increases. The actual primary rainbow observed is said to be the effect of superpositioning of a number of bows. If the red of the second bow falls on the green of the first, the result is to give a bow with an abnormally wide yellow band, since red and green lights when mixed form yellow. This is a very common type of bow, one showing mainly red and yellow, with little or no green or blue.

Source: From Fairbanks, G. (1960). *Voice and articulation drillbook.* New York, NY: Harper & Row; reprinted by permission.

Recording the Sample   The speech sample collected for analysis of an adult's speech communication may be audio or video recorded using standard audio and video recording equipment. Video recording offers the advantage of observing any extraneous movements or oral groping behaviors. Some clinical settings have instrumentation geared toward acoustic analysis of speech production, such as the KayPentax Computerized Speech Lab (CSL). In order to perform acoustic analysis of the adult client's speech, high-quality recordings in very quiet environments are necessary. Luckily, as technology advances, creation of high-quality recordings for acoustic analysis is possible with a computer with a high-quality sound card. Also, acoustic analysis software, such as Praat (Boersma & Weenink, 2012), is free and downloadable from the Internet, although it requires some practice to master for clinical purposes. Although acoustic analysis of the speech sample yields quantifiable, objective results, perceptual evaluation of the adult's speech behavior will suffice in most clinical contexts.

Analyzing the Sample   Perceptual analysis of the speech sample requires the clinician's judgments about the appropriateness of the client's respiration for speech, vocal quality, and articulatory precision, as well as resonance. All the procedures outlined in the articulation and phonology section of this chapter may be

Question	Answer	Degree
1. Are vowels and consonants produced clearly?	☐ Yes ☐ No	
2. Is the patient's rate of speech too slow? Or is it too fast?	☐ Yes ☐ No	
3. Does the patient show inappropriate silent intervals between words?	☐ Yes ☐ No	
4. Does the patient show hypernasality?	☐ Yes ☐ No	
5. Is nasal emission present?	☐ Yes ☐ No	
6. Does the patient vary loudness normally?	☐ Yes ☐ No	
7. If not, is there evidence of monoloudness?	☐ Yes ☐ No	
8. Is there evidence of tremor in the patient's voice?	☐ Yes ☐ No	
9. Does the patient show abnormal pitch variations?	☐ Yes ☐ No	
10. Does the patient's voice have a harsh vocal quality?	☐ Yes ☐ No	
11. Does the patient's voice have a strained-strangled vocal quality?	☐ Yes ☐ No	
12. Does the patient's voice have a breathy vocal quality?	☐ Yes ☐ No	
13. Does the patient speak in abnormally short phrases?	☐ Yes ☐ No	
14. Are there moments of involuntary inhalation or exhalation?	☐ Yes ☐ No	
15. Is inhalatory stridor present?	☐ Yes ☐ No	
16. Does the patient use normal stress on the appropriate syllables or words?	☐ Yes ☐ No	
17. If not, is there a reduction in normal stress?	☐ Yes ☐ No	
18. Or is there excess and equal stress?	☐ Yes ☐ No	

Figure 5.16. Questions the clinician should ask him- or himself when analyzing an adult speech sample. (From Freed, D. *Motor speech disorders*, 2E. © 2012 Delmar Learning, a part of Cengage Learning, Inc. Reproduced by permission. http://www.cengage.com/permissions)

applied to the adult speech sample as well. In addition, Figure 5.16 is a worksheet from Freed (2012) with a list of questions clinicians may ask themselves while analyzing the adult speech sample.

Resonance   Disorders of resonance in the adult are often due to neurological damage affecting the velopharyngeal apparatus or anatomical injuries resulting from trauma, such as a car accident. It is possible, however, that an adult with a history of cleft lip or palate (repaired or unrepaired) may seek services for inappropriate resonance. Evaluation of resonance may take place through clinical procedures such as counting or purposefully occluding the nares (i.e., holding one's nose) during production of phrases with and without nasal consonants. Yet, in the realm of communication sampling, the goal of assessment is to identify how any difficulties with resonance may affect the client's speech intelligibility.

Typically, the clinician will listen to the client's speech sample for aspects of **hyponasality** (too little nasal resonance) or **hypernasality** (too much nasal resonance, which may be accompanied by audible nasal emission of air during nonnasal phoneme production). The clinician may choose to assess the extent to which inappropriate resonance renders the client's speech unintelligible. To do so, the clinician may use the same procedures described for determining intelligibility at the word level in the school-age speech sampling section of this chapter.

Voice Quality   Like any other speech subsystem, voice quality may be negatively affected due to neurological damage. It may also be hindered by functional or behavioral disorders. **Functional disorders** of the voice are those problems resulting in impaired vocal quality that are derived from how the client uses or misuses the voice and are not a result of neurological or anatomical change or damage resulting, for example, from a stroke or partial laryngectomy due to head or neck cancer. Functional voice disorders may occur due to a child's misuse of voice as much as an adult's overuse of the voice, such as might occur in careers with a high vocal demand (e.g., teaching, acting, singing).

Disorders of phonation are most often diagnosed and characterized as part of an interdisciplinary evaluation. An otolaryngologist (ENT) is a team member who should be consulted in almost all cases in which impaired vocal quality is established. Misuse of the voice as well as disease can cause damage to the vocal folds, resulting in nodules, polyps, or cysts. Speech-language clinicians regularly perform an endoscopic evaluation of the voice in many areas of the United States, in collaboration with medical professionals, who have the primary responsibility to diagnose medical conditions, such as laryngeal cancer. SLPs use **endoscopy** to help understand the source of voice disorders that affect communication.

In addition to visual assessment of vocal function (i.e., endoscopy), the clinician often performs acoustic analysis of the client's voice. Just as with acoustic analysis of a speech sample, high-quality audio recordings are necessary for acoustic analysis of the voice. The same type of recording equipment and software is used for acoustic analysis of both articulation and voice. In acoustic analysis of the voice, sustained phonation of vowels and other nondiscourse tasks (Baken & Orlikoff, 2000) are often used. Although promising approaches to acoustic analysis of the voice in running speech are being developed and researched (e.g., Cepstral Analysis; Watts & Awan, 2011), they require that practitioners have advanced training in speech and voice science as well as knowledge of computer programs and are thus outside the scope of this text.

Assessment of a client's voice with only sustained phonation may provide some information through acoustic analysis, but it is less helpful for assessing how the client uses his or her voice in various contexts as well as to what extent the voice disorder may hinder the client's real-world communication. To get a better idea of the client's vocal use or quality in his or her everyday life, communication sampling is necessary.

Collecting the Sample   Elicitation and collection of the speech sample for perceptual voice quality analysis does not require any special techniques other than those previously described in the section on communication sampling for assessment of motor speech disorders. Formal perceptual assessments of voice, such as the Consensus Auditory-Perceptual Evaluation of Voice (CAPE-V; Kempster, Gerratt, Verdolini-Abbott, Barkmeier-Kraemer, & Hillman, 2009), are available and also have a communication sampling component, in addition to the use of sustained vowels and oral reading of sentences.

Recording the Sample   If the clinician is analyzing the speech sample strictly from a perceptual standpoint, a high-quality audio recording will suffice. It is essential, however, that the recording environment be close to free from background noise to provide the clinician with as clear a recording as possible. If the clinician suspects vocal misuse or other functional disorders as the culprit for impaired voice quality, a video-recorded sample may be used for analyzing any visible muscular tension in the neck and/or difficulties with respiration for speech (rise and fall of the thorax).

Analyzing the Sample   Perceptual analysis of a communication sample for voice quality will require the clinician to carefully listen to the audio or video recording and note any periods of voice quality that are considered to be atypical or suggestive of impairment. Since the clinician is using his or her ear, it is necessary to have a core vocabulary to describe the client's vocal quality that is consistent across clinicians as well as other voice professionals. Developing a consistent core vocabulary has been a matter of considerable attention in the voice professions. Although acoustic analysis of the voice gives the clinician objective, quantitative data about vocal function, it does little to illuminate the client's strengths and weaknesses in phonation for communication in various contexts. To help more easily standardize the vocabulary voice clinicians use, Kempster and colleagues (2009, p. 127) outlined six quality voice features that have appeared in the literature on perceptual voice assessment:

1.   *Overall severity:* global, integrated impression of voice deviance

2.   *Roughness:* perceived irregularity in the voicing source

3.   *Breathiness:* audible air escape in the voice

4.   *Strain:* perception of excessive vocal effort (hyperfunction)

5.   *Pitch:* perceptual correlate of fundamental frequency

6.   *Loudness:* perceptual correlate of sound intensity

Instructions: These are statements that many people have used to describe their voices and the effects of their voices on their lives. Circle the response that indicates how frequently you have the same experience.

F1.   My voice makes it difficult for people to hear me.
P2.   I run out of air when I talk.
F3.   People have difficulty understanding me in a noisy room.
P4.   The sound of my voice varies throughout the day.
F5.   My family has difficulty hearing me when I call them throughout the house.
F6.   I use the phone less often than I would like.
E7.   I'm tense when talking with others because of my voice.
F8.   I tend to avoid groups of people because of my voice.
E9.   People seem irritated with my voice.
P10.   People ask, "What's wrong with your voice?"
F11.   I speak with friends, neighbors, or relatives less often because of my voice.
F12.   People ask me to repeat myself when speaking face-to-face.
P13.   My voice sounds creaky and dry.
P14.   I feel as though I have to strain to produce my voice.
E15.   I find other people don't understand my voice problem.
F16.   My voice difficulties restrict my personal and social life.
P17.   The clarity of my voice is unpredictable.
P18.   I try to change my voice to sound different.
F19.   I feel left out of conversations because of my voice.
P20.   I use a great deal of effort to speak.
P21.   My voice is worse in the evening.
F22.   My voice problem causes me to lose income.
E23.   My voice problem upsets me.
E24.   I am less outgoing because of my voice problem.
E25.   My voice makes me feel handicapped.
P26.   My voice "gives out" on me in the middle of speaking.
E27.   I feel annoyed when people ask me to repeat.
E28.   I feel embarrassed when people ask me to repeat.
E29.   My voice makes me feel incompetent.
E30.   I'm ashamed of my voice problem.

Figure 5.17. Voice Handicap Index, Henry Ford Hospital. Note that the letter that precedes each item number corresponds to the subscale (E, emotional subscale; F, functional subscale; P, physical subscale). (From Jacobson, B.H., Johnson, A., Grywalski, C., Silbergleit, A., Jacobson, G., Benninger, M.S., et al. [1997]. The voice handicap index [VHI]: Development and validation. *American Journal of Speech-Language Pathology, 6*[3], 66–70; reprinted by permission. Copyright 1997 by American Speech-Language-Hearing Association. All rights reserved.)

To perceptually assess the client's speech sample, the clinician may use these six categories of perceptual voice assessment to describe any difficulties noted in the client's speech sample.

As additional information, the clinician may wish to use a functional measure of vocal use such as the Voice Handicap Index (VHI; Jacobson et al., 1997). Figure 5.17 details the VHI. Although communication sampling should take place in as many contexts or environments as feasible, it is unlikely that a clinician will be able to sample a client's communication in every type of context in which the client usually operates. Functional measures, such as the VHI, will give the clinician an idea of the client's self-reported vocal function in many areas not typically assessed in a clinical setting.

CONCLUSIONS

Communication sampling is the gold standard for determining to what extent, if at all, a client's impairment negatively affects his or her functioning in the real world. Use of communication sampling should be a part of every client's assessment and treatment plans if for no other reason than to document a client's progress in therapy and how that progress positively affects the client's functioning in life. Communication sampling is possible for very young children as well as with the elderly across all areas of communication. The knowledge and skills required to competently assess a client's communicative functioning in his or her life require development over a period of professional practice, yet they provide the backbone of client-centered speech and language services.

STUDY QUESTIONS

1. Why is communication sampling an important part of assessment?
2. What are the specific questions an assessment of nonverbal communication attempts to answer?
3. What types of devices can a clinician use to video record samples? What must a clinician do prior to recording to make sure that the recording will be successful?
4. What sampling contexts are appropriate for preschoolers? School-age children? Adults?
5. What are the advantages and disadvantages of computer-assisted analysis methods? Of manual methods?
6. How are utterances segmented in transcription of preschool language samples? School-age samples? Adult samples?
7. In addition to looking at syntax, what other areas need to be examined in communication samples of adults with acquired language disorders?
8. Discuss two methods for assessing speech intelligibility in children and adults.
9. Discuss the difference between cluttering and stuttering. How might analysis methods differ between the two? Why is this distinction important?
10. Discuss how communication sampling may be used in conjunction with formal tests of communication performance (standardized tests).
11. How are voice quality, resonance, and prosody typically assessed using communication sampling? How are these methods different from instrumental assessments of these areas?

REFERENCES

Aase, D., Hovre, C., Krause, K., Schelfhout, S., Smith, J., & Carpenter, L. (2000). *Contextual Test of Articulation*. Eau Claire, WI: Thinking Publications.

Ambrose, N.G., & Yairi, E. (1999). Normative disfluency data for early childhood stuttering. *Journal of Speech, Language, and Hearing Research, 42,* 895–909.

American Speech-Language-Hearing Association (ASHA). (n.d.). *Working with culturally and linguistically diverse (CLD) students in schools*. Retrieved from http://www.asha.org/slp/CLDinSchools

American Speech-Language-Hearing Association (ASHA). (2010). *Cultural Competence Checklist: Service Delivery*. Retrieved from http://www.asha.org/uploadedFiles/Cultural-Competence-Checklist-Service-Delivery.pdf#search=%22cld%22

American Speech-Language-Hearing Association. (2011). *Cultural competence in professional service delivery* [Professional issues statement]. Retrieved from http://www.asha.org/docs/html/PI2011-00326.html

Anderson, N. (2009, November). *Addressing appropriate diagnosis & educational disparities for CLD students*. Paper presented at the American Speech-Language-Hearing Association Annual Convention, New Orleans, LA.

Applebee, A. (1978). *The child's concept of a story: Ages 2 to 17*. Chicago, IL: University of Chicago Press.

Arbuckle, T., Gold, D., Frank, I., & Motard, D. (1989, November). *Speech of verbose older adults: How is it different?* Paper presented at the Gerontological Society of America, Minneapolis, MN.

Baken, R.J., & Orlikoff, R.F. (2000). *Clinical measurement of speech and voice* (2nd ed.). Clifton Park, NY: Delmar Learning.

Bankson, N.W., & Bernthal, J.E. (1990). *Bankson-Bernthal Test of Phonology*. San Antonio, TX: Special Press.

Bar-Adon, A., & Leopold, W. (1971). *Child language: A book of readings*. Upper Saddle River, NJ: Prentice-Hall.

Bauerlein, M. (2009, September 4). *Why Gen-Y Johnny can't read nonverbal cues*. Retrieved from the *Wall Street Journal* web site, http://online.wsj.com/article/SB10001424052970203863204574348493483201758.html#printMode

Berg, M.A. (2011). On the cusp of cyberspace: Adolescents' online text use in conversation. *Journal of Adolescent & Adult Literacy, 54*, 485–493. doi:10.1598/JAAL.54.7.2

Beukelman, D.R., & Mirenda, P. (2013). *Augmentative and alternative communication: Supporting children and adults with complex communication needs* (4th ed.). Baltimore, MD: Paul H. Brookes Publishing Co.

Biddle, K., McCabe, A., & Bliss, L.S. (1996). Narrative skills following traumatic brain injury in children and adults. *Journal of Communication Disorders, 29*(6), 447–469.

Bliss, L.S., McCabe, A., & Miranda, A.E. (1998). Narrative assessment profile: Discourse analysis for school-age children. *Journal of Communication Disorders, 31*(4), 347–363.

Boersma, P., & Weenink, D. (2012). Praat: Doing phonetics by computer (Version 5.3.04) [Computer software]. Retrieved from http://www.praat.org

Botting, N. (2002). Narrative as a tool for the assessment of linguistic and pragmatic impairments. *Child Language Teaching and Therapy, 18*(1), 1–21.

Brinton, B., & Fujiki, M. (2004). *Conversational management with language impaired children: Pragmatic assessment and intervention*. San Antonio, TX: PRO-ED.

Brown, R. (1973). *A first language, the early stages*. Cambridge, MA: Harvard University Press.

Buzolich, M.J. (2006). Augmentative and alternative communication (AAC) assessment: Adult aphasia. *Perspectives on Neurophysiology and Neurogenic Speech and Language Disorders, 16*(4), 4–12.

Calculator, S. (1997). Fostering early language acquisition and AAC use: Exploring reciprocal influences between children and their environments. *Augmentative and Alternative Communication, 13*, 149–157.

Capilouto, G., Wright, H., & Wagovich, S. (2005). CIU and main event analyses of the structured discourse of older and younger adults. *Journal of Communication Disorders, 38*, 431–444.

Chapman, R. (1978). Comprehension strategies in children. In J.F. Kavanaugh & W. Strange (Eds.), *Speech and language in the laboratory, school, and clinic* (pp. 308–327). Cambridge, MA: MIT Press.

Cheney, L., & Canter, G. (1993). Informational content in the discourse of patients with probably Alzheimer's disease and patients with right brain damage. *Clinical Aphasiology, 21*, 123–134.

Coelho, C., & Flewellen, L. (2003). Longitudinal assessment of coherence in an adult with fluent aphasia: A follow-up study. *Aphasiology, 17*, 173–182.

Costanza-Smith, A. (2010). The clinical utility of language samples. *Perspectives on Language Learning and Education, 17*(1), 9–15.

Craig, H., & Washington, J. (2002). Oral language expectations for African American preschoolers and kindergartners. *American Journal of Speech-Language Pathology, 11*, 59–70.

Crais, E.R. (2011). Testing and beyond: Strategies and tools for evaluating and assessing infants and toddlers. *Language, Speech, and Hearing Services in Schools, 42*(3), 341–364.

Crystal, D., Fletcher, P., & Garman, M. (1989). *Grammatical analysis of language disability* (2nd ed.). London, England: Cole & Whurr.

deVilliers, J., & deVilliers, P. (1973). A cross-sectional study of the acquisition of grammatical morphemes. *Journal of Psycholinguistic Research, 2,* 267–278.

Doyle, P., Goda, A., & Spencer, K. (1995). The communicative informativeness and efficiency of connected discourse by adults with aphasia under structures and conversational sampling conditions. *American Journal of Speech-Language Pathology, 4,* 130–134.

Doyle, P.J., McNeil, M.R., Park, G., Goda, A., Rubenstein, E., Spencer, K.A.,... Szwarc, L. (2000). Linguistic validation of four parallel forms of a story retelling procedure. *Aphasiology, 14,* 537–549.

Doyle J., Tsironas, D., & Goda, A. (1996). The relationship between objective measures and listeners' judgment of the communicative informativeness of the connected discourse of adults with aphasia. *American Journal of Speech-Language Pathology, 53,* 113–124.

Evans, J., & Craig, H. (1992). Language sample collection and analysis: Interview compared to freeplay assessment contexts. *Journal of Speech and Hearing Research, 35,* 343–353.

Fairbanks, G. (1960). Voice and articulation drillbook (2nd ed.). New York, NY: Harper & Row.

Farmer, S.F. (2000). *Coursebook: CSD 523 Assessment in Communication Disorders.* Las Cruces, NM: New Mexico State University.

Fey, M.E. (1986). *Language intervention with young children.* Boston, MA: College-Hill Press.

Fishman, I. (2011). Guidelines for teaching speech-language pathologists about the AAC assessment process. *Perspectives on Augmentative and Alternative Communication, 20*(3), 82–86.

Freed, D. (2012). *Motor speech disorders: Diagnosis and treatment* (2nd ed.). Clifton Park, NY: Delmar Learning.

Fudala, J.B. (2001). *Arizona Articulation Proficiency Scale* (3rd ed.). Los Angeles, CA: Western Psychological Services.

Gillam, R. (1999). Dynamic assessment of narrative and expository discourse. *Topics in Language Disorders, 20*(1), 33.

Gillam, R., & Pearson, N. (2004). *Test of Narrative Language.* Greenville, SC: Super-Duper Publications.

Gleason, J., Goodglass, H., Obler, L., Green, E., Hyde, M., & Weintraub, S. (1980).

Narrative strategies of aphasic and normal-speaking subjects. *Journal of Speech and Hearing Research, 23,* 370–382.

Gold, D., Andres, D., Arbuckle, T., & Schwartzman, A. (1988). Measurement and correlates of verbosity in older people. *Journal of Gerontology, 43,* 27–34.

Goldman, R., & Fristoe, M. (2000). *Goldman-Fristoe Test of Articulation–Second Edition* (GFTA-2). Circle Pines, MN: AGS Publishing.

Goodglass, H., & Kaplan, E. (1983). *The Boston Diagnostic Aphasia Examination.* Philadelphia, PA: Lea & Febinger.

Griffer, M.R., & Cheng, L. (2009, November). *Ourselves as diverse individuals: Implications for working with families.* Paper presented at the American Speech-Language-Hearing Association Annual Convention, New Orleans, LA.

Grunwell, P. (1985). *Phonological assessment of child speech.* San Diego, CA: College-Hill Press.

Guitar, B. (2005). *Stuttering: An integrated approach to its nature and treatment* (3rd ed.). New York, NY: Lippincott Williams & Wilkins.

Gummersall, D.M., & Strong, C.J. (1999). Assessment of complex sentence production in a narrative context. *Language, Speech, and Hearing Services in Schools, 30,* 152–164.

Halliday, M., & Hasan, R. (1976). *Cohesion in English.* New York, NY: Longman Publishers.

Halper, A., Cherney, L., Burns, M., & Mogil, S. (1996). *Clinical management of right hemisphere dysfunction* (2nd ed.). New York, NY: Aspen Publishers.

Hedberg, N., & Westby, C. (1993). *Analyzing storytelling skills: Theory to practice.* Tucson, AZ: Communication Skill Builders.

Hodson, B. (2004). *Hodson Assessment of Phonological Patterns* (3rd ed.). Austin, TX: PRO-ED.

Horton-Ikard, R. (2010). Language sample analysis with children who speak non-mainstream dialects of English. *Perspectives on Language Learning and Education, 17*(1), 16–23.

Hughes, D., McGillivray, L., & Schmidek, M. (1997). *Guide to narrative language: Procedures for assessment.* Eau Claire, WI: Thinking Publications.

Hunt, K. (1965). *Grammatical structures written at three grade levels* (Research Report No. 3). Urbana, IL: National Council of Teachers of English.

Jacobson, B.H., Johnson, A., Grywalski, C., Silbergleit, A., Jacobson, G., Benninger, M.S., & Newman, C.W. (1997). The Voice Handicap Index (VHI): Development and validation. *American Journal of Speech-Language Pathology, 6*(3), 66–70.

Justice, L.M., & Ezell, H.K. (2008). *The syntax handbook.* Austin, TX: PRO-ED.

Kempster, G.B., Gerratt, B.R., Verdolini-Abbott, K., Barkmeier-Kraemer, J., & Hillman, R.E. (2009). Consensus Auditory-Perceptual Evaluation of Voice: Development of a standardized clinical protocol. *American Journal of Speech-Language Pathology, 18,* 124–132.

Khan, L., & Lewis, N. (2002). *Khan-Lewis Phonological Analysis* (2nd ed.). Circle Pines, MN: AGS Publishing.

Labov, W., & Waletzky, J. (1967). Narrative analysis: Oral versions of personal experience. In J. Helm (Ed.), *Essays on verbal and visual arts* (pp. 12–44). Seattle, WA: University of Washington Press.

LaPointe, L.L. (2004). *Aphasia and related neurogenic language disorders.* New York, NY: Thieme New York.

Larson, V., & McKinley, N. (2003). *Communication solutions for older students: Assessment and intervention strategies.* Eau Claire, WI: Thinking Publications.

Lasker, J.P. (2009). *AAC language assessment: Specific considerations for adults with aphasia.* Paper presented at the American Speech-Language-Hearing Association Annual Convention, New Orleans, LA.

Leadholm, B., & Miller, J. (1992). *Language sample analysis: The Wisconsin guide.* Madison, WI: Wisconsin Department of Public Instruction.

Lee, L. (1974). *Developmental sentence analysis.* Evanston, IL: Northwestern University Press.

Lenhart, A. (2012, March 19). *Teens, smartphones, and texting.* Retrieved from the Pew Research Center web site, http://pewinternet.org/Reports/2012/Teens-and-smartphones.aspx

Liles, B., & Coelho, C. (1998). Cohesion analysis. In L. Cherney, B. Shadden, & C. Coelho (Eds.), *Analyzing discourse in communicatively impaired adults* (pp. 65–84). New York, NY: Aspen Publishers.

Lippke, B., Dickey, S., Selmar, J., & Soder, A. (1997). *Photo Articulation Test* (PAT-3). Austin, TX: PRO-ED.

Long, S. (2008). Computerized profiling (Version 9.7.0) [Computer software]. Retrieved from http://www.computerizedprofiling.org

Long, S., Fey, M., & Channell, R. (2000). Computerized profiling (Version 9.26) [Computer software]. Cleveland, OH: Case Western Reserve University.

Long, S., McKinley, N., Thormann, S., Jones, M., & Nockerts, A. (2005). *Language sample analysis II: The Wisconsin guide.* Madison, WI: Wisconsin Department of Public Instruction.

Lund, N., & Duchan, J. (1993). *Assessing children's language in naturalistic contexts* (3rd ed.). Upper Saddle River, NJ: Prentice Hall.

MacWhinney, B. (1996). The CHILDES system. *American Journal of Speech-Language Pathology, 5,* 5–14.

MacWhinney, B. (2000). *The CHILDES project: Tools for analyzing talk* (3rd ed.). Mahwah, NJ: Lawrence Erlbaum Associates.

MacWhinney, B. (2012a). *The Child Language Data Exchange System (CHILDES).* Retrieved from http://childes.psy.cmu.edu

MacWhinney, B. (2012b). *The CHILDES project: Tools for analyzing talk: Part 2. The CLAN programs* [Electronic edition]. Retrieved from http://childes.psy.cmu.edu/manuals/CLAN.pdf

McCabe, A., & Peterson, C. (1991). *Developing narrative structure.* Hillsdale, NJ: Lawrence Erlbaum Associates.

McCabe, A., & Rollins, P.R. (1994). Assessment of preschool narrative skills. *American Journal of Speech-Language Pathology, 3*(1), 45–56.

McLaughlin, K., & Cascella, P. (2008). Eliciting a distal gesture via dynamic assessment among students with moderate to severe intellectual disability. *Communication Disorders Quarterly, 29*(2), 75–81.

Merritt, D.D., & Liles, B.Z. (1989). Narrative analysis: Clinical applications of story generation and story retelling. *Journal of Speech and Hearing Disorders, 54,* 438–447.

Miller, J. (1981). *Assessing language production in children: Experimental procedures.* Boston, MA: Allyn & Bacon.

Miller, J., & Chapman, R. (2000). *SALT: Systematic analysis of language transcripts.* Madison, WI: Language Analysis Laboratory, Waisman Center, University of Wisconsin–Madison.

Miller, J., & Chapman, R. (2012). *SALT: Systematic analysis of language transcripts.*

Madison, WI: Language Analysis Laboratory, Waisman Center, University of Wisconsin–Madison. Retrieved June 4, 2012, from http://www.saltsoftware.com/resources-links/linksToSoftware.cfm

Miller, J., Freiberg, C., Rolland, M., & Reeves, M. (1992). Implementing computerized language sample analysis in the public school. *Topics in Language Disorders, 12*(2), 69–82.

Myers, P. (1979). Profiles of communications deficits in patients with right cerebral hemisphere damage. In R. Brookshire (Ed.), *Clinical aphasiology: Conference proceedings* (pp. 38–46). Minneapolis, MN: BRK.

Myers, S.C. (1986). Qualitative and quantitative differences and patterns of variability in disfluencies emitted by preschool stutterers and nonstutterers during dyadic conversations. *Journal of Fluency Disorders, 11,* 293–306.

Narration. (n.d.). Retrieved from http://www.cla.purdue.edu/english/theory/narratology/terms/narration.html

Nelson, N. (1998). *Childhood language disorders in context: Infancy through adolescence* (2nd ed.). Columbus, OH: Charles E. Merrill.

Nelson, N.W., & Van Meter, A.M. (2007). Measuring written language ability in narrative samples. *Reading & Writing Quarterly, 23*(3), 287–309.

Nicholas, L., & Brookshire, R. (1993). A system for quantifying the informativeness and efficiency of the connected speech of adults with aphasia. *Journal of Speech and Hearing Research, 36,* 338–350.

Nicholas, L., & Brookshire, R. (1995). Presence, completeness, and accuracy of main concepts in the connected speech of non-brain-damaged adults and adults with aphasia. *Journal of Speech and Hearing Research, 38,* 145–156.

O'Brien, M., & Nagle, K. (1987). Parents' speech to toddlers: The effect of play context. *Journal of Child Language, 14,* 269–279.

Ogletree, B.T., Fischer, M.A., & Turowski, B. (1996). Assessment targets and protocols for nonsymbolic communicators with profound disabilities. *Focus on Autism and Other Developmental Disabilities, 11*(1), 53–58.

Owens, R. (2004). *Language disorders* (4th ed.). Boston, MA: Allyn & Bacon.

Paul, R., & Norbury, C. (2012). *Language disorders from infancy through adolescence: Assessment and intervention* (4th ed.). St. Louis, MO: Mosby.

Peppé, S., & McCann, J. (2003). Assessing intonation and prosody in children with atypical language development: The PEPS-C Test and the revised version. *Clinical Linguistics and Phonetics, 17,* 345–354.

Plante, E., & Vance, R. (1994). Selection of preschool language tests: A data-based approach. *Language, Speech, and Hearing Services in Schools, 25,* 15–24.

Price, L.H., Hendricks, S., & Cook, C. (2010). Incorporating computer-aided language sample analysis into clinical practice. *Language, Speech, and Hearing Services in Schools, 41,* 206–222.

Proctor, L.A., & Oswalt, J. (2008). Augmentative and alternative communication: Assessment in the schools. *Perspectives on Augmentative and Alternative Communication, 17*(1), 13–19.

Prutting, C.A., & Kirchner, D. (1983). Applied pragmatics. In T.M. Gallagher & C.A. Prutting (Eds.), *Pragmatic assessment and intervention issues in language* (pp. 29–64). San Diego, CA: College-Hill Press.

Retherford, K. (2000). *Guide to analysis of language transcripts* (3rd ed.). Eau Claire, WI: Thinking Publications.

Riley, G. (1994). *Stuttering Severity Instrument* (3rd ed.). Austin, TX: PRO-ED.

Roberts, J.E., Burchinal, M., & Footo, M.M. (1990). Phonological processes decline from 2 ½ to 8 years. *Journal of Communication Disorders, 23*(3), 205–217.

Rojas, R., & Iglesias, A. (2009). Making a case for language sampling: Assessment and intervention with (Spanish-English) language learners. *The ASHA Leader, 14*(3), 10–13.

Rojas, R., & Iglesias, A. (2010). Using language sampling to measure language growth. *Perspectives on Language Learning and Education, 17*(1), 24–31.

Roth, F., & Spekman, N. (1984a). Assessing the pragmatic abilities of children: Part 1. Organizational framework and assessment parameters. *Journal of Speech and Hearing Disorders, 49,* 2–11.

Roth, F., & Spekman, N. (1984b). Assessing the pragmatic abilities of children: Part 2. Guidelines, considerations, and specific evaluation procedures. *Journal of Speech and Hearing Disorders, 49,* 12–17.

Scarborough, H. (1990). Index of productive syntax. *Applied Psycholinguistics, 11,* 1–22.

Scott, C. (2005). Learning to write. In H. Catts & A. Kamhi (Eds.), *Language and reading disabilities* (2nd ed., pp. 233–273). Boston, MA: Allyn & Bacon.

Scott, C., & Stokes, S. (1995). Measures of syntax in school-age children and adolescents. *Language, Speech, and Hearing Services in Schools, 26,* 309–317.

Scott, C., & Windsor, J. (2000). General language performance measures in spoken and written narrative and expository discourse of school-age children with language learning disabilities. *Journal of Speech, Language, and Hearing Research, 43,* 324–339.

Shadden, B. (1998). Sentential/surface level analyses. In L. Cherney, B. Shadden, & C. Coelho (Eds.), *Analyzing discourse in communicatively impaired adults* (pp. 35–64). New York, NY: Aspen Publishers.

Shipley, K.G., & McAfee, J.G. (2009). *Assessment in speech-language pathology: A resource manual* (4th ed.). Clifton Park, NY: Delmar Cengage Learning.

Shriberg, L.D., Austin, D., Lewis, B.A., McSweeney, J.L., & Wilson, D.L. (1997). The percentage of consonants correct (PCC) metric: Extensions and reliability data. *Journal of Speech-Language-Hearing Research, 40*(4), 708–722.

Shriberg, L., & Kwiatkowski, J. (1980). *Natural process analysis.* New York, NY: Macmillan/McGraw-Hill.

Shriberg, L., & Kwiatkowski, J. (1982). Phonological disorders III: A procedure for assessing severity of involvement. *Journal of Speech and Hearing Disorders, 47,* 256–270.

Shriberg, L., Paul, R., McSweeney, J., Klin, A., Cohen, D., & Volkmar, F. (2001). Speech and prosody characteristics of adolescents and adults with high functioning autism and Asperger syndrome. *Journal of Speech, Language and Hearing Research, 44,* 1097–1115.

Shriberg, L.D., Tomblin, J.B., & McSweeney, J.L. (1999). Prevalence of speech delay in 6-year-old children and comorbidity with language impairment. *Journal of Speech, Language, and Hearing Research, 42*(6), 1461–1481.

Smit, A.B., Hand, L., Freilinger, J.J., Bernthal, J.E., & Bird, A. (1990). The Iowa articulation norms project and its Nebraska replication. *Journal of Speech and Hearing Disorders, 55,* 779–798.

Spreen, O., & Risser, A. (2003). *Assessment in aphasia.* New York, NY: Oxford University Press.

St. Louis, K.O., Myers, F., Faragasso, K., Townsend, P.S., & Gallaher, A.J. (2004). Perceptual aspects of cluttered speech. *Journal of Fluency Disorders, 29,* 213–235.

Stein, N., & Glenn, C. (1979). An analysis of story comprehension in elementary school children. In R.O. Freedle (Ed.), *New directions in discourse comprehension* (Vol. 2, pp. 59–120). Norwood, NJ: Ablex.

Stockman, I. (1996). The promises and pitfalls of language sample analysis as an assessment tool for linguistic minority children. *Language, Speech, and Hearing Services in Schools, 27,* 355–366.

Strong, C. (1998). *Strong Narrative Assessment Procedure.* Eau Claire, WI: Thinking Publications.

Threats, T. T. (2009). Possible contributions of using the ICF in assessment. *Perspectives on Neurophysiology and Neurogenic Speech and Language Disorders, 19*(1), 7–14.

Tuttle, K. (2010). *I love you, now do your homework.* Retrieved from the Boston. Com web site, http://www.boston.com/community/moms/articles/2010/09/11/texting_can_distance_teens_from_parents_but_it_can_also_lead_to_better_communication

Tyack, D., & Gottsleben, R. (1974). *Language sampling, analysis, and training* (Rev. ed.). Palo Alto, CA: Consulting Psychologists Press.

Udvari, A., & Thousand, J. (1995). Promising practices that foster inclusive education. In R. Villa & J. Thousand (Eds.), *Creating an inclusive school.* Alexandria, VA: Association for Supervision and Curriculum Development.

Van Zaalen, Y.H., Wijnen, F., & De Jonckere, P.H. (2009). Differential diagnostic characteristics between cluttering and stuttering, Part One. *Journal of Fluency Disorders, 34,* 137–154.

Watts, C.R., & Awan, S.N. (2011). Use of spectral/cepstral analyses for differentiating normal from hypofunctional voices in sustained vowel and continuous speech contexts. *Journal of Speech, Language, and Hearing Research, 54,* 1525–1537.

Westby, C. (2005). Assessing and facilitating text comprehension problems. In H. Catts & A. Kahmi (Eds.), *Language and reading disabilities* (2nd ed., pp. 157–232). Boston, MA: Allyn & Bacon.

Wetherby, A.M., Allen, L., Cleary, J., Kublin, K., & Golldstein, H. (2002). Validity and reliability of the Communication and Symbolic Behavior Scales Developmental Profile with very young children. *Journal of Speech, Language, and Hearing Research, 45,* 1202–1218.

Wetherby, A.M., & Prizant, B.M. (2002). *Communication and Symbolic Behavior Scales: Developmental Profile.* Baltimore, MD: Paul H. Brookes Publishing Co.

World Health Organization. (2001). *International classification of functioning, disability and health.* Geneva: Author.

Yoder, P., & Davies, B. (1990). Do parental questions and topic continuations elicit replies from developmentally delayed children: A sequential analysis. *Journal of Speech and Hearing Research, 33,* 563–573.

Yorkston, K., & Beukelman, D. (1980). An analysis of connected speech samples of aphasic and normal speakers. *Journal of Speech and Hearing Disorders, 45,* 27–35.

CHAPTER **6**

Communication Intervention

Principles and Procedures

Froma Roth and Rhea Paul

CHAPTER OBJECTIVES

After reading this chapter, students will be able to

- Give three purposes for intervention
- State goals of intervention in behavioral terms
- Evaluate a range of intervention processes in light of the needs of particular clients
- Discuss where on the continuum of naturalness various intervention methods fall
- Explain the role of data collection in the intervention process

We would like to introduce you to some clients like those you may meet in your clinical practice:

1. Darrell, a preschooler with immature, unintelligible speech. Darrell's parents want him to improve his speech before he begins kindergarten next year.

2. Jonah, a 7-year-old with a severe bilateral sensorineural hearing loss. His school district referred him for reevaluation of his hearing, speech, and language and to determine whether his amplification equipment continues to be appropriate for him.

3. Anna, a seventh-grade student with significant learning disabilities.

4. Marlene, a 50-year-old woman with communication difficulty since her stroke 8 months ago.

5. Richard, aged 62, who recently underwent a total laryngectomy. He wants to use esophageal speech.

6. Thomas, a 27-year-old with a history of severe stuttering. Thomas feels that his speech disorder is interfering with his ability to advance in his career.

7. Mara, a 24-month-old toddler who attends a community-based social interaction program. Mara's grandparents, her primary caregivers, are concerned

that Mara is using only a very few words, although she "babbles a lot" and seems to understand what they say.

8. Leo, a 14-month-old baby was born deaf and received bilateral cochlear implants at age 12 months.

In the previous chapter we talked in some detail about assessment strategies for clients like these. Once the assessment is completed, though, a clinician is faced with implementing the recommendations made in the assessment. This phase of clinical practice is called *intervention*. The purpose of intervention is to effect change in communicative behavior in order to maximize an individual's potential to communicate effectively. The way we achieve this purpose varies according to the nature of the disorder, the age and therapy history of the client, the family situation, and the client's learning style and preferences. Whatever the methods of intervention are, though, intervention is designed to teach strategies for improving overall communication, rather than teaching specific behaviors. As such, all intervention involves the provision of *scaffolding* that varies along a continuum of type and intensity. Clinicians use these scaffolds to support the learning of a new skill or one that is beyond the client's current capacity. Scaffolds are gradually removed as the client demonstrates independent mastery of the target skill. Olswang and Bain (1991) discussed three basic purposes that intervention can serve:

1. In some cases, the purpose is to *eliminate the underlying cause* of the disorder. For example, the provision of amplification to a 9-month-old baby with a mild hearing impairment may prevent, or at least minimize, the emergence of developmental speech and language difficulties. For Jonah, audiological reevaluation might determine that his current speech and language difficulties are due to a change in hearing status that requires a change in amplification. In this case, the new intervention program, involving new hearing aids, may eliminate the underlying disorder.

2. In other cases, the purpose may be to teach a client *compensatory strategies* to improve functional communication. This purpose may be appropriate for Marlene, who needs to learn new ways to get her ideas across when her speech is unintelligible due to the motor neuron damage suffered during her stroke. Anna, too, may need to learn compensatory strategies to help her cope in the school setting. And Richard's desire to learn esophageal speech shows that he is eager to find a compensatory mechanism to allow him to communicate vocally despite the loss of his larynx.

3. A third purpose for intervention is to *modify the disorder* by teaching specific speech, language, or pragmatic behaviors that enable an individual to become a more effective communicator. Darrell, for example, may receive instruction on the correct production of his error sounds or sound classes to achieve improved speech production skills and better overall speech intelligibility. Thomas, the client with dysfluency, may not be able to entirely eliminate stuttering moments. If this is the case, he may need to learn to modify his stuttering so that it interferes less with his social communication.

There are a variety of approaches to planning intervention. The common thread among all these, however, is that communication intervention is a dynamic process that proceeds in a systematic progression. Following the diagnosis of a communication disorder, the clinician completes a detailed assessment of current strengths and needs and selects appropriate target behaviors for therapy. Intervention procedures are then developed and implemented to promote the acquisition of the target skills. The intervention process is completed when the client demonstrates mastery of these target behaviors. Periodic monitoring is often performed to ensure the retention and stability of the newly acquired behaviors (Roth & Worthington, 2011).

Essential to the selection of an intervention approach is the degree to which it is supported by the highest quality scientific research—in conjunction with the clinical expertise of a speech-language pathologist or audiologist and the values and perspectives of the client and the client's family (ASHA, http://www.asha.org/members/ebp; Sackett, Strauss, Richardson, Rosenberg, & Haynes, 2000; Schmitt & Justice, 2012). Using evidence-based practices (EBP) enables clinicians to critically appraise the available body of research as it applies to each client's needs, culture, and value system. Efficacy and effectiveness data are not currently available for all aspects of intervention or for all clinical populations. Still, it is the responsibility of the clinician to work within an EBP framework and approach intervention scientifically by providing specific rationales for intervention procedures and hypotheses about a client's responsiveness to those procedures. Of course, best practices change with evolving research and individual clinical experience, and so, EBP is best viewed as an ongoing, dynamic clinical decision-making process (Dollaghan, 2004). Schmitt, Fey, and Justice (Chapter 3) discuss ways clinicians can apply EBP to their daily activities.

Also essential is the provision of intervention services that adhere to the universal design for learning (UDL; Rose & Meyer, 2000). The UDL approach is based on three main principles:

1. Multiple means of representation (the "what" of learning): Various methods must be available to clients to access the targeted content, skills, or strategies (e.g., print textbooks, digital media, talk-to-text media).

2. Multiple means of expression (the "how" of learning): Several methods must be available for clients to express what they know (e.g., oral language, written expression, signs, gestures).

3. Multiple means of engagement (the "why" of learning): Clients must be provided with enough successful learning opportunities to maintain adequate motivation for learning.

When planning intervention, there are three aspects of a program that need to be considered: its products, processes, and contexts (McLean, 1998; Paul & Norbury, 2012). This chapter discusses the products and processes of intervention. The contexts, or the circumstances under which intervention takes place, are discussed in Chapter 10.

INTERVENTION PRODUCTS

The first step in planning intervention is the identification of the communicative behaviors to be acquired in the program. These are drawn from our assessment data and are usually called **long-term goals.** Long-term goals for a client are the relatively broad changes in communicative behavior to be achieved during a course of therapy. The achievement of these goals will be justification for terminating therapy.

For example, Marlene's stroke left her very limited in speech production, unable to verbalize her wants and needs, and depressed as a result of her frustration. Long-term goals for Marlene could include the following:

• Increasing the amount of intelligible speech

• Increasing her ability to communicate wants and needs

• Decreasing her frustration by providing alternative means of communication

Once general long-term goals have been identified, clinicians must decide how to help the client to progress toward them. This is accomplished by formulating the steps that will lead the client toward the long-term goal in such a way that progress can be observed and measured. To facilitate this, these steps are stated in a specific form as **behavioral objectives.** There are three components of a behavioral objective:

1.   The *do* statement identifies the action the client is to perform. This statement should contain verbs that name observable actions, such as *point, label, repeat, say, match, write, name,* or *ask.* Words to avoid in behavioral objectives are those that talk about processes that cannot be observed directly, such as *understand, know, learn, remember, comprehend,* or *discover.*

2.   The *condition* identifies the situation in which the target behavior is to be performed, such as when it will occur, where, in whose presence, and with what materials or cues. Some examples of condition statements include the following:

Following a clinician's model

In response to a question

Given a list of written words

In response to pictures

In the presence of other therapy group members

3.   The *criterion* specifies how well the target must be performed for the objective to be achieved. Typically used criteria include the following:

Achieve 90% correct

Have eight correct trials out of ten

Make fewer than four errors in three consecutive sessions

Do so consistently over a 10-minute period

At this point, you might try writing a behavioral objective for one of Marlene's long-term goals. The example in Box 6.1 will help you get started.

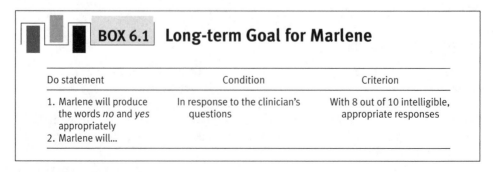

BOX 6.1 Long-term Goal for Marlene

Do statement	Condition	Criterion
1. Marlene will produce the words *no* and *yes* appropriately	In response to the clinician's questions	With 8 out of 10 intelligible, appropriate responses
2. Marlene will...		

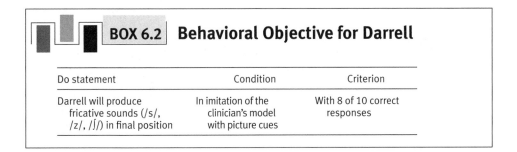

BOX 6.2 **Behavioral Objective for Darrell**

Do statement	Condition	Criterion
Darrell will produce fricative sounds (/s/, /z/, /ʃ/) in final position	In imitation of the clinician's model with picture cues	With 8 of 10 correct responses

Before beginning a therapy program, the clinician must be sure that the client cannot already perform the target behavior independently. This might seem obvious, but often a diagnosis is made on the basis of standardized tests that include only one item for a particular communication element, and a client may have missed that one item for a variety of reasons. Perhaps Darrell was given an articulation test, and he substituted a /t/ for the final /ʃ/ in the one item that tests final /ʃ/ (e.g., *dish*). Should we include final /ʃ/ as a therapy target? It is possible that Darrell would not say /ʃ/ in other final /ʃ/ words and did so in *dish* because he was influenced by the sound /d/ at the beginning of *dish*. This is an example of why potential therapy targets must be pretested before an intervention program is initiated. The **pretest** allows a clinician to establish that the client is not already consistently correct on a target behavior. When clinicians observe that a client is achieving target behaviors in most intervention activities, they administer a **posttest** to determine the client's consistency with target behavior. The pretest and posttest are usually the same; they consist of a set of 10–20 opportunities for the client to produce the target form when presented with minimal cues, prompts, or support from the clinician. The items in the pre- and posttest are different from the items used during instruction. Suppose one behavioral objective for Darrell were as listed in Box 6.2. Before beginning intervention, a pretest (e.g., the example that appears in Box 6.3) would be administered to ensure that a reasonable goal has been set. If the client fails to attain the criterion on the pretest, intervention on this target would be provided using the techniques described below. When the client achieves criterion levels of correct production in the intervention situation, a posttest is given to determine whether the objective has been met, using the same stimuli, responses, and criterion that were used in the pretest.

Once long-term and short-term objectives have been established and pretested, it is necessary to determine how to move the client toward achieving these objectives. This process usually involves **task analysis.** In a task analysis, a larger goal is broken down into small steps that can be followed to achieve it. To accomplish this breakdown, a clinician examines the input and output prerequisites necessary for completing the task. Consider Marlene's first long-term goal: increasing the amount of intelligible speech. The requirements of the goal could be analyzed this way:

Sensory: She must hear the speech spoken to her.

Motor: She must be able to make oral articulatory movements.

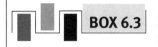

BOX 6.3 Pretest for Darrell, Based on Long-term Goal of Increasing Production of Final Fricatives

Stimulus	Response	Criterion
The client will view a picture card and will be given a prompting statement and question (e.g., "Here's a fish. What is it?").	*"fish"*	With 9 of 10 correct productions of final fricatives

Pretest: Show client 10 pictures of common items ending in fricative, such as:

Fish
Box
Kiss
Paws
Leaf
Sleeve
Garage
Jaws
Mouse
Rats

Incorporate long-term goal of increasing production of final fricatives if production of final fricatives in pretest is <80% correct.

Language: She must have some degree of semantic (word meaning) and syntactic (sentence structure) skill.

Cognitive: She must have some degree of conceptual and problem-solving ability; she must not be inordinately confused or demented.

A clinician would then proceed, by means of informal assessment, to determine whether Marlene has the requisite skills. If not, the clinician might revise the goal or work on developing its prerequisites. If Marlene does have the requisite abilities, however, the clinician would devise a series of steps, or a **task sequence,** through which Marlene will be guided in order to achieve the goal. The whole process, from establishing task prerequisites to sequencing steps to achieve goals, is the task analysis. Figure 6.1 presents a sequence of difficulty for verbal and nonverbal behaviors that are typically used in communication intervention. A task analysis encourages the clinician to move from the current form of response through a sequence of increasingly complex forms in the course of the intervention program. Table 6.1 gives an example of the sequence of steps a clinician might choose for Marlene to increase her production of intelligible speech. In summary, identifying the products or targets of intervention requires a clinician to

	Nonverbal	Verbal
Simple	Manipulated movement/gesture (clinician moves client's hand to form a gesture)	Immediate imitation (client repeats immediately after clinician)
	Imitated movement/gesture (clinician provides a model and asks client to imitate it)	Delayed imitation (clinician gives verbal model, some intervening speech, then asks client to imitate)
	Elicted movement/gesture (clinician asks client to produce gesture or movement without a direct model)	Partial imitation (clinician produces part of the target; client is asked to produce the whole target)
	Spontaneous movement/gesture (client produces movement/gesture appropriately without model or request for it)	Elicitation with object cue (clinician asks client for verbal response with an object as a cue)
		Elicitation with picture cue (clinician asks client for verbal response with a picture as a cue)
		Elicitation with written cue (clinician asks client for verbal response with a written word as a cue)
		Elicitation with question (clinician asks client for verbal response with a conversational question as a cue)
Complex		Spontaneous response (client produces target appropriately without model or request for it)

Figure 6.1. Task sequence for nonverbal and verbal clinician prompts.

1. Establish long-term goals

2. Identify short-term objectives that build toward the long-term goals

3. Use task analysis to create task sequences through which clients progress toward their goals

Once these steps have been accomplished, the next challenge is to find activities that facilitate this progress. To face this challenge, a clinician has a range of intervention processes.

INTERVENTION PROCESSES: THE CONTINUUM OF NATURALNESS

Intervention activities vary in their degree of naturalness. These variations have been described by Fey (1986) as falling along a **continuum of naturalness.** This continuum represents the degree to which intervention contexts correspond to everyday communication situations and interactions (see Table 6.2). This framework can be adapted for a broad range of communication disorders and ages. The continuum of naturalness also applies to clients who use **assistive technology** (AT) to augment their speech production capabilities or who rely completely on

Table 6.1. Task sequence for Marlene

1. Using sounds she can produce, Marlene will imitate simple words, such as *no, uh-huh, come, stop, hi.*
2. Marlene will produce these words without a direct imitative model (using delayed imitation—for example, "Hi, Marlene; nice to see you").
3. Marlene will practice using the words in scripts designed around daily activities, using picture cues. For example, with a series of pictures, tell Marlene a story about a woman's day, starting with greeting a friend, refusing a cigarette, agreeing with a colleague, and so forth. Marlene will produce the target word at an appropriate point in the story. The clinician will prompt her if necessary.
4. Marlene will practice using these words in conversations with family members, as the clinician coaches her with cues and prompts.

Table 6.2. Continuum of naturalness for a broad spectrum of communication disorders

Least natural	⟵————————————————⟶	Most natural
Clinician-directed	Hybrid	Client-centered
Drill	Organized activities	Daily activities
Drill play	Milieu teaching	Facilitative play
Modeling	Focused stimulation	Daily routines
	Script therapy	Vocational activities
	Role playing	
	Conversational coaching	
	More naturalistic modifications of clinician directed activities (e.g., structured scripts)	

Source: Fey (1986).

augmentative and alternative modes of communication (AAC) because speech is not a realistic communication mode.

According to Fey (1986), three factors affect naturalness: 1) the intervention activity itself, 2) the physical context in which the activity takes place, and 3) the individuals with whom the client interacts during intervention (see Table 6.3). Clinician-directed (CD) approaches and client-centered (CC) approaches denote the end points of this continuum, with hybrid approaches representing the midpoint.

Clinician-Directed Approaches

In CD approaches, or directive strategies, the clinician controls all aspects of the intervention: determining therapy goals, selecting stimulus materials, choosing the type and frequency of reinforcement, determining the order of activities, and identifying the specific target responses to be elicited.

Table 6.3. Factors affecting the degree of naturalness of intervention

Activity	Drill	Organized activities	Daily activities
	⟵————————————⟶		
Physical context	Clinic	School, workplace	Home
	⟵————————————⟶		
Social context	Clinician	Teacher, co-worker	Family members
	⟵————————————⟶		

Source: Fey, 1986.

Behavioral theorists (e.g., Roth & Worthington, 2011; Skinner, 1957) referred to these as antecedent, behavior, and consequence activities using the acronym ABC:

A: *Antecedent or stimulus:* The clinician provides a model of the desired behavior or a prompt to produce it.

B: *Behavior:* The client responds by producing a target behavior.

C: *Consequence:* The clinician provides reinforcement if the client's behavior was produced correctly. If not, the clinician provides feedback or correction or may ignore the incorrect behavior.

Behaviorist theory holds that all behavior occurs following some identifiable antecedent that prompts it and is maintained or discouraged by its consequences. What a clinician needs to do, in this view, is to manage the antecedents and consequences so that they facilitate the production of desired behaviors. To accomplish this management, behaviorists rely heavily on the operant procedures listed in Box 6.4. These approaches are not considered naturalistic because of the degree of clinician control and their lack of adherence to the conventions of genuine reciprocal communication.

 BOX 6.4 **Procedures Used in Operant Conditioning**

Cue: A verbal or nonverbal signal that tells the client when to produce the response; for example, the clinician taps Darrell on the hand to cue the response to each stimulus.

Delayed imitation: The clinician inserts an intervening statement after the stimulus, but the client still echoes the stimulus; for example, the clinician tells Darrell, "This is green. It's my favorite color. What color is it?" when working on /gr/.

Direct (immediate) imitation: The client echoes the clinician immediately after the stimulus is presented; for example, the clinician says, "This is green," and Darrell says, "Green."

Fading: A systematic withdrawal of reinforcement, either by decreasing the amount of reinforcement or by requiring more instances of the target behavior before reinforcement is given, after a behavior is established. For example, Mara is at first rewarded each time she names a toy after the clinician. Later, when she names more consistently, she is rewarded only every third time.

Prompt: A verbal or nonverbal hint, directive, or minimal guidance that assists the client in producing a behavior; for example, the clinician strokes his or her neck with a finger to remind Thomas to use easy onset.

Reinforcement: An item or activity that increases the frequency of a correct response; for example, a favorite food, a turn with a toy, or a monetary payment.

(continued)

BOX 6.4   *(continued)*

> For example, when playing with 14-month-old Leo, the clinician might tickle him each time he repeats the syllables in a back-and-forth babbling game.
>
> *Reinforcer:* An item or activity that is offered following a behavior to the increase or decrease of a particular behavior. Reinforcers can be
>
> * *Primary:* A biological necessity; for example, food or water.
> * *Secondary:* An item or activity that becomes important because it is linked to a primary reinforcer; for example, a bell that is rung when food is presented.
> * *Social:* The praise, approval, or attention that is given as a consequence for a behavior; for example, the clinician says, "You said everything clearly! That was a good job."
>
> *Reinforcement schedule:* The frequency with which reinforcement is given. Reinforcement schedules can be
>
> * *Continuous:* A reinforcement is given for every correct or target behavior.
> * *Intermittent:* A reinforcement is not given for every correct or target behavior; instead, behaviors are rewarded at certain intervals.
>
> *Shaping:* A reinforcement is provided contingent on successive approximations toward a target behavior; the clinician uses a series of reinforcements on different behavioral steps until the client's behavior at each step is consistent and, eventually, the target behavior is consistent as well. For example, Leo is first rewarded with a tickle for producing any sound in response to the clinician's playful babble. When Leo produces sounds consistently, the clinician withholds reinforcement until he produces a syllable that shares one consonant with the syllable the clinician has produced. Later, more accurate imitations are required in order to gain the reward.

The most common CD approaches are *drill* and *drill play.* Drill is considered the most highly structured format (Paul & Norbury, 2012; Roth & Worthington, 2011; Shriberg & Kwiatkowski, 1982). The clinician selects the training stimuli; explains the specific target response to the client; presents stimulus items in a predetermined order; and reinforces correct responses tangibly (e.g., with candy or a token), verbally (e.g., "Good job!"), or nonverbally (e.g., the client gets a high-five from the clinician). In drill play, the drill is embedded in a game format so that the client is motivated by the activity itself to produce the target forms as well as by the reinforcement that follows the production. For example, Darrell's clinician might have him play a game in which five paper bags are labeled with target words. Darrell is given a sponge ball to toss into one of the bags (motivating activity), and then he must say the word on the bag. He is reinforced only for correct production. Reinforcement may be tangible or may entail the chance to take another turn at the game.

It is important to note that CD approaches are thought to be most effective during the initial stages of intervention to establish a new target behavior. Once established, transitional activities can be introduced to provide the client with more naturalistic contexts in which to practice and use the new communicative behavior to achieve carryover or **generalization,** that is, the use of target behaviors outside the therapy situation without support from the clinician.

Client-Centered Approaches

Also referred to as responsive approaches, CC approaches emphasize the provision of communication therapy in authentic settings. The assumption underlying these approaches is that individuals will achieve therapy goals more readily and generalize newly learned behaviors more spontaneously when taught in the context of familiar experiences and activities with supportive communication partners who respond authentically to their communicative attempts. In CC activities, the client leads the intervention and determines the content, timing, and sequence of therapy. The key steps in naturalistic, or CC, approaches involve *waiting* for the client to initiate a behavior, *interpreting* the behavior as communicative (whether communication was intended), and *responding* to the behavior in a way that places it in a communicative context (Fey, 1986). In contrast to CD approaches, here the clinician does not attempt to elicit a predetermined set of responses from the client. Instead, the clinician follows the client's lead and offers consistent and meaningful responses that relate to the client's own actions or utterances. The CC approaches are considered highly naturalistic because the client is engaged in enjoyable and meaningful daily activities with a responsive, communicative partner.

The most common CC activity used with children is facilitative play. This is an indirect stimulation technique (Owens, 2010; Paul & Norbury, 2012). The clinician arranges the physical environment to encourage the child to generate target responses spontaneously during the natural course of a play sequence. The clinician uses several techniques to promote the child's communicative participation. Examples of some techniques are listed in Box 6.5.

Naturalistic CC intervention also can be used with adult clients. Two primary forms of naturalistic interventions are employed with adults: *functional therapy* and *conversational group therapy*. Functional therapy involves communicative activities of daily living, which the client practices with support and scaffolding from the clinician. Thomas, our fluency client, for example, may work on talking on the telephone with his clinician. The clinician may first conduct some structured activities to encourage easy onset. Thomas would then be asked to use easy onset in a role-playing activity with a telephone. In later phases of therapy, he would be asked to make real telephone calls, with prompts and cues from the clinician that would be systematically faded.

Conversational group therapy is often a form of treatment for adults with neurogenic disorders. Rather than (or in addition to) receiving individual, skill-focused therapy, group members engage in conversations with other clients and a clinician. As in all CC approaches, the clients determine the structure and topics of the conversation. They receive natural feedback on the relevance, intelligibility, and appropriateness of their turns from others in the group. The clinician takes advantage of a set of facilitative techniques, just as the young child's clinician does. These techniques were summarized by Ewing (2006) and are presented in Box 6.6.

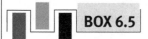 **BOX 6.5** | **Facilitative Play Techniques**

Self-talk: The clinician observes the child's behavior and engages in the same behavior while simultaneously engaging in an animated monologue that describes the clinician's ongoing actions. The monologue stays within the immediate attentional focus of the child.

Example: In the context building a sandcastle at the play table with Mara, the clinician builds a sandcastle as well and says "I'm making a castle. A big castle. See how big it is?"

Parallel talk: The clinician produces an ongoing commentary on the child's actions. The commentary stays within the immediate attentional focus of the child.

Example: In the context building a sandcastle at the play table with Mara, the clinician watches Mara's actions and says, "You're building a castle. It's really big. Look how big your castle is."

Expansions: The clinician reformulates the child's utterances into more grammatically complete versions.

Example:

Mara: "Kitty."

Clinician: "Yes, it *is* a kitty!"

Extensions or expatiations: The clinician enlarges on the child's utterances by adding new semantic information.

Example:

Mara: "Kitty drink."

Clinician: "Yes, the kitty is very thirsty today."

Recasts: The clinician expands the child's utterances into a different sentence type.

Example:

Mara: "Kitty drink."

Clinician: "Is the kitty drinking?"

Hybrid Approaches

Hybrid, or blended, approaches represent a midpoint between the two extremes of naturalness. Hybrid approaches use intervention activities that are highly natural, but the clinician maintains control over the therapy environment to maximize learning and generalization. There are three main characteristics of hybrid approaches:

1. Only one or a small number of goals are targeted for intervention.

2. The clinician selects therapy activities and materials, choosing those that promote the client's spontaneous use of the target behaviors.

3. The clinician produces utterance behaviors that are contingent to the client's communication but that also model and accentuate the target forms.

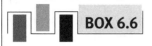

BOX 6.6 **Conversational Group Therapy Techniques**

Attending: Letting participants know that their messages are being received (e.g., "I heard Marlene say that she felt happy with that action.")

Facilitating questions: Encouraging participants to query each other (e.g., "Do you need to ask Thomas what he means?")

Negotiating goals: Providing tactful prompts that help participants decide what they want to accomplish, integrate new members, and renew goals (e.g., "Richard, our group has been working to decrease frustration in communication situations. Do you have any personal goals along those lines?")

Rewarding: Giving verbal praise to participants for their group interactions (e.g., "That's a very insightful thought, Marlene.")

Responding to feelings: Providing verbal or nonverbal reactions that show participants that their feelings are understood (e.g., "I can see that it really upsets Thomas to talk about his cancer.")

Focusing: Keeping the group discussion on track by reintroducing the target discussion topic as needed (e.g., "We were talking about using the telephone, though. Has anyone else had trouble with that?")

Summarizing: Stating a rendition of what the session has covered and providing the next step toward the group's goal (e.g., "It sounds as if everyone has felt frustrated about using the telephone. Should we plan to talk about suggestions to help on this front next time?")

Gatekeeping: Balancing participation among members so that one or a few participants do not dominate the discussion (e.g., "Richard, do you have a thought about what Marlene said?")

Modeling: Using demonstrations to teach conversational skills by example (e.g., "When I feel that way, I sometimes say, 'Hold on! I've got a thought on that!'")

Mediating: Resolving conflicts and encouraging conflict resolution among participants (e.g., "Thomas and Richard have a difference of opinion here; does anyone see some middle ground?")

According to Fey (1986), the four main types of hybrid instruction are as follows:

1. Focused stimulation

2. Milieu teaching

3. Script therapy

4. Conversational coaching

Focused Stimulation In focused stimulation, the clinician deliberately arranges the verbal and nonverbal environment to increase the likelihood that the client will spontaneously produce the target form. The clinician provides frequent models of the target behavior in meaningful and highly functional contexts to facilitate client success. Although a response is not required from the client, the environmental setup is conducive to the production of the target form. For example, the clinician can increase the salience of a target behavior by presenting it in sentence-final or stressed positions; to elicit the production of the copula *is*, the clinician may respond to Mara's utterance "*She big*" with "She *is*?" or "*Is* she big?"

There are a variety of language strategies that can be used to accomplish focused stimulation, many of which are given in Crystal, Fletcher, and Garman (1976); Fey, Cleave, Long, and Hughes (1993); Fey, Long, and Finestack, (2003); Owens (2010); and Paul and Norbury (2012). Some examples include the following:

- *False assertions:* The clinician makes a statement to elicit the copula from the client (e.g.,"That's not your hat!" "Yes, it is.").

- *Feigned misunderstandings:* The clinician pretends not to get the message sent by the client (e.g., "You want me to 'top'?").

- *Forced choices:* The clinician makes a statement to elicit the negative form from the client (e.g., "You do like it or you don't like it?" "I don't like it.").

- *Contingent query:* The clinician asks the client to clarify the message (e.g., "Want gween." "Which crayon do you want?").

- *Violating routines:* The clinician omits an expected action to elicit a response from the client (e.g., when greeting the 2-year-old late talker Mara, the clinician calls her by the wrong name).

- *Withholding objects and turns:* The clinician neglects to provide an expected object to elicit a response from the client (e.g., when playing with blocks, the clinician repeatedly "forgets" to give Mara some of the blocks).

Milieu Teaching *Milieu Teaching* stresses the use of ongoing activities as the basis for intervention and incorporates the operant principles of imitation, modeling, and reinforcement into naturalistic settings. Incidental Teaching and the Mand-Model method are two specific milieu teaching techniques. The steps involved in the Incidental Teaching approach (Hart & Risley, 1975; Warren & Kaiser, 1986; Yoder & Warren, 2002) are outlined in Box 6.7.

The Mand-Model method (Rogers-Warren & Warren, 1980; Warren, 1991) is similar to Incidental Teaching with two exceptions. First, it does not require the client to initiate communication before teaching begins. Rather, the clinician observes the client carefully, and when the client displays interest in an object or some aspect of the environment, the clinician *mands* a response (e.g., "Tell me what you need."). Second, the goals are general (e.g., elicit two-word utterances, elicit well-formed sentences) rather than specific (e.g., elicit agent–object

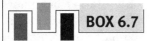 **BOX 6.7** **Steps in Incidental Teaching**

1. The clinician arranges the environment so that desired objects or items are visible to the client but out of reach (e.g., a toy, a newspaper).

2. The client initiates the interaction verbally or nonverbally (e.g., pointing to the desired item).

3. The clinician selects the target response to be evoked from the client (e.g., "I want the newspaper so I can read it").

4. The clinician uses cues to obtain a more elaborated response. The first cue is focused attention, which involves physically approaching the client, making eye contact, or issuing an expectant look. If the client does not respond after a brief waiting period, the clinician then offers a second cue such as a general question (e.g., "What do you want?"). If the client's response to the question contains the target response, the clinician provides a confirmation that includes a model of the target form (e.g., "Yes, you want the newspaper so you can read it?").

5. If the question does not elicit the target response, the clinician issues a prompt in the form of a general request (e.g., "You need to tell me"), a request for partial imitation (e.g., "Say, 'I want the newspaper so...'"), or a request for complete imitation (e.g., "Say, 'I want the newspaper so I can read it'"). If the client does not generate the target response even after the prompts, the clinician gives one additional prompt.

6. If the client achieves the target behavior, the clinician provides confirmation that the communicative intent was achieved (e.g., the client is given the newspaper).

7. If the client does not produce the target response, the clinician gives the client the desired item and determines the type of cue that may be more effective for the next session.

utterances, elicit conjoined sentences). If the client produces an appropriate response, the clinician presents verbal reinforcement and presents the desired item (e.g., "Great! You told me why you wanted the newspaper, and here it is."). If the client's response is inappropriate, the clinician offers prompts such as those used in Incidental Teaching.

Both of these milieu approaches extend the operant procedures of imitation, prompting, and reinforcement to naturalistic activities in which the client accomplishes authentic communication goals with the behaviors being trained. In addition, the reinforcement received is a natural outcome of the communication interaction.

Script Therapy   *Script therapy* is an approach in which target behaviors are taught within the context of a familiar routine or script (Olswang & Bain, 1991; Weismer & Evans, 2002). A script is an ordered sequence of events that depicts a familiar activity such as making dinner, going to a birthday party, or ordering a meal in a restaurant (Nelson, 1985). The clinician and client enact the script, during which the clinician can violate the sequence of activities (e.g., in the birthday party script, the clinician might eat the cake before blowing out the candles), providing a natural opportunity for the client to communicate verbally or gesturally. Other violations may include hiding props necessary for the script and introducing broken or incomplete materials (e.g., using unwrapped gifts in the birthday party script). Once a script is overlearned, the clinician can use it to introduce more complex forms. For example, the client can be told to pretend that the birthday party was yesterday or will be tomorrow to encourage the production of past and future tense markers. The clinician also can have the client pretend that the person who had the birthday received at least two copies of every gift to promote the use of plural tense forms.

Social stories (Gray, 1995), originally developed for high-functioning children with autism, are a form of script therapy that provide written scaffolds for clients who can read. The "stories" are written as explanations of social situations and are tailored to a client's level of comprehension. Most stories contain descriptive statements and directive statements. The descriptive statements help the client understand the particular situation and give words for situations that the client cannot generate independently. The directive statements script what the client should do in a situation that would be more socially appropriate than his or her current responses.

Video modeling is another variation of script therapy, one that has been found to be particularly effective with individuals with autism spectrum disorders (Prelock, Paul, & Allen, 2011). Here, a script exemplifying a problem social situation is enacted, either by the client or by peers. The enactment is recorded and then viewed by the client and clinician, who discuss, verbally rehearse, and then reenact the script in a therapy setting. Later, the client is coached to utilize the script with peers in a more naturalistic setting.

Interrupted-behavior chain strategy (Caro & Snell, 1989) is an additional variation of script therapy. It utilizes authentic contexts to introduce new intervention targets with structured instructional techniques. In this approach, a new behavior is inserted into an already established behavioral sequence. For instance, Marlene, the adult client with aphasia, may have mastered an instructional strategy for walking her dog, which includes getting the leash, collaring the dog, retrieving house keys, locking the front door, and walking the dog around the block. In the middle of this sequence, the clinician interrupts the behavior chain and asks Marlene to state the dog's name and the address of the dog's owner. If necessary, the clinician models the correct response, prompts Marlene to produce it, and reinforces her attempt.

Conversational Coaching   *Conversational coaching* was developed by Holland (1995) to facilitate functional communication skills of adults with aphasia and

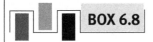

BOX 6.8 | **Sample Script and Procedures for Conversational Coaching**

1. I have to change my hairdresser.

2. She always cuts my hair too short.

3. And I always have to wait.

4. This time she made my hair uneven.

5. I need to find someone else.

has been extended to intervention with children who have autism spectrum disorders or other social communication difficulties (Bellini, 2013). This technique simulates conversational interaction in a structured context. The clinician prepares a short written script based on the client's interests, experiences, and level of communication skills. According to Holland (1995), the scripts should be written in a communicative style, consist of short sentences to promote successful communication, and emphasize target communication behaviors. A sample script followed by a summary of the recommended procedures is presented in Box 6.8.

The client reads the script aloud one sentence at a time. Self-cuing strategies are suggested by the clinician when the client evidences difficulty expressing the scripted information. Common self-cuing strategies include chunking utterances into shorter units and using gestures to communicate meaning. The clinician records the client reading the script to a familiar listener who is unaware of the script's contents. The listener is coached to glean the gist of the script, rather than trying to understand each word. The three participants then evaluate the recording to determine the success level of the scripted interaction, the aspects that the listener found most and least helpful, and alternative strategies the client and the listener might have used to improve the interaction. The coaching and evaluation format is repeated with increasingly unfamiliar listeners, and new target behaviors are scripted into conversations.

USING THE CONTINUUM OF NATURALNESS

Research evidence supports the use of both naturalistic and structured intervention approaches with a broad range and severity of speech, language, and communication disorders for children (e.g., Conture, 1996; Geirut, 1998; Hemmeter, Ault, Collins, & Meyer, 1996; Kim, Yang, & Hwang, 2001; Kouri, 2005; McCauley & Fey, 2006; Swanson, Fey, Mills, & Hood, 2005; Yoder & Warren, 2001) and adults (Conture, 1996; Holland, Fromm, DeRuyter, & Stein, 1996; Ramig & Verdolini, 1998; Robey, 1998). Some therapy goals are most effectively accomplished through naturalistic strategies, though others are more amenable to highly structured CD approaches.

The degree of naturalness to use in intervention must be determined by the nature and severity of a client's communication impairment and the client's responsiveness to different intervention strategies. Highly naturalistic activities are preferred only if they bring about improved communication abilities. Less naturalistic activities should be chosen only if they are more effective in eliciting a target behavior. For example, children with language impairments may have difficulty inducing linguistic rules from natural interactions and may require more focused and explicit language input. Some adults with fluency disorders may benefit from more naturalistic strategies that provide opportunities to engage in genuine communication interactions.

The approaches that form the continuum are not mutually exclusive. A combination of strategies may be appropriate for a particular client. For example, one communicative objective may be accomplished most efficiently using a highly structured CD strategy, whereas another objective may be met more efficiently through naturally occurring activities. Often, programming for the same objective may make use of several activities that can range in naturalness from highly structured to highly natural. Fey (1986) reminded clinicians that if two activities are equally effective in eliciting a particular linguistic structure or communicative function, the naturalistic one is preferred because it will more likely promote the use of the newly acquired target behavior in everyday speaking situations. Following are examples of intervention activities at various points along the continuum of naturalness for some of the children and adults we have been discussing.

DARRELL, A PRESCHOOLER WITH UNINTELLIGIBLE SPEECH

Target behavior: Increase ability to produce three-syllable words correctly.

Drill: The clinician names a set of picture cards with three-syllable words (e.g., tomato, banana). After each label, Darrell is cued to repeat the word. Each time all three syllables are produced, he receives a token. With 20 tokens, he can "buy" a turn throwing darts at a dart board.

Hybrid: The clinician and child play the game I Spy with a picture of fruits and vegetables that Darrell has practiced saying. Darrell chooses which one to name on his turn; the clinician points to the one he names.

Daily: The clinician and Darrell make a Thanksgiving collage together. The cutouts include many of the fruits and vegetables Darrell has been practicing naming. As they work, the clinician names some of these or asks Darrell to name them. The clinician praises Darrell when he names them correctly, in imitation, in response to the request to name, or spontaneously.

JONAH, A SCHOOL-AGE CHILD WITH HEARING IMPAIRMENT

Target behavior: Improve classroom listening skills using appropriate amplification.

Drill: Jonah imitates the clinician's instructions (drawn from those typically used by his classroom teacher) and acts each instruction out as he imitates. The clinician reinforces correct actions.

Hybrid: The clinician and Jonah play "Army," taking turns being "Sarge." Sarge gives instructions (written on slips of paper, following teacher instructions, and drawn from an army hat). The partner must correctly follow the instruction.

Daily: The clinician works with Jonah in class during an instructional activity. Using prompts and cues, the clinician encourages him to write down the instructions, ask questions about what he does not understand, adjust his hearing aid if needed, and so forth.

ANNA, A SEVENTH-GRADER WITH LEARNING DISABILITY

Target behavior: Use of *because*, *if*, and *so* to produce cause–effect complex sentences.

Drill: The clinician explains the use of conjunctions, such as *because*, *if*, and *so*, to link ideas in sentences. The clinician presents simple sentences on cards, along with the conjunctions written on paper "hooks." Anna combines each pair with the given conjunction, following the clinician's model.

Hybrid: The clinician reads Anna a cause–effect selection from a classroom textbook. The clinician provides several models of retelling the passage, using sentences with the conjunctions practiced. Anna is then asked a question that she can answer with a similar conjoined sentence.

Daily: The clinician runs a study group with Anna and some other students who are struggling with a classroom textbook selection that discusses cause and effect. The students are encouraged to discuss the selection. The clinician occasionally models sentences using the target conjunctions within the context of the discussion.

MARLENE, AN ADULT WITH APHASIA

Target behavior: Improve the use of the self-cuing strategy of sentence completion for retrieving verbal labels.

Drill: The clinician presents a list of incomplete sentences, such as "We use a broom to sweep the _____," for Marlene to imitate and complete.

Hybrid: The clinician collects several identical pairs of cards depicting objects necessary to perform daily activities and demonstrates the sentence completion strategy for Marlene to imitate. After imitative practice of the strategy, Marlene, the clinician, and some other people play a card game. The clinician shuffles the deck and gives each player five cards. The clinician explains that the goal of this activity is to make pairs for all the cards in the player's hand by taking turns asking one another, "Do you have a _____?"

Daily: Marlene selects three daily activities (e.g., brushing teeth, making coffee, watering the plants). Marlene and the clinician make a list of items necessary to perform each task. Marlene uses the sentence completion self-cuing strategy "I need a _____" to request each item.

RICHARD, AN ADULT WHO WANTS TO USE ESOPHAGEAL SPEECH

Target behavior: Increase the use of appropriate prosody.

Drill: The clinician writes pairs of sentences that contain the same subject, verb, and object. Each sentence is written on a separate card with a different word underlined for emphasis (e.g., I want coffee; I want coffee). The clinician points to one card at a time and produces each sentence for Richard to imitate.

Hybrid: Using the same set of cards as above, the clinician places a pair of cards face up on the table and asks a question for Richard to answer using the prosodically appropriate sentence with exaggerated stress (e.g., Q: *Who* wants coffee? A: *I* want coffee. Q: *What* do you want? A: I want *coffee*).

Daily: Richard chooses reading passages from magazines or newspapers that interest him or from which he wants to learn new information. The clinician highlights the words that receive primary stress. The client reads aloud each passage concentrating on emphasizing the appropriate words.

THOMAS, AN ADULT WHO HAS A FLUENCY DISORDER

Target behavior: Decrease stuttering moments and reduce anxiety associated with dysfluencies.

Drill: The clinician reads a presented passage and engages in voluntary stuttering on predetermined words. Thomas imitates each of the voluntary stutters.

Hybrid: The clinician introduces a board game such as *Jeopardy!* and explains that Thomas is the contestant. After reviewing the technique of pull-outs (Van Riper, 1973), Thomas is instructed to use one or more pseudo- or real dysfluencies in response to game questions and to modify stuttering moments using pull-outs.

Daily: Thomas's task is to enter a situation that has previously been identified as mildly fearful and use the pull-out technique. Examples of situations include calling a family member on the telephone, making an appointment for a haircut, and asking for directions.

MARA, A 2-YEAR OLD WITH FEW WORDS

Target behavior: Produce five names for clothing items in the context of a play interaction with an adult.

Drill: The clinician presents several pieces of doll clothing and a doll. He or she names each piece, and when Mara imitates an approximation of the name, the clinician helps Mara put the clothing on the doll. This process is repeated with other dolls and stuffed animals.

Hybrid: The clinician works with Mara to make a clothes collage. Mara chooses (by pointing) pictures of clothing in a magazine; the clinician excitedly names the piece Mara chooses, providing focused stimulation. He or she waits to provide Mara a chance to repeat the name. Whether Mara repeats or not, the clinician cuts out each picture Mara chooses and allows her to paste it on paper.

Daily: Consult with classroom teachers to encourage them to ask Mara to name each item she needs to put on in order to go outside to play at outdoor time each day.

LEO, A 14-MONTH-OLD WITH A COCHLEAR IMPLANT

Target behavior: Identify family members by name

Drill: The clinician presents photos of Leo's parents, brother, sister, and dog, either printed out or on an iPad. She names a family member and asks Leo to point to the one she names. When he points correctly, she tickles him or sings a snatch of a favorite song; when he points incorrectly, she ignores the response and provides the stimulus (family name) again.

Hybrid: The clinician tapes pictures of family members onto cars in a toy train. As Leo plays with the cars, she casually suggests he "put Mom's car here. Then let's put Rover's car next," and so forth. As he plays, she names the people on the cars and responds with enthusiasm when he touches the car with the named person on it.

Daily: Encourage family members to name each other as they play with or care for Leo and to look at the named family member when they do ("Oh, look, there's Daddy!"). Urge them to show excitement when Leo looks at the family member named and to repeat the activity often throughout the day.

DEVELOPING INTERVENTION ACTIVITIES THAT MAXIMIZE LEARNING

Bayles (2011) and Gillam and Loeb (2010) identified several essential ingredients that enhance intervention, regardless of the goals or procedures. These principles are drawn from evidence based on randomized controlled trials of a range of intervention procedures, as well as from literature on neuroplasticity, which highlights conditions associated with the brain's ability to reorganize after an injury. They are summarized in Box 6.9. As clinicians plan intervention activities, they try to keep these principles in mind and attempt to incorporate as many as possible into each clinical encounter.

DATA COLLECTION

An important aspect of intervention is tracking a client's progress within the program. This data collection has several functions within an intervention program.

1. It permits the clinician to track the client's progress from one session to another.

2. It provides documentation of the efficacy of a particular intervention strategy or set of strategies.

3. It maximizes clinician effectiveness.

BOX 6.9	**Strategies for Maximizing Learning in Intervention**

Principle	Description
Intensity	Engaging in daily sessions for a period of weeks
Active engagement	Sustaining a client's active involvement in intervention tasks by monitoring and guiding attention through cueing, and choosing activities that are appealing enough to sustain client engagement
Feedback	Giving information about the accuracy of client response
Reinforcement	Delivering a reward following a correct response that increases the rate or likelihood of the appearance of the target behavior
Repetition	Providing many opportunities for clients to use or process a new target
Distributed practice	Engaging in short, intense periods of practice for new forms, interspersed with practice on other forms or instruction in new targets
Specificity	Providing instruction and practice on the specific skill targeted, not on skills thought to be prerequisite or related to it
Control complexity	Providing activities the client can do with the clinician's support but cannot do without it
Minimize error responses	Providing adequate cueing and scaffolding so the client's responses are correct almost all the time
Work within schemas	Embedding practice of new forms and functions within familiar sequences of actions

Sources: Paul and Norbury (2012); Gillam and Loeb (2010); and Proctor-Williams (2009).

For naturalistic intervention approaches, video recording is the data collection procedure of choice because it permits a permanent audio and visual record. Frequently, repeated viewing of an interaction or session is necessary to fully describe and analyze the client's verbal and nonverbal communicative behaviors. Video recording may not be possible at all times and in all settings, though. Alternative data collection methods include the development of checklists, rating scales, graphs, and audiotapes and use of multiple observers, each focusing on a different behavioral component. Data-recording forms can be developed for group as well as individual sessions.

The type of notation system used to chart data yields different kinds of information. A binary system records whether a behavior is correct (i.e., appropriate) or incorrect (i.e., inappropriate). An interval rating scale gives more qualitative information because behaviors are rated on a continuum (e.g., degree of accuracy or appropriateness). It is also desirable to code whether the client's behavior is gestural, vocal, or verbal, or a combination thereof. In addition, data collection procedures should allow the clinician to distinguish between imitative, prompted, self-corrected, and spontaneous responses. Figures 6.2 and 6.3 present two examples of charts that can be used to track client behaviors. You may want to try coming up with your own to track the behaviors elicited in some of the examples we reviewed previously.

CONCLUSION

The aim of all intervention is to improve communicative behavior. This means that even though clinicians structure therapy to achieve specific, measurable

Name: _____				Behavioral objective: _____						
Clinician: _____				Reinforcement type/schedule: _____						
Date: _____				Materials: _____						
Trials											
Task	1	2	3	4	5	6	7	8	9	10	Percent correct

Figure 6.2. Example of a data log.

goals, the true objective is to increase clients' overall ability to use communication in authentic, functional settings. When clinicians assess the effectiveness of intervention, it is this larger goal that needs to be kept in mind. In addition, we need to remember that our job is to help clients communicate better, not to adopt a philosophy of therapy or join a "school" of intervention. We should, in other words, take advantage of all the intervention approaches available to us and match each goal for each client to the most effective technique for that particular objective. Chances are, the appropriate technique will change over time. Although very structured CD intervention may work for some clients early in the course of intervention, the clients are likely to need more naturalistic approaches later. Other clients may require a naturalistic approach early on, while they are still becoming familiar with their clinicians, and may be more willing to tolerate structured formats later. Whatever activities or sequences clinicians decide to employ, the goal is always to maximize communicative effectiveness for the client. Part of the way clinicians do this is by being aware of the range of therapeutic options available and choosing the most appropriate for each situation. Another part is by carefully monitoring the efficacy of the intervention by collecting and analyzing data throughout the course of the therapy. Tracking client behaviors allows us to know

Block 1

Client				Objective						Number of responses					Number of correct responses						Percent correct			
1	2	3	4	5	6	7	8	9	10	11	12	13	14	15	16	17	18	19	20	21	22	23	24	25
26	27	28	29	30	31	32	33	34	35	36	37	38	39	40	41	42	43	44	45	46	47	48	49	50

Block 2

Client				Objective						Number of responses					Number of correct responses						Percent correct			
1	2	3	4	5	6	7	8	9	10	11	12	13	14	15	16	17	18	19	20	21	22	23	24	25
26	27	28	29	30	31	32	33	34	35	36	37	38	39	40	41	42	43	44	45	46	47	48	49	50

Block 3

Client				Objective						Number of responses					Number of correct responses						Percent correct			
1	2	3	4	5	6	7	8	9	10	11	12	13	14	15	16	17	18	19	20	21	22	23	24	25
26	27	28	29	30	31	32	33	34	35	36	37	38	39	40	41	42	43	44	45	46	47	48	49	50

Block 4

Client				Objective						Number of responses					Number of correct responses						Percent correct			
1	2	3	4	5	6	7	8	9	10	11	12	13	14	15	16	17	18	19	20	21	22	23	24	25
26	27	28	29	30	31	32	33	34	35	36	37	38	39	40	41	42	43	44	45	46	47	48	49	50

Figure 6.3. Sample group therapy data sheet.

when our intervention strategies have achieved their goals so that we can move on to other goals or even, if we are very fortunate, have clients "graduate" from intervention. Performance data also tell us when our strategies are not working and need to be changed to provide a better match to the client's needs. We need to be aware of the standards for EBP and continually update our knowledge of what research tells us about which intervention procedures meet these standards. Communication intervention, then, involves continual and thoughtful monitoring. That is why it takes a clinician, not a technician, to do it.

STUDY QUESTIONS

1. What are the three basic purposes of intervention?
2. What are the three components of a behavioral objective?
3. Discuss the sequence of steps used to do a task analysis.
4. Describe three points along the continuum of naturalness of intervention activities.
5. Describe a drill activity to teach correct /s/ production to a 5-year-old client.
6. Describe three types of language used in facilitative play.
7. Name six steps involved in Incidental Teaching.
8. Create an activity for a client with aphasia, using a conversational coaching approach.
9. Name three functions of clinical data collection.
10. When are naturalistic approaches preferred over other methods?

REFERENCES

Bayles, C. (2011). *Cognitive communication.* Workshop presented at the Connecticut Speech-Language-Hearing Association State Convention, New Britain, CT.

Bellini, S. (2013). Social skills training. In F. Volkmar, R. Paul, K. Pelphrey, & S. Rogers (Eds.), *Handbook of autism spectrum disorders.* New York, NY: Wiley.

Caro, P., & Snell, M. (1989). Characteristics of teaching communication to people with moderate and severe disabilities. *Education and Training in Mental Retardation, 24,* 63–77.

Conture, E.G. (1996). Treatment efficacy: Stuttering. *Journal of Speech and Hearing Research, 39,* 19–26.

Crystal, D., Fletcher, P., & Garman, M. (1976). *The grammatical analysis of language disability: A procedure for assessment and remediation.* London, England: Edward Arnold.

Dollaghan, C. (2004, April 13). Evidence-based practice: Myths and realities. *The ASHA Leader, 12,* 4–5.

Ewing, S. (2006). Group process, group dynamics, group techniques with neurogenic communication disorders. In R. Elman (Ed.), *Group treatment of neurogenic communication disorders* (2nd ed., pp. 9–17). Boston, MA: Butterworth-Heinemann.

Fey, M. (1986). *Language intervention with young children.* San Diego, CA: College-Hill Press.

Fey, M., Cleave, P., Long, S., & Hughes, D. (1993). Two approaches to the facilitation of grammar in children with language impairment: An experimental evaluation. *Journal of Speech and Hearing Research, 36,* 141–157.

Fey, M., Long, S., & Finestack, L. (2003). Ten principles of grammar facilitation for children with specific language impairments. *American Journal of Speech-Language Pathology, 12,* 3–15.

Geirut, J. (1998). Treatment efficacy: Functional phonological disorders in children. *Journal of Speech, Language, and Hearing Research, 41,* 85–100.

Gillam, R., & Loeb, D. (2010). Principles for school-age language intervention: Insight from a randomized controlled trial. *The ASHA Leader, 15*(1), 10–13.

Gray, C.A. (1995). Teaching children with autism to "read" social situations. In K.A. Quill (Ed.), *Teaching children with autism strategies to enhance communication and socialization* (pp. 219–241). Albany, NY: Delmar.

Hart, B., & Risley, T. (1975). In vivo language intervention: Unanticipated general effects. *Journal of Applied Behavioral Analysis, 13*, 411–420.

Hemmeter, M., Ault, M., Collins, B., & Meyer, S. (1996). The effects of teacher-implemented language instruction within free time activities. *Education and Training in Mental Retardation and Developmental Disabilities, 31*, 203–212.

Holland, A. (1995, April). *Current realities of aphasia rehabilitation: Time constraints, documentation demands and functional outcomes.* Paper presented at Mid-America Rehabilitation Hospital, Voerland Park, KS.

Holland, A.L., Fromm, D.S., DeRuyter, F., & Stein, M. (1996). Treatment efficacy: Aphasia. *Journal of Speech and Hearing Research, 39*, 27–39.

Kim, Y., Yang, Y., & Hwang, B. (2001). Generalization effects of script-based intervention on language expression of preschool children with language disorders. *Education and Training in Mental Retardation and Developmental Disabilities, 36*, 411–423.

Kouri, T. (2005). Lexical training through modeling and elicitation procedures with late talkers who have specific language impairment and developmental delays. *Journal of Speech, Language, and Hearing Research, 48*, 157–172.

McCauley, R., & Fey, M. (2006). *Treatment of language disorders in children.* Baltimore, MD: Paul H. Brookes Publishing Co.

McLean, L. (1998). A language-communication intervention model. In D. Berstein & E. Tiegerman (Eds.), *Language and communication disorders in children* (pp. 208–228). Boston, MA: Allyn & Bacon.

Nelson, K. (1985). *Making sense: The acquisition of shared meaning.* San Diego, CA: Academic Press.

Olswang, L., & Bain, B. (1991). Intervention issues for toddlers with specific language impairments. *Topics in Language Disorders, 11*, 69–86.

Owens, R. (2010). *Language disorders: A functional approach to assessment and intervention* (5th ed.). Boston, MA: Allyn & Bacon.

Paul, R., & Norbury, C. (2012). *Language disorders from infancy through adolescence: Listening, speaking, reading, writing, and communicating* (4th ed.). St. Louis, MO: Mosby.

Prelock, P., Paul, R., & Allen, E. (2011). Evidence-based treatments in communication for children with autism spectrum disorders. In F. Volkmar & B. Reichow (Eds.), Evidence-based treatments for children with ASD (pp. 93–170). New York, NY: Springer.

Proctor-Williams, K. (2009). Dosage and distribution in morphosyntax intervention. *Topics in Language Disorders, 29*, 294–311.

Ramig, L.O., & Verdolini, K. (1998). Treatment efficacy: Voice disorders. *Journal of Speech, Language, and Hearing Research, 41*, 101–116.

Robey, R.R. (1998). A meta-analysis of clinical outcomes in the treatment of aphasia. *Journal of Speech, Language and Hearing Research, 41*, 172–187.

Rogers-Warren, A., & Warren, S. (1980). Mands for verbalization: Facilitating the generalization of newly trained language in children. *Behavior Modification, 4*, 230–245.

Rose, D.H., & Meyer, A. (2000). Universal design for individual differences. *Educational Leadership, 58*, 39–43.

Roth, F.P., & Worthington, C.K. (2011). *Intervention resource manual for speech-language pathology* (4th ed.). Clifton Park, NY: Thomson Delmar Learning.

Sackett, D., Strauss, S.E., Richardson, W.S., Rosenberg, W., & Haynes, R.B. (2000). *Evidence-based medicine: How to practice and teach EBM* (2nd ed.). Edinburgh, Scotland: Churchill Livingstone.

Schmitt, M.B., & Justice, L.M. (2012). Evidence-based practice: A retrospective overview and proposal for future directions. *Evidence-Based Briefs, 7*, 1–6.

Shriberg, L., & Kwiatkowski, J. (1982). Phonological disorders III: A conceptual framework for management. *Journal of Speech and Hearing Disorders, 47*, 242–256.

Skinner, B.F. (1957). *Verbal behavior.* New York, NY: Appleton-Century-Crofts.

Swanson, L., Fey, M., Mills, C., & Hood, S. (2005). Use of narrative based language intervention with children who have specific language impairment. *American Journal of Speech-Language Pathology, 14*, 131–143.

Van Riper, C. (1973). *The treatment of stuttering*. Upper Saddle River, NJ: Prentice Hall.

Warren, S. (1991). Enhancing communication and language development with milieu teaching procedures. In E. Cipani (Ed.), *A guide to developing language competence in preschool children with severe and moderate handicaps* (pp. 68–93). Springfield, IL: Charles C. Thomas.

Warren, S.E., & Kaiser, A.P. (1986). Incidental language teaching: A critical review. *Journal of Speech and Hearing Disorders, 51*, 291–299.

Weismer, S., & Evans, J. (2002). The role of processing limitations in early identification of specific language impairment. *Topics in Language Disorders, 22*, 15–29.

Yoder, P.J., & Warren, S. (2001). Relative treatment effects of two prelinguistic communication interventions on language development in toddlers with developmental delays vary by maternal characteristics. *Journal of Speech, Language and Hearing Research, 44*, 224–237.

Yoder, P.J., & Warren, S. (2002). Effects of prelinguistic milieu teaching and parent responsivity education on dyads involving children with intellectual disabilities. *Journal of Speech, Language, and Hearing Research, 45*, 1158–1175.

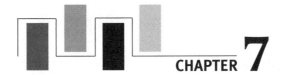

CHAPTER 7

Interviewing, Counseling, and Clinical Communication

Kevin M. McNamara

CHAPTER OBJECTIVES

After reading this chapter, students will be able to

- Identify strategies for engaging in effective oral and written clinical communication
- Recognize cultural factors that influence effective communication
- Describe effective and appropriate counseling in the clinical practice of audiologists and speech-language pathologists
- Differentiate among different written clinical documents and their purposes

As audiologists and speech-language pathologists (SLPs), we are called on to share information during a variety of clinical activities, including interviewing and counseling clients, documenting evaluation findings, developing intervention plans, recording treatment outcomes, and educating caregivers. We must convey information clearly to a wide variety of people, among them clients, families, educators, health care providers, and administrators. To accomplish this task successfully, we need to employ sensitive and efficient strategies for sharing information with the people that we serve. Our effectiveness in communicating information will affect the quality of the therapeutic relationships that we establish with our clients. It will influence our ability to advocate and obtain funding for appropriate services and resources for those whom we serve. Haynes and Pindzola (2012), in speaking of the diagnostic process, note that a written clinical document is an extension of the clinician, whose competence will be evaluated by the quality of the writing. Poorly written clinical documentation can compromise a clinician's professional credibility (Roth & Worthington, 2011), and a poor oral communication style can negatively influence the ability of a clinician to establish trusting relationships with clients and to relate vital clinical information to them. As clinicians for people with communication disorders, we are obligated to be skilled communicators ourselves.

EVIDENCE-BASED PRACTICE AND
ITS RELATION TO CLINICAL COMMUNICATION

Our professional literature continues to reflect the importance of counseling in the clinical management of a variety of communication disorders, including hearing loss (Luterman, 2008; Nelson-Crowell et al., 2009), geriatric–related communication impairment (Rao, 2003), aphasia (Cunningham, 1998), laryngectomy (Blood et al., 1994), stuttering (Shapiro, 2011), and language impairment (Wolter et al., 2006). In our ensuing discussion of clinical communication, as it pertains to interviewing, counseling, and clinical documentation, it will be particularly important to think about how our ability to communicate effectively is an essential factor in providing best clinical practice. Our ability to listen actively and nonjudgmentally, our capacity for empathy and perspective taking, and our skill in absorbing and sharing information will serve as the linkage between research, experience, and client perspective.

BASIC PRINCIPLES OF ORAL AND WRITTEN CLINICAL COMMUNICATION

As clinicians, we rely on a set of principles fostering effective communication in order to exchange information with those whom we serve in a manner that is sensitive and appropriate to their needs. Information shared either orally or in writing should be presented in a way that is concise, well organized, and related to a clearly stated topic. Sensitivity must be shown to issues such as a client's language style, emotional needs, and level of familiarity with the topic being discussed. In the case of written reports, audiologists and SLPs write for a mixed and sometimes unknown audience of readers, many of whom will differ from the author in terms of educational backgrounds, language styles, and cultural perspectives. Unlike direct verbal exchanges, in which a listener has an opportunity to provide verbal and nonverbal feedback in order to clarify or expand the information being presented, there is not always an immediate opportunity for readers to ask for clarification or to confirm their understanding of written information. To increase our effectiveness in both oral and written communication, there are some general principles of effective clinical communication to follow.

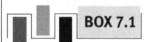 **BOX 7.1** **Principles of Effective Clinical Communication**

In both oral and written presentations, use these strategies:

- Organize all information in a logical, cohesive manner by subtopic.
- Clearly introduce the topic about which you are writing or speaking.
- Avoid using technical language whenever possible. Use vocabulary and a language style easily understood by a wider audience.
- When you cannot avoid using technical terms, explain them parenthetically or by stating examples.

BOX 7.1   *(continued)*

- Whenever possible, use objective terms such as *observed*, *completed*, or *demonstrated*; avoid vague or subjective terms such as *appears* or seemed.
- Avoid redundancy unless you are summarizing key concepts.
- Use "person first-language" (e.g., "a man with aphasia," "a person who stutters") rather than referring to people as disabilities (e.g., "an aphasic," "a stutterer").

During direct verbal exchanges, also use these strategies:

- Attend to the comfort of your listener.
- Explain the purpose of your discussion.
- Establish trust by being an active, empathetic, and nonjudgmental listener.
- Allow the people with whom you are communicating to be active participants in the conversation, ensuring opportunities for them to respond to questions, make comments, and ask questions.
- Remember that individuals comprehend information differently. Provide sufficient time for your listener to process and react to your statements.
- Be sensitive to and respectful of cultural differences and their impact on interpersonal communication. Avoid imposing your own cultural values, especially if they appear to conflict with those of your listener.
- Watch for both verbal and nonverbal cues from your listener to see if you are presenting your message in a way that is understandable and culturally acceptable. Rephrase, expand, or eliminate statements and questions based on these cues.
- Enlist the assistance of interpreters to assist in situations in which you must verbally communicate with people who speak a language different from yours. Exercise extra caution in these situations to ensure that your message is being translated appropriately and that you accurately comprehend the information being conveyed to you via an interpreter.

The information that you, as a clinician, will convey to people may at times be difficult or even painful for them to hear. Shames (2006) reminds us that people's communication problems are integrated into how they see and define themselves and how they feel, think, and act as total human beings. As a new clinician, you may be tempted to avoid confronting your clients with "bad news" regarding their prognoses for improvement or limited achievements in therapy. In addition, clients or administrators may ask you to provide information that you do not have or pressure you into saying or writing statements that you do not believe or cannot substantiate through research or clinical data. Above all else, clinicians are bound by ethical practice to be honest in all interactions with their clients, as well as with those people and agencies that support their clients. The code of ethics of the American Speech-Language-Hearing Association (ASHA, 2010) and the American Academy of Audiology (2011) clearly emphasize your responsibility for truthfulness in all aspects of your clinical practice. The ASHA Code of Ethics states, "Individuals shall not engage in dishonesty, fraud, deceit, or misrepresentation" (ASHA, 2010; see also Appendix 2A). It is possible, however, to share difficult information with your clients in a manner that is supportive, sensitive, and truthful if you employ the principles of effective clinical communication.

MAINTAINING CONFIDENTIALITY OF INFORMATION

Clients, or their legal guardians, ultimately control to whom information is released, and the principle of confidentiality applies to both oral and written communication between clients and clinicians (Silverman, 2003). The Health Insurance Portability and Accountability Act (HIPAA) of 1996 (PL 104-191) requires that all health care organizations, including speech-language pathology and audiology providers, that engage in electronic billing adopt and maintain rigorous standards and procedures to ensure the protection and restriction of client information. The HIPAA law levies severe financial and legal consequences on organizations that fail to keep confidentiality. This public law legally mandates what had been standard ethical practice in our profession for many years, namely, that the information we obtain and record about our clients be kept confidential and restricted to the people directly working with those clients unless our clients provide us with written permission to release such information to others. Principle I, Rule M of the ASHA Code of Ethics states, "Individuals shall adequately maintain and appropriately secure records of professional services rendered, research and scholarly activities conducted, and products dispensed, and they shall allow access to these records only when authorized or when required by law" (ASHA, 2010). As SLPs and audiologists, it is essential that you become knowledgeable of and adhere to the information protection policies of the facilities in which you practice.

STRATEGIES USED TO GATHER AND CONVEY CLINICAL INFORMATION

It is essential to gather as much pertinent background information regarding your clients as you can when you start the process of evaluating their communication needs. You may acquire information through a combination of methods, such as reviewing existing records, conducting interviews, and using written questionnaires. You should be as thorough as possible in exploring all relevant sources of information to which you have been granted access.

Reviewing Existing Records

You have an obligation as a clinician to consider the needs of the clients you serve in the context of their home, school, work, family, and social interactions (Tomblin, 2000). A review of existing records can provide vital clues revealing clients' communication needs in those settings. Other audiologists or SLPs, as well as other health care providers, therapists, or educators, may have already seen the clients who now seek your assistance. These previous encounters may yield medical reports, educational records, previous speech-language and audiological evaluations, and documents summarizing past interventions. You can gain knowledge of previous medical, cognitive, psychological, or psychiatric diagnoses, as well as information regarding clients' social, adaptive, and educational functioning. This information can allow you to make more appropriate decisions relating to evaluation and intervention strategies and avoid recommending interventions that may have been contraindicated by medical status or previously unsuccessful therapies. Remember that clients or their guardians ultimately control to whom information is released. Silverman (2003) reminds us that confidentiality applies to both oral and written communication with and on behalf of our clients.

CASE EXAMPLE 1

Mr. Rodrigues, a 78-year-old man, has just been transferred from an acute care unit in a local hospital to a short-term rehabilitation unit of a skilled nursing facility. He experienced a stroke approximately 2 weeks ago and was evaluated and received speech therapy in the hospital setting prior to his transfer. He has been admitted to the rehabilitation unit with doctor's orders for speech therapy evaluation and intervention to address residual communication and swallowing problems secondary to his stroke.

If you were the SLP evaluating Mr. Rodrigues in the skilled nursing facility, you could, theoretically, assess both his communication and his swallowing status without first looking at the information available from his previous stay in the hospital acute care unit. By doing so, though, you would miss vital information essential to the safe and effective management of this client. For example, it would be important for you to review information regarding his ability to swallow safely, as determined by a modified barium swallow study performed in the hospital setting, prior to initiating dysphagia (swallowing) therapy. Implementing therapy procedures, diet modifications, or feeding protocols based on insufficient information about the client's functioning in this area may put him at risk for aspiration and other related and potentially life-threatening medical complications such as pneumonia. Specific information regarding the nature of the client's brain damage, as revealed through a computed topography scan, and more general medical information regarding the client's overall health status will help you to determine treatment goals and a realistic prognosis for improvement. Access to this information will allow you to better understand the origin of the client's impairment and to make more appropriate intervention decisions that are consistent with his medical status and potential for improvement.

CASE EXAMPLE 2

Susan, a 7-year-old girl with a severe bilateral sensorineural hearing loss, has recently moved with her family to a new home in a different state. She currently wears two behind-the-ear hearing aids. She has been referred to a local audiologist's office for an audiological reassessment and to explore the possibility of being fitted with a frequency modulation (FM) amplification system to enhance her classroom listening skills.

In Susan's example, it is essential that the new audiologist has an opportunity to review previous findings regarding this client's hearing status in order to monitor for potential deterioration of hearing across time. A review of previous audiological evaluations, recommendations for hearing aids and other assistive listening devices, and follow-up documentation of audiological intervention will allow the audiologist to make better decisions regarding the assessment and management of the client's audiological needs. In addition, reviewing related educational and speech-language pathology records will allow the audiologist to understand the functional, social, and academic communication needs of the client and to offer recommendations for equipment and audiological management strategies that are appropriate for those needs and settings.

As you review existing records, you must remember that "information from other professionals can potentially lead to a biased view of your client's condition" (Shipley & McAfee, 2009, p. 73). Similarly, Groopman (2007) cautions against the phenomenon of "availability," in which your own recent or frequent past experiences influence your clinical decision making. When you make clinical decisions, it is essential that you balance your own current clinical observations and findings with the information reported from other sources and be vigilant for thought biases based on prior experiences.

Conducting Interviews

One of the most useful ways to gain insight into the needs and backgrounds of clients is by directly interviewing them and the people who know them. An **interview** is a flexible and multifaceted process that is guided by the clinician and constructed by all participants (see Figure 7.1). It is a vehicle for gathering relevant information and educating people on issues related to communication disorders. Often, it is the first opportunity to begin to establish a trusting and cooperative relationship with clients and their families. Interviewing is a task that requires you to employ active listening skills (Luterman, 2008; Shames, 2006); to be sensitive to individual personal, cultural, and linguistic styles (Battle, 2011; Coleman, 2000); and to exercise flexibility in questioning

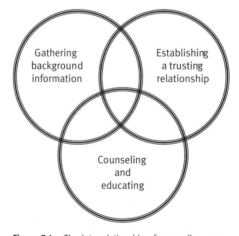

Figure 7.1. The interrelationship of counseling, questioning, and trust building in a clinical interview.

and responding to the information being shared. In addition to interviewing your clients and their families, you may interview doctors, nurses, caregivers, classroom teachers, special educators, social workers, vocational counselors, and clinicians from other disciplines, including physical and occupational therapists and psychologists.

Establishing Trust

Shapiro (2011), when discussing interviews related to stuttering assessment, noted the importance of clinicians, clients, and families first recognizing and respecting each other as people in order to interact effectively in a professional domain. Rollin, in his discussion of facilitating a counseling relationship, encouraged us to value our clients as individuals first and to "separate the disorder from the person" (2000, p. 24). Being sensitive to differences in cultural styles can help clinicians better establish understanding, respect, and trust during an interview (Lynch & Hanson, 2011; Shipley & McAfee, 2009). For example, Latino clients and their families may view an initial period of informal talking as an appropriate prelude to more serious discussions, whereas an attempt to discuss such issues immediately may be considered rude (Anderson & Fenichel, 1989; Zungia, 2011). Conversely, members of many other cultural groups may find it disrespectful if too casual an approach is taken during an interview, as may African Americans, whose cultural traditions often call for a high level of formality, especially when addressing seniors (Goode, Jones, & Hopkins Jackson, 2011).

Maintaining Appropriate Professional Boundaries

As we clinicians establish trusting and empathetic relationships with our clients through effective interview and counseling strategies, we may set the stage for our clients to engage in the process of *transference*. From a psychodynamic standpoint, this concept refers to the process by which "the counselor becomes the object for, target of, and the symbol of the client's emotional expressions" (Shames, 2006, p. 84). Shames (2006) noted that this transference was a natural result of establishing a trusting relationship between client and clinician. These emotional expressions from a client can take many forms, from personal questions to romantic inclinations, and Shames cautioned clinicians to try to understand the function of these expressions and not to view them as necessarily a personal threat. In addition, Flasher and Fogle (2012) reminded us, as clinicians we may engage in *countertransference*, in which our responses will be influenced by the emotions and past experiences that are evoked during our interaction with our clients. By identifying what in our relationship with a client may have triggered these emotions, we may develop insight into the factors affecting that therapeutic relationship. Clinicians, however, may share their own personal feelings only if the expression of those feelings will facilitate the therapeutic process. Stone and Olswang (1989) noted the importance of establishing limitations on the content, focus, and style of the counseling efforts of SLPs and audiologists. They suggested that the expression of attitudes and questions relating to the presenting communication disorder is within an appropriate content boundary for audiologists and SLPs, but other topics not related to communication disorders are out of bounds and may necessitate referring the client to other sources of support.

Using Appropriate Question Formats to Elicit Information

Clinicians rely on a variety of question types to elicit information during an interview. Open-ended questions, or comments, are typically used to initiate an interview, allowing the person being questioned to establish the direction of the interview and express issues that he or she holds as priorities. These questions encourage the client to be an active participant rather than a passive respondent in the interview process. Hall and Morris (2000) noted that by using open-ended questions, clinicians, though controlling the general background areas being explored, do not control the range of responses elicited from the client or how extensively he or she responds. Such questions or statements as "How can I help you today?" or "Tell me about the trouble you're having hearing" allow the clinician to relinquish to the respondent some of the control held in an interview, leading to increased trust and willingness to share information about sensitive and important issues.

After the client has had an opportunity to express priority concerns by responding to open-ended questions, the clinician may find it necessary to use closed questions that narrow the range of responses and elicit more specific information. There are a finite number of possible answers to such questions as "How much did your son weigh when he was born?" or "When was your last hearing evaluation?" The use of such question forms allows the interviewer to regain more control of the interview and focus on specific clinical issues. A particularly narrow form of closed questions is one that requires only a yes or no response. This type of question requires the respondent to confirm or deny statements made by the clinician and allows the client no control over the intent or direction of the question. Closed questions are, by design, limiting. Shipley and Roseberry-McKibbin remind us that though useful, "relying on too many closed questions ... can be detrimental to a relationship or can result in clinicians not understanding some of an interviewee's major areas of concern or interest" (2006, p. 76).

As with all interpersonal interactions, cultural values and styles may affect how people respond to certain question forms. For African American clients, direct questions may, at times, be seen as rude or overly personal (Shipley & McAfee, 2009), and disagreement by an African American listener may be conveyed through silence. Latino clients, out of respect for people in professional roles, may refrain from openly expressing disagreement with a clinician's statements even though they may not agree with the clinician (Langdon & Cheng, 1992). Members of some Asian cultures, to avoid offending a person, may say what they think the listener wants to hear, rather than what they themselves believe (Shipley & McAfee, 2009; Roseberry-McKibbin, 2008). Gender differences also play a part in how a respondent may answer questions, and this may especially be the case with some Middle Eastern cultures that place restrictions on the content and format of interactions between people of different genders (Sharifzadeh, 2011). Even within the broader collective American culture, differences in communication styles often demonstrated by both genders may lead to miscommunication. This difference can be seen in a woman's affirmative head nod to indicate active listening and empathy and a man's use of the same gesture to convey agreement (Maltz & Borker, 1982). A more comprehensive discussion of multicultural issues related to communication disorders can be found in Chapter 10.

Case History Questionnaires

A written **case history questionnaire** is a tool that is used to gather and organize information regarding the nature of speech, language, and hearing concerns; general developmental and health history; educational background; and history of related support services. By presenting both general and specific questions, it attempts to elicit a client's opinion of the communication disorder and its effect on daily communication. Case history questionnaires may be broad in their scope of questions related to communication or may be customized to include questions related to specific issues such as hearing loss, auditory processing disorder, fluency or voice disorders, and augmentative communication needs. Separate formats are typically used for adults and children (see Figure 7.2 for an adult format).

Name: _____   D.O.B: _____

Examiner: _____   Date: _____

1. How old were you when your hearing loss was first identified?

2. What have you done about your hearing loss?

3. What do you feel is the cause of your hearing problem?

4. Has a physician examined your ears?

   Who?   Date of last exam?

5. Have you experienced pain in either of your ears?   When?

   Describe.

6. Have you ever had ear infections (running ears)?

   Which ear?   When?

7. Have there been any changes in your hearing in the last six months?

   Last year?

   Last 2 years?

8. Do you have any allergies?   Describe.

9. Do you ever feel dizzy?   How often?

10. Does your hearing seem better on some days than on others?

11. Have you ever worn a hearing aid?

Figure 7.2. Sample questions found on an audiological case history form for adults.

In some practice settings, clients or caregivers are asked to complete a case history questionnaire prior to arriving or a few minutes before the start of their initial diagnostic evaluation. As clinicians, you must be cautious, however, that you do not make your clients' first task the completion of a long, jargon-filled, and often confusing and intimidating questionnaire form, thereby creating a barrier for people who are attempting to gain access to clinical services. Alternatively, case history questionnaires may serve as a flexible guide for topics during person-to-person diagnostic or intake interviews. You may find the structure offered by such forms useful as you develop skills in the areas of interview and evaluation, but you should not rely too much on the rigid format of written case history questionnaires during client interviews, which can serve as a barrier to more spontaneous and meaningful communication (Haynes & Pindzola, 2012).

FORMATS FOR CONVEYING CLINICAL INFORMATION

The formats you use to share information with your clients and those individuals and agencies that support them are influenced by a number of factors. The type of information being conveyed, as well as the audience with whom the information is being shared, may in part determine whether you use a structured versus informal or written versus oral format. Specific speech-language pathology or audiology programs or facilities may follow policies that dictate the use of particular formats for documenting evaluation results, intervention programs, and outcome data. For example, early intervention programs for children birth to 3 years of age, school-based services for children 3 to 21 years of age, and geriatric speech-language pathology and audiology services funded by Medicare all have documentation requirements, formats, and time lines influenced by federal, state, and local policies.

Electronic Medical Records

Increasingly, medical and rehabilitation settings in which audiologists and SPLs work are employing **electronic medical records** (EMRs) to expedite the management, storage, and exchange of patient information. In this mode of record keeping, patient information is entered into standardized electronic templates accessed through desktop computers or handheld tablets and digitally archived in an access-restricted server. Different templates may exist for the type of assessment done, service provided, or setting in which service was delivered. These templates will allow you to record evaluation and therapy findings, diagnoses, recommendations, and diagnostic coding for billing purposes, among other pertinent information. The purported advantages to EMRs are numerous and include reduced cost and space associated with record storage, efficiency in collating and disseminating patient information, ease and immediacy of updating, ease and accuracy of billing, and the reduction of medical errors due to incomplete documentation or illegible records; disadvantages include potential breech of privacy through unauthorized electronic access, as well as fixed reporting formats that may restrict content and interpretation of information (Jha et al., 2009; Loomis, Reis, Saywell, & Thakker, 2002; Salomon et al., 2010; Wright et al., 2010). Figure 7.3 provides a sample EMR.

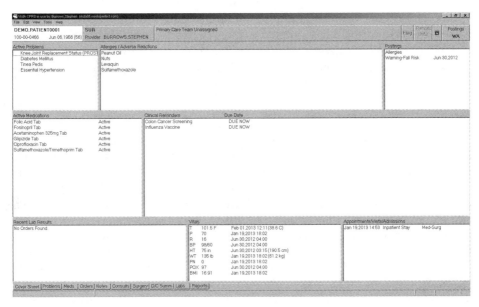

Figure 7.3. Sample electronic medical record. (*Source:* Neehr Perfect® networked educational EHR featuring WorldVistA. Courtesy of Archetype Innovations, LLC 2013.)

Regulations set forth in HIPAA address the concern over the security and privacy of EMRs by evoking clear mandates regarding the restriction of access to authorized entities only, with substantial legal and monitory penalties levied for both accidental and willful unauthorized dissemination of protected information. The adoption of EMRs in rehabilitation and health care settings is a work in progress at the time of this writing. The Health Information Technology for Economic and Clinical Health Act, enacted under Title XIII of the American Recovery and Reinvestment Act (ARRA) of 2009 (PL 111-5), however, provides financial incentives from the Centers for Medicare and Medicaid Services for the adoption of EMRs and, starting in 2014, penalties for not doing so.

Evaluation Reports

Written **diagnostic evaluation reports** are used to summarize information obtained in both audiological and speech-language evaluations. These reports serve as an official record of assessment findings, diagnoses, and recommendations (Meitus, 1983) and as a written description of the hearing and communication profiles of the individuals who are being evaluated. They are legal documents that may, as is the case with all written documentation, be called into legal proceedings to determine service provision and liability issues. The actual format for an evaluation report will vary across settings and sometimes by individual clinician. The format may include specific outlines for individually written reports or, in some cases, prewritten paper or electronic forms or checklists into which the details and interpretations from a client's evaluation are inserted. Regardless of the format, most evaluation reports contain specific sections summarizing background information, a summary of test results and diagnostic observations, interpretations of findings, prognosis for improvement, and recommendations. A well-formulated diagnostic report is one that presents all information in an organized and sequential manner and efficiently integrates all diagnostic data, interpretations, and recommendations. The structure of a diagnostic report is examined in greater detail later in this chapter.

Oral Reports and Conferences

Interactions with clients may involve sharing information orally as well as in writing. You will answer questions from your clients, their family members, and their caregivers on an ongoing basis regarding intervention procedures and outcomes. With their written permission, you may share with teachers, program administrators, and insurers information concerning your clients' communication needs in order to advocate for the materials, resources, or funding necessary for adequate intervention of the clients' communication disorders. The expanding role that SLPs and audiologists play in providing collaborative intervention has increased the frequency and importance of orally reporting information regarding clients' communication needs (ASHA, 1991, 2002; National Joint Committee for the Communication Needs of Persons with Severe Disabilities, 2003).

Case conferences are focused opportunities to present information to or about your clients. During these exchanges, you may follow a more systematic approach to sharing information than you do in more casual oral reports. The specific content may be dictated by the purpose of the conference as well as by the needs of the participants. Examples of formal case conferences include individual meetings with clients and their families and conferences with teachers to discuss their students' communication needs in the classroom setting. Clinicians working in hospitals or rehabilitation centers may meet with other therapists, medical personnel, caregivers, and family members to discuss their clients' progress in therapy and service needs. Regardless of the setting, audiologists and SLPs are responsible for presenting information in a succinct and organized manner that is easily understood by clients as well as those individuals who support them.

Intervention Plans

After an initial assessment of speech, language, and/or hearing, the need for intervention is determined. This decision is based on evaluation findings, client and family priorities, program eligibility requirements, and other related factors. Once the decision is made to begin an intervention, a formal intervention plan is developed. The formats and required terminology for intervention plans may be determined by both federal and state regulations governing a particular type of service delivery program. Examples of comprehensive intervention plans that outline a broad range of supports and outcomes include school-based **individualized education programs** (IEPs) and **individualized family service plans** (IFSPs) for children from birth to 3 years of age who are enrolled in early intervention programs. In medically based rehabilitation settings funded by Medicare, specific intervention plans outline the skilled services that only a certified SLP may perform, although **functional maintenance plans** are developed to identify nonskilled communication supports that are provided by noncertified support staff, family members, and other caregivers.

In your initial clinical training, you may be asked to develop intervention plans that outline individual sessions of speech, language, and audiology intervention in detail. These plans usually include long-term goals and short-term objectives related to speech, language, hearing, and other communication needs. Targeted communication behaviors are identified, as well as the conditions under which they are expected to occur, and measurable criteria for success are stated for each behavior. Intervention techniques, activities, and materials are listed as well. Such plans serve as a guide from which clinicians organize and implement individual therapy sessions and are similar in purpose to the lesson plans developed by classroom teachers. During your clinical training, you may be asked to develop intervention plans that offer a large amount of detail in order to facilitate your understanding of intervention and documentation processes.

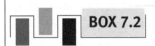 **BOX 7.2** | **Individual Intervention Plan for Speech-Language Therapy**

Long-term Goal(s)

José will increase his recognition and use of picture communication symbols in order to express needs and participate in classroom activities.

Short-term Objective(s)

1. José will match 10 newly introduced picture symbols depicting classroom materials with the actual objects they represent.

2. José will point to the above-mentioned picture symbols presented on a picture symbol communication board when named by the clinician.

3. José will request a minimum of two items needed during a classroom activity by pointing to an appropriate picture symbol on a picture symbol board with no more than verbal prompting from the clinician.

Procedures

Verbal instruction, visual modeling of the targeted behavior, physical cuing, verbal reinforcement

Activities

1. Object–picture matching using the "Treasure Hunt" game

   Short-term objective(s) targeted during activity: 1

   Materials needed: picture symbol cards, corresponding objects

2. Arts and crafts project based on curriculum-based reading theme

   Short-term objective(s) targeted during activity: 2, 3

   Materials needed: picture communication board, corresponding objects, craft material, storybook

SOAP Notes

Therapeutic intervention is a dynamic process in which continual changes to therapy objectives and activities are made in response to a client's performance and to new information revealed through ongoing assessment. The **SOAP note**—with the acronym standing for Subjective, Objective, Assessment, and Plan—is a format often used in medical and other settings to record and analyze data specific to a client's ongoing performance in therapy (Golper, 1998). SOAP notes are documents summarizing the clinician's observations regarding the conditions affecting a client's level of attention and participation in therapy (i.e., subjective), specific data regarding performance on therapy tasks (i.e., objective), interpretation of those subjective observations and objective data (i.e., assessment), and recommendations for future action based on that interpretation (i.e., plan). These notes may be quick handwritten entries in a client's chart in a hospital or rehabilitation setting or may take the form of more extensive reports summarizing a client's progress in therapy. The SOAP note format may also be used for reporting more detailed diagnostic findings.

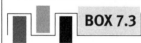 **BOX 7.3**   **A Brief Progress Report in a SOAP Format**

Subjective: Mr. Smith was alert and oriented during today's session. Nursing staff reported an increase in the number of hours he was awake and in his general orientation to surroundings since yesterday evening. Mrs. Smith (his wife) was present during the last half of therapy and reported that he was frustrated the night before at his inability to "find the right words."

Objective: Mr. Smith pointed to pictures of familiar household items with 75% accuracy (15/20) when named by the clinician and with 80% accuracy (8/10) by function. He named 20% (2/10) of the same pictures with maximum cuing from the clinician. Severe dysarthria persisted, negatively affecting speech intelligibility. Imitation of lingual movements (tongue tip elevation, lateralization, and tongue retraction) was slow and labored.

Assessment: Mr. Smith continues to demonstrate severe word-finding problems negatively influencing functional communication, as well as limited speech intelligibility secondary to oral motor weakness. An increase in word recognition and overall alertness and orientation to communication partners was noted since the last intervention session.

Plan: Continue speech therapy for 30 minutes per day, targeting increased word finding and speech intelligibility. Provide a picture board of common objects to facilitate Mr. Smith's word finding when he is conversing with his wife and the staff. Counsel Mrs. Smith regarding strategies to facilitate word finding and to repair communication breakdowns.

Progress Reports

At periodic intervals throughout the course of your clients' intervention, you will be required to summarize and document their cumulative progress toward achieving targeted intervention goals and to make recommendations regarding their need for continued therapy. These intervals are typically determined by the regulations governing the specific program in which the service is provided and the funding source requirements, and these intervals may vary from 1 month or less to 1 year or more. In these days of increasing demands on clinicians' time and increasingly limited funding for clinical services, it has become critical for clinicians to make carefully documented decisions regarding the continued need for intervention based on client outcome data. Progress reports are used as vehicles to summarize and review a client's cumulative achievement of intervention goals and objectives across a specific period and to outline the future direction of intervention. Typically, such reports contain brief background information, a summary of specific goals and objectives, a data-based analysis of the client's progress, an interpretation of the data, a prognosis for change, and a recommendation regarding the need for and direction of future intervention.

Discharge Summaries

Discharge from audiology and speech-language pathology services is based on a number of interrelated factors. These may include a client's progress (or lack of progress) toward targeted objectives, achievement of functional communication status, successful fitting and use of hearing aids or other assistive listening devices, and changing priorities regarding communication intervention (ASHA, 2004). A **discharge summary** is a written report of a client's cumulative progress from the initiation of therapy to his or her discharge. As in the case of a progress report, a summary and interpretation of a client's accomplishments and continued needs are made based on a review of cumulative client performance data, the clinician's judgment regarding the client's prognosis for further change, and other related variables. Recommendations for necessary postintervention supports or services are typically offered.

Professional Correspondence

Audiologists and SLPs often exchange information regarding clients with other professionals serving those same individuals. A variety of written correspondence formats are used to share client information, including **referral letters** to other service providers, **follow-up letters** to those professionals referring clients, and requests for the release of information from other service providers. At times, clinicians write **letters of justification** to advocate for diagnostic or therapy services, hearing aids, FM systems, communication devices, and other supports for their clients. In accordance with HIPAA regulations and the ASHA Code of Ethics (ASHA, 2010), written permission must be obtained from a client before any information can be released among practitioners or agencies, and clients have the final decision about what information, if any, may be released and to whom.

REPORTING DIAGNOSTIC FINDINGS

It is essential for SLPs and audiologists to share diagnostic assessment findings in a manner that is efficient, well organized, and clearly understood by all who need access to this information. This process may begin with a verbal review shared with your client and his or her family or caregivers immediately after the completion of the evaluation and continues with a written summary of findings that becomes a permanent record of this information.

Evaluation Feedback

Anyone seeking the help of professionals generally expects to have at least some feedback regarding findings immediately following an evaluation. Think about your last trip to your doctor for a comprehensive physical examination. Although you know that your doctor will not have the results of blood tests, throat cultures, or other lab tests immediately following your examination, you expect him or her to take a few minutes to summarize the general findings and their implications regarding your overall health status. Failure to do so would certainly leave you in a state of uncertainty and anxiety, potentially reducing your confidence in the physician's ability to effectively evaluate and manage your health needs. Individuals who seek a clinician's help in diagnosing hearing loss, swallowing, speech, language, and other communication disorders have a similar need for immediate feedback, and they experience many of the same concerns if a summary of the findings at the conclusion of the evaluation is not provided.

How can you immediately summarize your evaluation findings before you have had time to score tests, transcribe language samples, or carefully analyze the relationship between all the diagnostic data collected during the course of an evaluation? First, clearly state that all comments made during follow-up counseling sessions are only your first impressions of diagnostic findings and will be subject to possible revision after you have had time to carefully analyze the information that you have collected. Second, review the purpose of the assessment activities and your initial impression of the outcomes of each in order to help the client begin to understand both the reasons for those activities and their implications concerning his or her communication status. Such a review provides you with a systematic and sequential structure through which to begin to relay your findings and helps you to convey information in smaller segments more easily processed by your client.

In addition to providing a mechanism to summarize evaluation results, engaging in postevaluation feedback presents an opportunity for audiologists and SLPs to continue the process of educating clients about communication disorders that began during the preassessment interview, a very important step in developing a partnership between the client and clinician. As is the case during an initial interview, the style in which you present information when counseling a client after an evaluation is as important as the content. Haynes and Pindzola cautioned, "Refrain from being didactic; do not lecture your clients. Focus on sharing options rather than giving advice" (2012, p. 44). You should begin your discussion with a summary of strengths demonstrated by the client and transition to areas of weakness in measured increments based on your perceptions of his or her ability to accept and process that information. Incorporate information about normal processes of hearing and communication; also, relate this information to the profile of communication strengths and needs that you have identified for your client.

Again, as in all clinical interactions, use language that is readily understood by clients, their family, and their caregivers. You must be alert to both verbal and nonverbal signals from your listeners regarding their level of understanding, and you should paraphrase or modify the style and content of your statements accordingly. Remember that the counseling following a diagnostic assessment often takes place immediately after a long and sometimes arduous evaluation session that may leave the participants fatigued and emotionally drained. Too much technical information, information presented in a rapid and confusing manner, or information that is presented in a style inconsistent with the clients' cultures may be difficult to understand. For example, in a 2010 survey of 84 patients receiving in-hospital medical services, Olson and Windish noted that significant differences exist between patients' and physicians' impressions about information and care provided, highlighting the potential miscommunication between patient and health care provider. Margolis (2004) noted that information presented in a clear, easy-to-understand format to clients about their communication disorders is remembered better than information presented in a more complex manner. Because some individual and cultural interaction styles may preclude listeners from letting you know that they do not understand what you are saying (Shipley & McAfee, 2009), you must not assume that your clients have comprehended your message simply because they nodded their heads or verbally agreed. You should allow opportunities for follow-up questions, and you should listen carefully to these questions to judge the listeners' comprehension of the information that you have presented.

By maintaining a flexible style in which you encourage ongoing comments and questions from your clients as you present diagnostic findings, you will create a two-way flow of communication that fosters a trusting therapeutic relationship. Remember that counseling remains an ongoing dynamic process woven into the continuum of clinical activities and does not end with the reporting of diagnostic findings. You must be prepared to develop and maintain an appropriate counseling role throughout the entire course of intervention.

Diagnostic Evaluation Reports

A diagnostic evaluation report serves as a tool for organizing, integrating, and interpreting information regarding a client's hearing and communication skills. A thorough report summarizes background information pertaining to a client's presenting concern, gives results of evaluation measures and observations, and allows for a discussion of the implication of those findings as related to the person's communication needs and potential. As do all clinical records, diagnostic reports serve as legal documentation of assessment activities and findings long after the diagnostic event has passed. Both audiology and speech-language pathology reports are divided into subsections to more clearly organize information. The exact format and section headings of reports may vary from setting to setting but typically include background information, test results and other diagnostic data and observations, a summary, and recommendations based on the findings of the evaluation. In some settings, these sections follow the SOAP format. Figure 7.4 shows an example of a format for a speech-language diagnostic report from a university speech-and-hearing clinic.

Name: D.O.B: C.A.:
Address:
Phone(s): (H):   (W):   (C):
Parent/guardian/spouse: Relationship to client:
Referral source:
Date of evaluation:
Supervisor: Clinician:

Background:

- State referral information/reason for evaluation.
- Summarize birth/developmental history as appropriate.
- Identify primary language(s).
- Comment on findings of previous communication evaluations, other related evaluations.
- List medical/developmental diagnoses which relate to presenting communication disorder.
- Identify educational placement/modifications (children).
- Summarize history of past and current speech and language intervention; contacts made with other service providers.

Evaluation Conditions:

- Describe testing conditions (location, length of time, use of interpreter, augmentative communication, etc.).
- Describe client behavior during evaluation (attentiveness, cooperation, etc.).
- State your level of confidence in your findings, based on the above factors.

Results:

- List standardized tests used, describe their purpose, and list scores obtained.
- List observed and derived data from non-standardized evaluation tasks (MLU, frequency of stuttering, summary of language strengths and weaknesses, etc.).

Interpretation:

- Describe findings related to presenting communication concerns (receptive language, expressive language, oral-motor skills, speech production, voice, fluency, hearing, etc.).
- Synthesize data listed in the *Results* section.
- Answer diagnostic questions you posed when planning the evaluation.
- Conclude with a short statement summarizing findings, diagnosis, and contributing factors.
- State prognosis for improvement.

Recommendations:

- State all recommendations as options to consider, not mandates to follow.
- Present menus of options to achieve same result, if possible.
- Include suggestions for additional evaluations, related services, when appropriate.
- Provide suggestions for therapy goals and objectives, as well as frequency and duration of therapy, when appropriate.

_____   _____
John Doe, B.A.   Jane Smith, M.A. CCC/SLP
Graduate Student Clinician   Supervising Speech-Language Pathologist

Figure 7.4. Speech-language evaluation format.

Identifying Information All reports begin with a section identifying the client who was evaluated, as well as providing other pertinent information regarding the type, setting, and date(s) of evaluation. The name of the clinician who conducted the evaluation, as well as his or her credentials, must be clearly listed. Other identifying information includes the client's address and telephone number, primary languages, parents or guardians if appropriate, and referral source. It is extremely important to list complete and accurate identifying information to facilitate record keeping and assure confidentiality.

Background History Most diagnostic evaluations are at best a snapshot in time, reflecting the test data and observations collected during a limited period and often under conditions that do not represent the typical communication environments of the person being tested. One way that you can attempt to compensate for this partial view of your client's communication skills is to summarize background information collected through written case histories, record reviews, and personal interviews with the client and his or her family members, educators, or other caregivers. This summary should be a succinct overview of medical and developmental diagnoses related to the presenting communication concerns; findings of previous speech, language, and audiological evaluations; and evaluations from other disciplines and reviews of any past or current speech, language, or audiological intervention. In the case of children, background summaries typically include a birth and developmental history and information regarding educational placement and related support services. In the case of adults, educational and vocational history is usually summarized. The individual's primary and any secondary languages should be identified, as well as any other considerations unique to the person that may influence the interpretation of evaluation findings. Caution should be taken to include only information relevant to the assessment being completed, with heightened sensitivity to the confidential nature of some of the information that may have been shared with you.

Evaluation Conditions and Results In the results section of a diagnostic report, all standardized tests and nonstandardized assessment procedures are listed, along with a brief explanation of what each test or procedure attempted to accomplish. Normative test scores, data from nonstandardized evaluation tasks, and behavioral observations are listed in a brief narrative or table format. In speech-language evaluation reports, this section may contain a summary of communication strengths and weaknesses, whereas an audiological evaluation might report the results of a client's response to trial fittings of hearing aids, FM systems, and other assistive listening devices. A description of the testing conditions, duration of testing, adaptations to standardized test administration protocols, and level of cooperation and attention demonstrated by the individual being assessed is typically included to assist in appropriately interpreting evaluation results. Detailed analysis of evaluation findings, however, is usually reserved for the *interpretation* section of the report.

Interpretation Once the clinician has successfully summarized all the data, he or she must then interpret those data to draw conclusions regarding the communication status of the individual. Similar to research projects, all communication evaluations begin with the evaluator framing a series of questions regarding the client's communication and hearing status (Tomblin, 2000). These questions guide the evaluator and provide the foundation for interpreting all evaluation results. In the interpretation section of an evaluation report, the clinician compares and interprets the data collected in relation to these questions or hypotheses. Because the data collected during an evaluation do not always point to the same conclusions, as clinician you must consider these data in relation to client behavior, evaluation conditions, pertinent background information, and other related factors in order to make a thoughtful interpretation of their meaning and draw conclusions relevant to your initial questions. You will not always be able to definitively answer the questions that you initially set out to explore during the evaluation. Based on careful interpretation of diagnostic data, however, you should be able to integrate and summarize the knowledge you have gained through the evaluation process and identify diagnostic questions that remain fully or partially unanswered, if any. Based on this summary, you must also include a statement of prognosis, estimating the likelihood that the individual can improve (or maintain) communication or hearing skills.

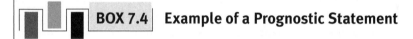

BOX 7.4 **Example of a Prognostic Statement**

Prognosis for improvement of Jon's speech intelligibility through the elimination of speech sound errors appears fair to good, given his ability to imitate developmentally appropriate speech sounds and his strong family and educational support systems.

Recommendations The recommendations section of a diagnostic report is often the first, and sometimes the only, section to be read by the numerous individuals who will review this document. In this section, recommendations regarding the need for follow-up intervention are stated, based on the data collected during the evaluation and the conclusions outlined in the preceding interpretation section. The recommendations section reflects the culmination of the diagnostic process and serves as an important tool for determining an individual's need and eligibility for service. You may make recommendations for additional testing, either within the domain of the current evaluation or by professionals in other disciplines. Recommendations for equipment such as hearing aids and other assistive listening devices, augmentative and alternative communication devices, or educational materials can be stated. Recommendations can also be included for modifications to home, educational, and vocational routines to better enhance communication skills in those settings. Potential intervention goals and objectives and the suggested frequency, duration, and mode of intervention may be outlined. Realistic recommendations should be offered based on the individual client's needs and the priorities and values held by the client, his or her family members, and their community. Other factors necessary to implement the recommendations include the client's health status and the availability of time, money, and other resources. Recommendation statements usually take the form of numbered or bulleted statements but may at times include more narrative descriptions of recommended intervention strategies, adaptive equipment, or environmental or educational modifications.

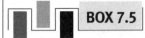 **BOX 7.5   Examples of Recommendation Statements**

1. Anita will benefit from speech-language intervention targeting the development of age-appropriate language and speech skills necessary for her successful participation in academic tasks and social routines. Specific focus should be placed on

    •   Increased speech intelligibility through the elimination of the sound error patterns of fronting and final consonant deletion

    •   Increased use of age-appropriate syntax, including auxiliary verb forms, prepositions, and the possessive marker /s/

    •   Increased comprehension of vocabulary related to curricular and social demands

2. Anita should continue to be monitored regularly for signs of middle-ear infection and receive medical intervention as needed to minimize the risk of transient hearing loss due to middle-ear infection.

3. The SLP should collaborate with the classroom teacher to develop intervention activities that can be supported in the context of classroom-based activities.

CONTRIBUTING TO COMPREHENSIVE SERVICE PLANS

Audiologists and SLPs often serve as contributing members of interdisciplinary and/or transdisciplinary service teams composed of service providers from multiple disciplines, as well as clients, families, and other stakeholders. In this capacity, you will be called on to assist in the development of comprehensive service plans outlining the educational or rehabilitative supports offered to your clients. The formats of these plans will vary based on the age of the client and the service delivery setting. Regardless of their format, all such plans serve as a legal mechanism for detailing the supports to be offered to a client, the time lines for delivery of these services, the people responsible for providing these supports, and the mechanisms for evaluating outcomes.

Individualized Family Service Plans

When the Education for All Handicapped Children Act of 1975 (PL 94-142) was reauthorized as the Education of the Handicapped Act Amendments of 1986 (PL

99-457), it introduced Part H in order to create a federally supported mechanism for the provision of early intervention services for children from birth to 3 years of age who demonstrated substantial and measurable delays in key developmental areas. More recently, the Individuals with Disabilities Education Improvement Act (IDEA) of 2004 (PL 108-446) reauthorized that legislation, continuing a mechanism for early intervention as Part C. Early intervention services include adaptive and self-help skills (e.g., bathing, feeding, dressing), cognitive skills, physical development (e.g., gross and fine motor skills, hearing, vision), social and emotional development, and receptive and expressive communication skills. Services provided through this program are based on the concept of family-centered practice (see Chapter 12), with the child's family members serving as key team members and determiners of the type and focus of the intervention services. Assessment and intervention are implemented in the child's natural environment, and a major focus is placed not only on the specific developmental needs of the child but also on the needs of the child's family members.

Upon referral, a child undergoes a transdisciplinary developmental evaluation by members of the birth-to-3 team. If the child meets eligibility requirements, team members will meet with the family to develop an IFSP. A written IFSP document is developed to capture information about a child's needs and how the child's family and their birth-to-3 service providers will work together to address those needs. This document contains outcomes identified by the family for their child, actions to take to achieve these outcomes, and strategies for assessing progress (see Figure 7.5).

Child/Family Outcomes

Outcome #:	1	of	4	

What we want to see for our child or family is:
That he will be able to use words to tell us what he wants

How will we know when we are making progress or we are done? (i.e., how to measure it or when do we hope to see it) These are the next steps or objectives we will work toward.   Timeline

He will make more different sounds.	May 2014
He will use syllables with one consonant and one vowel.	July 2014
He will start to repeat words people say to him.	September 2014

What will we do to accomplish this? (i.e., Describe how the child / family will participate in a routine by doing activities-specific behaviors.) Strategies we'll all use include:

We will talk to our child about what we are doing during bath time, dressing, dinner, and other things we do every day.

We will read picture books to our child, naming pictures and describing what is happening in them.

When our child makes sounds, we will repeat them back playfully, adding new sounds to the mix.

When our child reaches or points to something, we will name it and when appropriate help him get it.

Figure 7.5. Summary of child and family outcomes on a birth-to-3 individual family service plan (IFSP). (*Source:* Connecticut Birth-to-Three System, 2013.)

Name: _Tonya Williams_   **DOB:** _2/3/11_   **Date:** _2/18/14_

What is going to happen	Delivered by (discipline responsible)	Location	How often	How long	Start date	End date
Instructional home visit	Early intervention specialist (teacher)	Family's home	Once a week	1 hour	3/5/14	2/2/15
Speech therapy consultation	Speech-language pathologist	Family's home	Once a month	1 hour	3/1/14	1/12/15
Nursing consultation	Nurse	Family's home	Twice a month	1 hour	3/10/14	2/10/15

Figure 7.6.   Early intervention services and supports. (*Source:* Connecticut Birth-to-Three System, 2013.)

More global family needs, such as access to health care or adequate shelter or the needs of other siblings, are also discussed in recognition of the influence that such considerations have on the child's development. Early intervention specialists assist the family in identifying their priorities for support and then aid in developing a plan to meet those needs, helping the family to access needed services both within and outside of the birth-to-3 program. At times, the priorities stated by the family may differ from the priorities set by other team members, including the SLP and audiologist, but family-generated priorities always take precedence. Once the child's strengths and needs and the family's priorities are identified, a plan of services and supports is developed. The team outlines in the plan the type of supports needed, the service provider's responsibilities, and the location and schedule of the intervention services (see Figure 7.6). The completed IFSP document becomes the working guide to the child and family's participation in the birth-to-3 program. The document will be reviewed by the early intervention team periodically throughout the period that the child is enrolled in the program and revised as needed. As is the case with all the clinical intervention and documentation formats, you must rely on a style of presenting information that is clear, supportive, and respectful to the needs of the families with whom you are working.

Individualized Education Programs

The Education for All Handicapped Children Act (PL 94-142) was passed in 1975, ensuring a free and appropriate public education and related services for all children regardless of their disability. This act has been amended and reauthorized several times over the ensuing years and is currently encompassed in IDEA 2004, which specifies that educators develop an annual IEP for children ages 3–21 who are determined eligible for special education services. An IEP is a comprehensive written document identifying the specialized resources needed to maximize the academic success of students who have met eligibility requirements due to academic-based learning impairments, such as speech, language, and hearing disorders. The process leading to the development of an IEP begins with the informal identification of children with special needs by classroom teachers, parents, family members, or such specialists as SLPs, psychologists, or social workers. A prereferral screening process is used to estimate the nature and extent of the child's problems and their potential influence on academic success. If, after an initial period in which trial strategies and modifications to academic tasks and classroom routines are implemented, the child continues to exhibit problems that are likely to have a negative influence on academic success, a more formalized evaluation process is initiated. In this phase, the SLP serving the school may be asked to complete and document a more comprehensive speech-language evaluation if communication problems appear to contribute to the child's academic difficulties. This evaluation may include both standardized testing and nonstandardized assessment and observation of the student communicating in classroom or other social settings. An interdisciplinary **planning and placement team** (PPT) reviews the results of this evaluation, along with the results from evaluations by educators and professionals in other disciplines who may have been called in to the process. The PPT determines the appropriateness of special education services based on state and federal eligibility criteria. If eligible, an IEP is developed at a PPT meeting to outline specific educational services and modifications designed to meet the student's individualized learning needs. The IEP document is typically entered on a prepared fill-in-the-blank form and ideally is completed by the conclusion of the PPT meeting.

The components of an IEP are clearly specified in IDEA 2004. The IEP document begins with a cover sheet with identifying information regarding the child, his or her family members, the participating team members, and the reason for the PPT meeting. Subsequent sections summarize the child's present level of educational performance in the areas of health and development (e.g., vision, hearing); academic, cognitive, and social, emotional, and behavioral skills; motor and communication abilities; activities of daily living; and vocational domains. These summaries are generated from observations of classroom performance, parent reports, and direct assessment results. Not all domains may be reviewed, given the age and presenting concerns of the child. The SLP participating on the PPT may be called upon to contribute both formalized evaluation findings and more incidental observations of the child's communication skills. As part of this discussion, the SLP should employ the principles of effective oral and written communication discussed earlier in this chapter. Based on this cumulative information, the team ultimately decides if the child's disability affects his or her involvement and progress in the general academic or preschool curriculum and if the child's intervention may be eligible for federally funded special education services.

Once eligibility has been determined, the team proceeds to formulate and record annual goals and short-term objectives based on the child's needs. Broad-based goals, including those in the communication domain, are written in functional terms that directly relate to the child's success in an academic environment and are followed by measurable short-term objectives that support those goals. Methods of evaluating progress and a schedule and place for reviewing and recording the child's outcomes are also included in this section (see Figure 7.7).

The team then documents the specific education resources allocated to the child. These include services such as speech-language therapy, physical therapy or

☐ Academic/cognitive ☐ Social/behavioral **X** Communication ☐ Gross/fine motor	☐ Employment/postsecondary education**	Enter dates for evaluating and reporting progress in boxes below		
☐ Self-help ☐ Community participation*** ☐ Independent living*** ☐ Health	☐ Other (specify)			

☐ Check here if the student is 15 years of age. (Note: Page 6, Transition Planning must be completed if this box is checked)

		9/30	10/31	11/28	1/5
		2/2	3/3	4/30	6/1

Measurable annual goal* (linked to present Levels of performance)

Eric will demonstrate improved receptive language skills allowing him to participate in grade level curricular activities

		Report progress below (use reporting key)			
Eval. procedure:	10	1 S	2 S	3 S	4
Perf. criteria:	A	5	6	7	8
(%, trials, etc.)	75%				

Short-term objectives/benchmarks (linked to achieving progress toward annual goal)

Objective #1 Eric will demonstrate understanding of two-step directions related to academic routines by listening to each complete direction, restating the direction, and correctly following the instruction

		Report progress below (use reporting key)			
Eval. procedure:	1,3	1 S	2 S	3 M	4
Perf. criteria:	A	5	6	7	8
(%, trials, etc.)	75%				

Objective #2 Eric will demonstrate comprehension of later developing "wh" questions "when", "why", and "how" by producing correct verbal responses to targeted question forms in the context of curriculum-based activities

		Report progress below (use reporting key)			
Eval. procedure:	1,3	1 S	2 S	3 S	4
Perf. criteria:	A	5	6	7	8
(%, trials, etc.)	75%				

Objective #3 Eric will demonstrate comprehension of prepositions "under", "behind", "in front of", and "next to" by pointing to appropriate picture stimuli or manipulating objects during classroom-based activities

		Report progress below (use reporting key)			
Eval. procedure:	1,3	1 NI	2 S	3 S	4
Perf. criteria:	A	5	6	7	8
(%, trials, etc.)	75%				

Evaluation procedures

		Performance Criteria	
1. Criterion-referenced/curriculum-based assessment	7. Behavior/performance rating scale	A. Percent of Change	F. Duration
2. Pre- and poststandardized assessment	8. CMT/CAPT	B. Months Growth	G. Successful Completion of Task/Activity
3. Pre- and postbaseline data	9. Work samples, job performance, or products	C. Standard Score Increase	H. Mastery
4. Quizzes/tests	10. Achievement objectives *(note: use with goal only)*	D. Passing Grades/Score	I. Other: (specify)
5. Student self-assessment/rubric	11. Other (specify)	E. Frequency/Trials	J. Other: (specify)
6. Project/experiment/portfolio	12. Other (specify)		

Progress reporting key: (indicating extent to which progress is sufficient to achieve goal by the end of the year)

U = unsatisfactory progress – unlikely to achieve goal	N = no progress – will not achieve goal	S = satisfactory progress – likely to achieve goal
M = mastered	NI = not introduced	O = other (specify)

Figure 7.7. Example of goal and objective documentation on an individual education program (IEP). (*Key:* Eval., evaluation; Perf., performance; Obj., objective; %, percentage; CMT, Connecticut Master Test; CAPT, Connecticut Academic Performance Test.) (*Source:* Connecticut State Department of Education, 2013.)

227

SPECIAL EDUCATION, RELATED SERVICES, AND REGULAR EDUCATION

Special Education Services	Goal(s) #	Frequency	Responsible Staff	Service Implementer	Start Date (mm/dd/yyyy)	End Date (mm/dd/yyyy)	Site*	If needed, description of Instructional Service Delivery (e.g., small group, team taught classes, etc.)
Reading Instruction	5, 6	5 hrs/wk	Reading Specialist	Reading Specialist	9/15/14	6/5/15	2	Individual and small group instruction
Related Services								
Speech-Language Pathology	1,2,3	1.5 hrs/wk	Speech-language pathologist	Speech assistant	9/15/14	6/5/15	1, 2	Small group instruction
Occupational Therapy	4	30 min/wk	Occupational Therapist	Occupational Therapist	9/15/14	6/5/15	5	Individual instruction
*Instructional Site:	1. Regular Classroom	2. Resource/Related Service Room	3. Self-Contained Classroom	4. Community-Based	5. Other: Gym			
Description of participation in General Education	Susan will participate in the 6th grade classroom for 80% of her weekly schedule, with curricular supports and modifications as stated.							

Figure 7.8. Identifying educational support services on an individual education program (IEP). (*Source:* Connecticut State Department of Education, 2013.)

Program Accommodations and Modifications - INCLUDING NONACADEMIC AND EXTRACURRICULAR ACTIVITIES/COLLABORATION/SUPPORT FOR SCHOOL PERSONNEL

Accommodations and Modifications to be provided to enable the child: – To advance appropriately toward attaining his/her annual goals; – To be involved in and make progress in the general education curriculum; – To participate in extracurricular and other non-academic activities; and – To be educated and participate with other children with and without disabilities. **Accommodations may include Assistive Technology Devices and Services**	**Sites/Activities Where Required and Duration**
Materials/Books/Equipment: Supplementary visuals; FM listening system, laptop computer with word processing	Regular classroom, resource room
Tests/Quizzes/Assessments: Alternative tests, extra time, preview test procedures; simplify test wording; allow extra response time.	Regular classroom, resource room
Grading: Base grade on ability.	Regular classroom, resource room
Organization: Provide study outlines; give one paper at a time; assist student to make daily assignment and homework lists; post routines and assignments near student's work areas.	Regular classroom, resource room
Environment: Preferential seating away from sources of noise and visual distractions.	Regular classroom
Behavioral Interventions and Support: Daily feedback to student regarding performance; visual progress charts, alert student prior to transitions.	All settings
Instructional Strategies: Check work in progress; use manipulatives; employ a multi-sensory learning approach with emphasis on visual information; verbal and visual reinforcement; pre-teach content with emphasis on key vocabulary.	Regular classroom, resource room
Other:	
Frequency and Duration of Supports Required for School Personnel to Implement This IEP Include: Speech-language pathologist to train classroom teachers and instructional aid in use of FM listening system during the first 2 weeks of term. Special education teacher, speech-language pathologist and regular classroom teacher will meet weekly to adapt curriculum and identify multi-modality teaching strategies.	

Figure 7.9. Educational modifications as outlined on an individual education program (IEP). (*Source:* Connecticut State Department of Education, 2013.)

TRANSITION PLANNING

1. ☐ **Not Applicable:** Student has not reached the age of 15 and transition planning is not required or appropriate at this time.

   ☒ This is either the first IEP to be in effect when the student turns 16 (or younger if appropriate and transition planning is needed) or the student is 16 or older and transition planning is required.

2. **Student Preferences/Interests – document the following:**
   a) Was the student invited to attend her/his Planning and Placement Team (PPT) meeting?   ☒Yes   ☐No
   b) Did the student attend?   ☒Yes   ☐No
   c) How were the student's preferences/interests, as they relate to planning for transition services, determined?
   ☒Personal Interviews   ☒Comments at Meeting   ☒Functional Vocational Evaluations   ☒Age appropriate transition assessments   ☐Other _____
   d) Summarize student preferences/interests as they relate to planning for transition services: *Jamal's preferences include physical activities, social interactions and being outdoors.*

3. **Age Appropriate Transition Assessment(s) performed: (Specify assessment(s) and dates administered)** *4/12/13: community-based communication needs and skills assessment* _____

4. **Agency Participation:**
   a) Were any outside agencies invited to attend the PPT meeting?   ☒ Yes with written consent   ☐ No   (If No, MUST specify reason as listed in the IEP Manual) _____
   b) If yes, did the agency's representative attend?   ☒ Yes   ☐No
   c) Has any participating agency agreed to provide or pay for services/linkages?   ☐ Yes   ☒ No   (If Yes, specify) _____

5. **Post-School Outcome Goal Statement(s) and Transition Services recommended in this IEP**
   a) Post-School Outcome Goal Statement - **Postsecondary Education or Training:**   *N/A*
   ☐ Annual goal(s) and related objectives regarding Postsecondary Education or Training have been developed and are included in this IEP
   b) Post-School Outcome Goal Statement – **Employment:** *Jamal will participate in an adult day program with a focus on community-based social and volunteer activities.*
   ☒ Annual goal(s) and related objectives regarding Employment have been developed and are included in this IEP
   c) Post-School Outcome Goal Statement - **Independent Living Skills (if appropriate):** *With appropriate supports, Jamal will engage in activities of daily living including: shopping, cooking, caring for his home, maintaining personal hygiene, and participating in preferred leisure activities.*
   ☒ Annual goals and related objectives regarding Independent Living have been developed and are included in this IEP (may include Community Participation)

6. **Please select ONLY one:**
   ☒ **The course of study** needed to assist the child in reaching the transition goals and related objectives **will include** (including general education activities): *Social communication skills, functional math skills, community awareness and access skills, pre-vocational skills* _____

   ☐ **Student has completed academic requirements:** no academic course of study is required – student's IEP includes **only** transition goals and services.

7. **At least one year prior to reaching the age of 18, the student must be informed of her/his rights under IDEA which will transfer at age 18.**
   ☒ NA (Student will not be 17 within one year)   ☐ The student has been informed of her/his rights under IDEA which will transfer at age 18   ☐ No IDEA rights will transfer

8. **For a child whose eligibility under special education will terminate the following year due to graduation with a regular education diploma or due to exceeding the age of eligibility, the Summary of Performance will be completed on or before: (specify date)** _____

Figure 7.10. Individual transition plan (ITP). (*Key:* NA, Not applicable; PPT, planning and placement team; IEP, individual education program; IDEA, Individuals with Disabilities Education Improvement Act of 2004 [PL 108-4660].) (Based on the Connecticut State Department of Education IEP forms. [2010]. *IEP manual and forms.* Retrieved from http://www.sde.ct.gov/sde/lib/sde/PDF/DEPS/Special/IEPManual.pdf.)

other supports, the hours each week that those services will be delivered, beginning and ending dates, and the parties responsible for implementing the service (see Figure 7.8). The instructional site (e.g., regular classroom, resource room, related services office) for each service is identified, and the need for assistive technology (e.g., communication devices, FM systems) is identified as well. Any modifications to the child's academic schedule are listed, as are accommodations for hearing and vision impairments, behavior challenges, or limited English proficiency.

A placement summary outlines the rationale for the type and location of educational placement chosen, as well as exit criteria from special education. According to the IDEA 2004 mandate, school systems must provide education for all students in the least restrictive environment. Modifications and adaptations in general education settings are indicated, including specialized instructional strategies; organizational supports; behavior management support; testing procedures; and adaptations to materials, books, and equipment (see Figure 7.9).

Individualized Transition Plans

Under IDEA 2004, the focus of educational goals and objectives for students 16–21 years of age who receive special education services shifts to include training in independent living and employment-related skills. An effort is made to involve members from the client's educational team and representatives from adult support agencies in this transitional planning process. An **individual transition plan** (ITP) may be developed as an integrated component of the client's IEP and is designed to identify the specific skills and supports that the client will need to make a successful transition. The focus of goals and objectives may shift somewhat at this point from academic development to independent living, community participation, and prevocational skills. The transition plan is recorded as part of the overall IEP document (see Figure 7.10).

An SLP's role in the IEP process continues after the development of the initial plan and involves subsequent implementation and review of the components of the IEP. Audiologists, though not always physically present during PPT meetings, also contribute to the development and implementation of IEPs through consulting with the team, writing diagnostic reports, and communicating with the team via the school-based SLP.

CONCLUSION

The act of obtaining, relaying, and documenting clinical information is a multifaceted task that requires you to integrate writing abilities, interpersonal skills, cultural sensitivity, and clinical knowledge in order to serve clients, their families, and their caregivers effectively. It is a process in which form does not follow function but, rather, blends with it to foster effective information sharing. It is a process that we refine throughout the entire course of our clinical education and subsequent professional practice as audiologists and SLPs. We will serve our clients most effectively if we remember that in addition to increasing their communication skills, we have an obligation to refine our own.

STUDY QUESTIONS

1. Describe at least four principles of effective oral and written communication.
2. Discuss the advantages of using an in-person interview rather than a written case history questionnaire to gain background information from your clients.
3. Name three cultural factors that may influence a person's responses to interview questions.
4. Explain the importance of follow-up counseling as a component of diagnostic assessment.
5. What criteria are used to determine if a particular topic is appropriate for an audiologist or SLP to address during a clinical counseling session?
6. Describe the components of an individual intervention plan for speech-language therapy.
7. Compare and contrast the purpose of the following documents: individual intervention plan, SOAP note, progress report, and discharge summary.

TEST QUESTIONS

1. A primary purpose of an initial interview between an audiologist or speech-language pathologist and their client is to

    a. Complete the paperwork necessary for billing or administrative purposes.
    b. Establish a trusting rapport between client and clinician.
    c. Establish the authority of the clinician.
    d. Gain enough information about the client's situation to eliminate the need for further discussion.

2. To engage in effective oral and written clinical communication, we should

    a. Avoid using technical language whenever possible.
    b. Label people by terms that describe their impairment, such as *stutterer* or *aphasic.*
    c. Use objective terms, such as *observe* or *completed*, rather than subjective terms such as *appears* or *seemed.*
    d. a. and c.

3. It is essential that you consider your and your client's cultural perspectives in order to

    a. Help your clients learn the correct way to respond to your questions.
    b. Correctly interpret your clients' verbal and nonverbal responses.
    c. Establish your own cultural values as the framework for your relationship with your clients.
    d. Identify the limitations of your clients' belief systems.

4. The written document summarizing your client's progress during a therapy session is a

    a. SOAP note.
    b. Treatment plan.

    c. Individual educational plan (IEP).

    d. Individual family service plan (IFSP).

5. An *individual transition plan*

    a. Documents the termination of speech-language therapy services.

    b. Identifies the steps needed to become an effective first-time hearing aid user.

    c. Is the component of an IEP for students 16 to 21 years old that identifies services and supports needed to develop independent living and vocational skills.

    d. Lists services and supports needed to help a preschooler with special needs enter kindergarten.

FURTHER READING

Goldfarb, R., & Serpanos, Y.C. (2009). *Professional writing in speech-language pathology and audiology.* San Diego, CA: Plural Publishing.

Luterman, D.M. (2008). *Counseling persons with communication disorders and their families.* Austin, TX: PRO-ED.

Lynch, E.W., & Hanson, M.J. (2011). *Developing cross-cultural competence: A guide for working with children and their families* (4th ed.). Baltimore, MD: Paul H. Brookes Publishing Co.

Shipley, K.G., & Roseberry-McKibbin, C.X. (2006). *Interviewing and counseling in communication disorders* (3rd ed.). Austin, TX: PRO-ED.

REFERENCES

American Recovery and Reinvestment Act (ARRA) of 2009, Title XIII, Health Information Technology for Economic and Clinical Health Act, PL111-5, 123 Stat. 227. Retrieved from http://www.hhs.gov/ocr/privacy/hipaa/understanding/coveredentities/hitechact.pdf

American Speech-Language-Hearing Association (ASHA). (1991). *A model for collaborative service delivery for students with language-learning disorders in the public schools* [Relevant paper]. Available from www.asha.org/policy

American Speech-Language-Hearing Association. (2002). *A workload analysis approach for establishing speech-language caseload standards in the schools: Guidelines.* Retrieved from www.asha.org/policy

American Speech-Language-Hearing Association. (2004). *Preferred practice patterns for the profession of speech-language pathology.* Retrieved from www.asha.org/policy

American Speech-Language-Hearing Association. (2010). *Code of ethics.* Retrieved from www.asha.org/policy

Anderson, P.P., & Fenichel, E.S. (1989). *Serving culturally diverse families of infants and toddlers with disabilities.* Washington, DC: National Center for Clinical Infant Programs.

Battle, D.E. (2011). *Communication disorders in multicultural and international populations* (4th ed.). St. Louis, MO: Elsevier Mosby.

Blood, G.W., Simpson, K.C., Raimondi, S.C., Dineen, M., Kauffman, S.M., & Stagaard, K.A. (1994). Social support in laryngeal cancer survivors: Voice and adjustment issues. *American Journal of Speech-Language Pathology, 1,* 37–44.

Coleman, T.J. (2000). *Clinical management of communication disorders in culturally diverse children.* Boston, MA: Allyn & Bacon.

Connecticut Birth-to-Three System. (2013). *Individual family service plan form.* Retrieved from http://www.birth23.org/files/procedures/forms/3-1-ifsp.pdf

Connecticut State Department of Education. (2013). *IEP manual and forms.* Retrieved from http://www.sde.ct.gov/sde/lib/sde/PDF/DEPS/Special/IEP Manual.pdf

Cunningham, R. (1998). Counseling someone with severe aphasia: An explorative study. *Disability and Rehabilitation: An International Multidisciplinary Journal, 20,* 346–354.

Education for All Handicapped Children Act of 1975, PL 94-142, 20 U.S.C. §§ 1400 *et seq.*

Education of the Handicapped Act Amendments of 1986, PL 99-457, 20 U.S.C. §§ 1400 *et seq.*

Flasher, L.V., & Fogle, P.T. (2012). *Counseling skills for speech-language pathologists and audiologists* (2nd ed.). Clifton Park, NY: Thompson Delmar Learning.

Golper, L.G. (1998). *Sourcebook for medical speech pathology* (2nd ed.). San Diego, CA: Singular Publishing Group.

Goode, T.D, Jones, W., & Hopkins Jackson, V. (2011). Families with African American roots. In E.W. Lynch & M.J. Hanson (2011). *Developing cross-cultural competence: A guide for working with children and their families* (4th ed., pp. 140–189). Baltimore, MD: Paul H. Brookes Publishing Co.

Groopman, J. (2007). *How doctors think.* New York, NY: Houghton Mifflin.

Hall, P.H., & Morris, H.L. (2000). The clinical history. In J.B. Toblin, H.L. Morris, & D.C. Spriestersbach (Eds.), *Diagnosis in speech-language pathology* (2nd ed., pp. 65–82). San Diego, CA: Singular Publishing Group.

Haynes, W.O., & Pindzola, R.H. (2012). *Diagnosis and evaluation in speech pathology* (8th ed.). Upper Saddle River, NJ: Pearson Education.

Health Insurance Portability and Accountability Act of 1996, PL 104-191, 42 U.S.C. §§ 201 *et seq.*

Individuals with Disabilities Educational Improvement Act of 2004, PL 108-466, 20 U.S.C. §§ 1400 *et seq.*

Jha, A.K., DesRoches, C.M., Campbell, E.G., Donelan, K., Rao, S.R., Ferris, T.G., … Blumenthal, D. (2009). Use of electronic health records in U.S. hospitals. [Electronic version]. *New England Journal of Medicine, 360,* 1628–1638.

Langdon, H.W., & Cheng, L.L. (1992). *Hispanic children and adults with communication disorders: Assessment and intervention.* New York, NY: Aspen Publishers.

Luterman, D.M. (2008). *Counseling persons with communication disorders and their families.* Austin, TX: PRO-ED.

Loomis, G.A., Reis, J.S., Saywell, R.M., & Thakker, N.R. (2002). If electronic records are so great, why aren't family physicians using them? [Electronic

version]. *Journal of Family Practice, 51*(7), 636–641.

Lynch, E.W., & Hanson, M.J. (2011). *Developing cross-cultural competence: A guide for working with children and their families* (4th ed.). Baltimore, MD: Paul H. Brookes Publishing Co.

Maltz, D., & Borker, R. (1982). A cultural approach to male–female miscommunication. In J.J. Gumperz (Ed.), *Language and social identity: Studies in international sociolinguistics* (pp. 146–216). New York, NY: Cambridge University Press.

Margolis, R.H. (2004, August 11). Boosting memory with informational counseling: Helping patients understand the nature of disorders and how to manage them [Electronic version]. *The ASHA Leader.* Retrieved from http://www.asha.org/leaderissue.aspx?year=2004&id=2004-08-03

Meitus, I.J. (1983). Clinical report and letter writing. In I.J. Meitus & B. Weinberg (Eds.), *Diagnosis in speech-language pathology* (pp. 287–301). Boston, MA: Allyn & Bacon.

National Joint Committee for the Communication Needs of Persons with Severe Disabilities. (2003). *Position statement on access to communication services and supports: Concerns regarding the application of restrictive "eligibility" policies.* Retrieved from http://www.asha.org/policy/TR2002-00233.htm

Nelson-Crowell, R.L., Hanenburg, J., & Gilbertson, A. (2009). Counseling adolescents with hearing loss using a narrative therapy approach. *Perspectives on Administration and Supervision, 19*(2), 72–78.

Olson, D.P., & Windish, D.M. (2010). Communication discrepancies between physicians and hospitalized patients [Electronic version]. *Archives of Internal Medicine, 170*(15), 1302–1307.

Rao, P.R. (2003). Counseling elders with communication disorders and families/related professionals. *Perspectives on Gerontology, 8*(1), 16–21.

Rollin, W.J. (2000). *Counseling individuals with communication disorders psychodynamic and family aspects* (2nd ed.). Boston, MA: Butterworth-Heinemann.

Roseberry-McKibbin, C. (2008). *Multicultural students with special language needs: Practical strategies for assessment and intervention* (3rd ed.). Oceanside, CA: Academic Communication Associates.

Roth, F.P., & Worthington, C.K. (2011). *Treatment resource manual for speech-language pathology* (4th ed.). Clifton Park, NY: Delmar Cengage Learning.

Salomon, R.M., Blackford, J.U., Rosenbloom, S.T., Seidel, S., Clayton, E.W., Dilts, D.M., & Finder, S.G. (2010). Openness of patients reporting with use of electronic records: Psychiatric clinician's views [Electronic version]. *Journal of the American Medical Information Association, 17,* 54–60.

Shames, G.H. (2006). *Counseling the communicatively disabled and their families: A manual for clinicians* (2nd ed.). Mahwah, NJ: Lawrence Erlbaum Associates.

Shapiro, D.A. (2011). *Stuttering intervention: A collaborative journey to fluency freedom* (2nd ed.). Austin, TX: PRO-ED.

Sharifzadeh, V. (2011). Families with Middle Eastern roots. In E.W. Lynch & M.J. Hanson (2011), *Developing cross-cultural competence: A guide for working with children and their families* (4th ed., pp. 392–436). Baltimore, MD: Paul H. Brookes Publishing Co.

Shipley, K.G., & McAfee, J.G. (2009). *Assessment in speech-language pathology: A resource manual* (4th ed.). Clifton Park, NY: Delmar Cengage Learning.

Shipley, K.G., & Roseberry-McKibbin, C. (2006). *Interviewing and counseling in communication disorders* (3rd ed.). Austin, TX: PRO-ED.

Silverman, F.H. (2003). *Essentials of professional issues in speech-language pathology and audiology.* Long Grove, IL: Waveland Press.

Stone, J.R., & Olswang, L.B. (1989). The hidden challenge in counseling. *ASHA, 31,* 27–31.

Tomblin, J.B. (2000). Perspectives on diagnosis. In J.B. Tomblin, H.L. Morris, & D.C. Spriestersbach (Eds.), *Diagnosis in speech-language pathology* (2nd ed., pp. 3–33). San Diego, CA: Singular Publishing Group.

Wright, A., Soran, C., Jenter, C.A., Volk, L.A., Bates, D.W., & Simon, S.R. (2010). Physician attitudes toward health information exchange: Results of a statewide survey [Electronic version]. *Journal of the American Medical Information Association, 17,* 66–70.

Wolter, J.A., DiLollo, A., & Apel, K.(2006). A narrative therapy approach to counseling: A model for working with adolescents and adults with language—literacy deficits. *Language, Speech and Hearing Services in Schools, 37,* 168–177.

Zuniga, M.E. (2011). Families with Latino roots. In E.W. Lynch & M.J. Hanson (Eds.), *Developing cross-cultural competence: A guide for working with children and their families* (4th ed., pp. 190–233). Baltimore, MD: Paul H. Brookes Publishing Co.

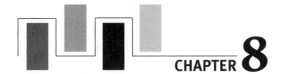

CHAPTER **8**

Public Policies Affecting Clinical Practice

Michele A. Anderson and Nickola W. Nelson

After reading this chapter, students will be able to

- Define basic terms related to public policy
- Understand how current policy can effect the delivery of speech-language pathology and audiology services
- Advocate on behalf of clients and our profession to influence policy decisions

To a newly graduated clinician eager to begin a career, "policy issues" may not be front and center when anticipating client assessment and treatment planning. Policies influence clinical practice in many ways, however. They play a significant role in determining how clinical decisions are made for clients of all age levels, from early infancy through late adulthood, where and when services are provided, and how (and if) costs are reimbursed. Public policies are related to the broader systems in which clients are assessed and treated, including home, school, and health care settings. Moreover, public policies may be changed at any time, which is both good and bad news. The good news is that ineffective policies can be modified, which can be reassuring when a policy has negative or unintended outcomes. The bad news is that effective policies also can be changed, which means that advocates for people with communication disorders must remain vigilant for the need for advocacy at all times.

What makes a policy good? A good policy can be described as one that is effective for addressing the rights and needs of people with disabilities, including access to services and participation opportunities for individuals with communication disorders that put them at risk for educational, vocational, or social disadvantage. Policies that limit the access of individuals to interventions may be viewed as short-sighted, ineffective, or even harmful, with possible negative effects on the potential for recovery from acute or chronic conditions. For example, **Medicare** Part B regulations have placed a $1,880 reimbursement limit on fees for speech-language pathology and physical therapy services combined (http://www.medicare.gov/coverage/pt-and-ot-and-speech-language-pathology.html). This "therapy cap" limits access to two services that might be equally important in a person's recovery from stroke. Although from a societal perspective a reimbursement limit on services may be an essential step toward keeping Medicare solvent, from the perspective of access to care for a person with aphasia, the policy is a bad one, possibly forcing a choice about whether walking or talking should be the priority for treatment. Intense advocacy efforts by the American Speech-Language-Hearing Association (ASHA; http://www.asha.org/advocacy/federal/cap) and others have made it possible to renew provisions for exceptions to the therapy cap repeatedly since it was written into law. Without changes to the original policy, however, these adjustments are only temporary.

As this example shows, criteria for evaluating whether a given policy is effective or "good" vary depending on one's values and point of view. Another example of a policy with controversial provisions is the No Child Left Behind (NCLB) Act (PL 107-110). This law, which was passed in 2001, raised expectations for all children to develop literacy abilities and to learn the general education curriculum—both admirable goals in themselves. Among many problems with the law's implementation, however, have been conflicts between requirements under NCLB for aggregate assessment of children with disabilities and requirements under the Individuals with Disabilities Education Improvement Act (IDEA) of 2004 (PL 108-446) for individualized assessment and service delivery for these children (Etscheidt, 2012). Responding to advocacy efforts by representatives of state departments of education and others, President Obama had granted waivers to the full accountability requirements of the NCLB Act to 34 states and the District of Columbia by the close of 2012. States could apply for waivers by submitting alternate "rigorous and comprehensive state-developed plans" for improving educational outcomes for all students, closing achievement gaps, increasing equity, and improving the quality of instruction (see U.S. Department of Education, n.d., http://www.ed.gov/esea/flexibility).

Whether a policy is judged good, bad, or neutral with respect to certain criteria depends on the standards and value system one applies to evaluate it. Before policies can be evaluated, however, they need to be understood. This chapter provides an overview of key public policies that have implications for clinical service provision by professionals in speech-language pathology and audiology. Clinicians who are knowledgeable about policies can implement them with fidelity, recognize when variations are allowable within policy boundaries, and decide when and how to advocate actively for changes if necessary. This overview emphasizes each policy's major features rather than its specific details. Because public policies change frequently, it is recommended that professionals review updated policy versions, which are readily accessible on web sites that are maintained by policy-making agencies, professional associations such as ASHA, and other advocacy groups. In this chapter, we first provide definitions of basic terms necessary for understanding discussions of public policy. We then review several aspects of current policy that relate to communication disorders. Finally, we discuss ways in which professionals can influence important policies that affect our clients.

DEFINING PUBLIC POLICY

Public policy has been defined as any action (or lack thereof) taken by local, state, or federal officials to address a given problem or set of problems (Dye, 1998). Public policies may be established at federal, state, and local levels. They can occur in many forms, including laws, regulations, guidelines, and court decisions, as well as in the form of local policies governing local practices within a confined region or agency.

Laws begin as bills that move through legislative committees (state or federal). After they are passed by legislative bodies, different versions are reconciled as necessary and signed into law (or vetoed) by executive officials (states' governors or the U.S. President), who become responsible for implementing any current acts.

Regulations are generated by executive agencies charged with interpreting and implementing particular laws. Before passage, proposed regulations are generally opened for a period of public comment. Both laws and regulations require action by the regulatory and legislative bodies that originated them before they can be changed.

Guidelines or other local policies may be developed by such entities as communities, school districts, health care agencies, hospitals, or professional associations to provide interpretations of how legislative and regulatory mandates are to be implemented in specific settings. Guidelines carry less legal weight than do laws and regulations, but they are easier to change.

Case law refers to the outcomes of litigation. Court decisions set precedents that influence how policies are interpreted and implemented. This occurs when disputes are taken to court and decisions are issued that have implications broader than the single case.

PUBLIC POLICIES AFFECTING
INDIVIDUALS WITH COMMUNICATION DISORDERS

Early Hearing Detection and Intervention

In 1999, the U.S. Congress passed the Newborn and Infant Hearing Screening and Intervention Act (PL 93-406), which authorized grants to states to provide early hearing detection and intervention programs. Congress reauthorized the grants in 2000 through the Children's Health Act of 2000 (PL 106-310), which included provisions related to early hearing screening and evaluation of all newborns, coordinated intervention, rehabilitation services, and research. By 2007, there were 40 of 50 U.S. states with early hearing detection and intervention laws and 5 had voluntary compliance programs to screen the hearing of 95% or more of newborns, compared with only about 40% of infants being screened in 2000. By 2012, there were 43 states with programs that had been approved, but only 28 of them required screening of all babies. Challenges were still noted in following children who failed newborn-screening tests (National Center for Hearing Assessment and Management, 2012). The Early Hearing Detection and Intervention Act of 2010 (PL 111-337), therefore, added two primary provisions: to expand the newborn and infant hearing loss program to include diagnostic services (beyond newborn screening) and to add programs through the Health

Resources and Services Administration for building an adequate supply of qualified personnel to meet the screening, evaluation, and early intervention needs of
children with hearing loss.

No Child Left Behind Act of 2001

On January 8, 2002, President George W. Bush signed into law the NCLB Act of
2001 (PL 107-110), reauthorizing the Elementary and Secondary Education Act
(ESEA; PL 89-10), which was first passed in 1965. The NCLB Act aimed at making schools accountable for providing "high-quality" education. It established a
goal of promoting adequate educational achievement for all children, including
demonstration of proficiency in selected areas, among them English literacy and
math, by 100% of students by 2013–2014. The NLCB comprised four primary
components, described as addressing accountability, flexibility, effective methods,
and parental choice (U.S. Department of Education, 2002).

Accountability was defined by NCLB as the legal requirement of educational
agencies to ensure that all students achieve academic proficiency, including students in all racial and ethnic groups, English language learners, students with
disabilities, and students affected by socioeconomic disadvantage. Accountability
provisions require annual statewide testing of all students in third through eighth
grade to determine whether schools have met goals defining adequate yearly
progress (AYP). Schools and school districts that meet AYP are eligible for State
Academic Achievement Awards; those that do not meet AYP goals are targeted
for corrective action and improvement. The student population that provides the
scores on which the AYP is based includes many subpopulations. Of the subpopulations that are classified as high risk, the scores of at least 95% of students within
those subpopulations must contribute to the AYP. The subpopulations classified as
high risk are economically disadvantaged students, students from major racial or
ethnic groups, students with disabilities, and students who are English language
learners. The U.S. Secretary of Education (U.S. Department of Education, 2005)
issued an interpretation in April 2005 in which she indicated that 3% (a revision of the originally specified 1%) of students with disabilities (largely students
with intellectual developmental disabilities) would be allowed to take alternative
annual assessment tests without penalizing the AYP result of the school or school
district. Further, accommodations, modifications, or alternative assessment tests
for students with disabilities must be consistent with the requirements of the current version of IDEA'04 (Annett, 2003).

Flexibility is defined within NCLB as school districts' ability to use up to 15%
of federal special education funds to support general education activities. Flexibility, for example, allows schools to assign speech-language pathologists (SLPs)
who are paid with special education dollars to provide, as part of their workload,
preventive and identification activities for students in general education who are
struggling (Annett, 2003).

Effective methods are those that have been satisfactorily demonstrated to have
a positive effect on student education. The NCLB Act identifies five essential components that are effective methods for reading instruction: 1) *phonemic awareness*,
which involves noticing, thinking about, and working with individual sounds in
spoken words; 2) *phonics instruction*, which involves associating written language
letters (graphemes) with spoken language speech sounds (phonemes); 3) *fluency*,

which involves reading the words of a text both quickly and accurately; 4) *vocabulary*, which involves applying knowledge of word meanings for listening, speaking, reading, and writing; and 5) *text comprehension*, which involves purposeful and active construction of text meaning. Federal funding through NCLB is also available for a variety of special programs: Reading First, Early Reading First, Even Start Family Literacy, and Even Start Migrant Education. Grants for these initiatives can be obtained through competitive federal and state application processes (Moore-Brown & Montgomery, 2005).

Parental choice permits parents of students who are attending schools that fail to meet AYP for 2 consecutive years to elect to send their children to different schools of their choice. In such instances, school districts are required to spend up to 20% of their Title I monies (part of NCLB) to provide alternative school options for qualified families.

Concerns about the provisions of NCLB have included that the law is underfunded; that testing in a one-size-fits-all model focuses on limited skills; that English language tests, which are required under the law, "leave behind" students who are English language learners; and that there is a heightened potential for bias in interpreting research results when policy makers, research funders, and test and curriculum developers are closely related (e.g., Metcalf, 2002; Meyer, 2004). An even more basic concern is that schools in impoverished communities are unlikely to achieve AYP goals without extensive changes in unequal socioeconomic structures.

Another controversial aspect of the NCLB Act is that it has influenced schools to move toward a standards-based curriculum and away from a functional curriculum for students with disabilities. Some authors (e.g., Ayres, Lowrey, Douglas, & Sievers, 2011) have argued that a functional curriculum (i.e., one that teaches daily living skills needed for independence in adulthood) might better serve the needs of students with disabilities, particularly severe disabilities, than would a standards-based curriculum. Others (e.g., Courtade, Spooner, Browder, & Jimenez, 2012) have countered that a standards-based curriculum might have advantages even for these students. Courtade et al. (2012) cite a number of reasons for focusing on academic learning, including that functional skills are not a prerequisite to academic skills and that a standards-based curriculum need not be a replacement for a functional curriculum. Blosser et al. (2012) provided examples of how SLPs might target Common Core State Standards (National Governors Association Center for Best Practices, Council of Chief State School Officers, 2010) for students with a range of disabilities.

Moores (2011) discussed evidence from the 2009 National Assessment of Educational Progress (NAEP), which is known as the "Nation's Report Card," that suggested that the NCLB was not working. According to the NAEP report, only 38% of high school seniors demonstrated proficiency in reading and 26% in math after almost a decade of enforcement of the NCLB Act. Further, no progress had been made in closing achievement gaps that historically have separated white students from black and Hispanic students. Moores observed that, in fact, achievement has essentially declined since the imposition of federal mandates with NCLB. He noted, "True transformation at the federal level would involve starting from scratch in regular education, special education, and education of the deaf, not making minor revisions of present ineffective legislation and regulations" (Moores, 2011, p. 525). Indeed, noted previously, the extent of the concerns had led a majority of states to seek and be granted waivers to many of the NCLB requirements by December 2012 (http://www.ed.gov/esea/flexibility). This is one example of how advocacy can lead to changes in policies that seem not to be working the way they were intended.

Individuals with Disabilities Education Improvement Act of 2004

In the 1970s, the previous laws and amendments of laws governing students with special needs were united into one act, which became known as Part B of the Education of the Handicapped Act (EHA) of 1970 (PL 91-230). It was the antecedent to the Education for All Handicapped Children Act (EAHA) of 1975 (PL 94-142), which was the predecessor to IDEA, the Individuals with Disabilities Education Act (PL 101-476), as it was renamed in the 1990 reauthorization. In 2004, the act was reauthorized once again, this time as the Individuals with Disabilities Education Improvement Act (PL 108-446), although it still carries the official designation, IDEA. This law took effect July 1, 2005, but the code of federal regulations, with implementation specifications for the revised act, was not approved until the summer of 2006. The term *improvement* in the title of the law signaled the lawmakers' goal to align IDEA with provisions of NCLB (Moore-Brown & Montgomery, 2005).

From the law's inception, the purpose of IDEA has been to ensure that all children with disabilities have access to a *free appropriate public education (FAPE)* in the *least restrictive environment (LRE)*. Whereas ESEA–NCLB targets group accountability for learning the general curriculum, IDEA provides for assessment and intervention at the individual level to improve outcomes and help students with disabilities succeed (Etscheidt, 2011). It is the definition of "success" that raises controversy.

IDEA has four major parts. Part A includes definitions and general provisions. Part B specifies how services are to be provided to school-age students under an **individualized education program** (IEP). Preschool-age children 3–5 years of age also may receive services under an IEP under Section 619 of Part B of IDEA. Part C specifies requirements for service provision to infants and toddlers and their families to receive services under an **individualized family service plan** (IFSP). If parents elect, their preschool-age children may continue to be served under an IFSP rather than transitioning to an IEP at 3 years of age. Part D includes provisions for supporting research, personnel preparation, technical assistance, support, and dissemination of information for improving the education of children with disabilities.

Individualized Family Service Plans For infants and toddlers, IFSPs define the service unit as the family rather than the child. Development of IFSPs for infants and toddlers requires decisions to be made about a family's service needs and mandates family representation in the decision-making process. These plans include statements about 1) the present development level of the infant or toddler; 2) the family's resources, priorities, and concerns; 3) the major outcomes expected; 4) the specific early intervention services; 5) the natural environments in which services shall occur; 6) the projected dates of initiation of services and length thereof; 7) the identification of the service coordinator; and 8) the steps to be taken to support the transition to preschool or other educational levels. Figure 8.1 contains an example of an abbreviated IFSP.

Today's date _2-12-13_

Agency initiating IFSP _Anytown Public School_

Child information

Child's legal name	Janna Johnson		Nickname	_Janna_	Date of birth _11-1-11_	Sex: M/F
Address	123 Main Street				Phone (home) _555-5555_	Phone (daycare) _555-5554_
Address	Anytown, USA				Medical insurance # _123456789_	
School district of residence	Anytown Schools		County _Any County_	Ethnic heritage _African Am._	Native language _English_	

Name	Relationship to child	Birth date (optional)	Address	Phone (home)	Phone (work)
Mike Johnson	Father		Same as above	Same	555-1212
Sharika Johnson	Mother		Same as above	Same	555-1234
Issac Johnson	Brother		Same	Same	-----

If parent/guardian needs an interpreter, give language:

Agencies and persons working with the family (fill in anytime)

Start date	Agency	Contact person(s)	Phone	Type of service or title	End date	Send copy of IFSP?
11-5-11	University Hospital	Isabel Jones	222-2222	Audiologist		X
1-5-12	Anytown Public School	Diane Smith	333-3333	Speech-language pathologist		

Child's strengths and needs

Child's name _Janna Johnson_		Birth weight _7.2_	Birth date _11-1-11_	Number of weeks premature _NA_	

Area	Present level of development		Date	Name/type of evaluation	Person doing evaluation	Agency
	Parent input	Professional input				
General	Very expressive, and "laid back." A good baby.	Continued hearing impaired services after a cochlear implant.	1-15-04	Developmental screening	Developmental psychologist	Anytown Schools
Hearing	Failed newborn screening. Follow-up testing showed profound hearing loss. Doesn't respond to sound but does to gestures.	Profound bilateral hearing imp scheduled for cochlear implant 2-20-13.	11-2-11 12-15-11 12-15-12	Neonatal screening ABR	Audiologist	University Hospital
Communication	Follows eyes, coos, and makes sounds	Age appropriate so far Communicative & interactive	12-10-12	Rossetti Infant-Toddler Scale	Speech-language pathologist	Anytown Schools

Figure 8.1. Sample individualized family service plan. (*Key:* ABR, auditory brainstem response audiometry; IDEA, Individuals with Disabilities Education Improvement Act [PL 108-446].) © 2013 by N.W. Nelson, D. Chamberlain, and S. Sexton.

(continued)

Child eligibility

Part C of IDEA	X Yes	□ No	□ Unknown	(Based on: Established condition _hearing impaired_	Developmental delay _____

Service Plan

Service coordinator _D. Smith_ Services coordinator phone # _333-0300_

□ Interim | X Initial | □ Review | □ Annual | □ Transition (90 days before entry into new program or third birthday – whichever comes first.)

OUTCOMES	WHO & WHAT	WHERE, WHEN & HOW	DATE SERVICE		PAYOR	REVIEW *
What would we like to have happen, by when, and how will we know when it happens?	What service or activity is needed? Who will do it?	When will the services occur? How often? How long each time? Individual or group?	Begins	Ends	Who will pay for it?	Date/ rating/ comments
1) Cochlear implant scheduled (2-20-13) 2) Understand and say words by age 2.0 (11-1-13) (at least 50) 3) Use spoken language and listening to participate in conversation and play by age 3.0 (make comments, express intent, ask and answer questions, etc.)	1) Univ. Hospital 2) Speech-language pathologist, speech language therapy 3) Hearing-impaired consultant 4) Early intervention coordinator	1) Implant programming 2) Parent-toddler group 60 min. 2x/week; 20-30 min Tx with family in Center for Early Childhood Development 3) Home visit 1x/month by consultant for hearing impaired children	2-20-13 2-15-13 2-18-13	When complete Ongoing	Private insurance + Medicaid Anytown Schools Anytown Schools	

Figure 8.1. (continued)

Individualized Education Programs For students with disabilities, IEPs must include statements about the following areas: 1) the child's present levels of academic achievement and functional performance; 2) the measurable annual academic and functional goals designed to meet needs that result from the child's disability, support the child's progress in the general education curriculum, and meet each of the child's other educational needs resulting from the disability; 3) the special education, related services, modifications, and supports that are designed to help the child advance toward attaining the annual goals, be involved in and make progress in the general education curriculum, participate in extracurricular and other nonacademic activities, and participate with other children with and without disabilities; 4) to the extent practicable, an explanation of how special education, related services, and supplementary services are based on peer-reviewed research; 5) the accommodations necessary for state- and districtwide assessments and, as needed, an explanation for how benchmarks and short-term objectives are aligned to the alternate achievement standards on the IEP; 6) the transition goals and services that must be implemented by the time the child is 16 years old; and 7) the plans for periodic reports of the child's progress toward annual goals provided concurrent with report cards. Changes in IDEA in 2004 also specified procedures for excusing selected professionals from IEP meetings (e.g., if their area or service is not being reviewed or if their written input is deemed sufficient) and for modifying IEPs in writing rather than in periodic face-to-face meetings if team members agree that such procedures are acceptable at the annual meeting.

In developing each student's IEP, the team members must consider evaluation data, the strengths of the student, concerns of the student's parents, and information from state and district testing. The LRE requirements of Part B of IDEA specify that whenever appropriate, children with disabilities must be educated with children without disabilities. The IEP team should consist of one or both parents, at least one general education teacher, and at least one special education teacher or service provider. One of these latter two also may fill the role of the local education agency's representative who is knowledgeable about the general curriculum. A sample portion of an IEP appears in Figure 8.2.

Identification of Students with Disabilities and Response to Intervention Identification of school-age students with disabilities under Part B of IDEA must involve consideration of whether the child has had appropriate instruction in reading, including the essential components of reading instruction as defined in NCLB. In determining eligibility, the IEP teams must review existing evaluation data, including local and state assessments. A major change in the 2004 reauthorization of IDEA, when identifying specific learning disability, was that states must not require IEP teams to consider a severe discrepancy between achievement and intellectual ability. The regulations for IDEA allow school districts to use other procedures as long as the procedures are research based (IDEA Regulations, 34 C.F.R. § 300.307). As an alternative, school teams could now use a process called "response to intervention" (RTI) to determine if a student who is struggling might respond to early intervention services. The wording related to RTI in

Sample

Individualized education program: Measurable annual goal with benchmarks

Student: _Sam Johnson_   DOB: _7/25/2004_   Date: _10/2/2012_

☒ Academic/cognitive   ☐ Social/behavioral   ☒ Communication   ☐ Gross/fine motor   ☐ Health   ☐ Self-help   ☐ Other (specify) _____

☐ **Check here if the student is 13 or older.** (If checked, **IEP** Transition Planning Summary must be completed.)

Measurable annual goal #1	Method of evaluation	Performance criteria	Report of progress*			
			Nov.	Jan.	April	June
Sam will show story reading, writing, and retelling abilities that are comparable to those of his 2nd grade general education classmates.	Probe stories and stories produced in language arts	Demonstration of new behaviors independently				
Benchmarks for annual goal #1						
#1a: *Sam will use a planning template to organize a story with characters, a problem, and cause and effect when writing and for stories written by others to use in retelling.*						
#1b: *Sam will show ability to combine sentences using a variety of structures to yield average lengths that exceed his baseline levels (mean length of T-unit at baseline was 3.5; 2 sentences were simple incorrect; 3 were simple correct; 0 complex).*	Same	MLTU of <4.0 At least 1 complex sentence				
#1c: *Sam will increase the number of different words in his written and retold stories from baseline levels (10 different words; 20 total words) and, with scaffolding help, will add at least 2 novel "interesting words" when editing.*	Same	New stories will average 25+ words and include 15+ different words				

Evaluation Procedures

1 = Criterion-references/curriculum-based assessment
2 = Pre- and poststandardized assessment
3 = Pre- and postbaseline data
4 = Quizzes/tests
5 = Student self-assessment rubric
6 = Observation
7 = Work samples/project/experiment/portfolio
8 = Job performance or products
9 = Behavior/performance rating scale
10 = Statewide achievement test
11 = Achievement of objectives (specify)
12 = Other (specify)

Performance criteria

A = 100%
B = 90%
C = 80%
D = 70%
E = Standard score increase: _____
F = Months growth increase: _____
G = Passing grades/score: _____
H = Frequency/trials: (e.g., 9/10) _____
I = Duration: (e.g., 15 min, 1 per) _____
J = Successful completion of task/activity
K = Other (specify) _Meet benchmarks in goals_ **(Note: Use with goal only)**
L = Other (specify) _____

Report of progress key*

M = Mastered
S = Satisfactory progress (likely to achieve)
U = Unsatisfactory progress (unlikely to achieve)
NP 1 = No progress (will **not** achieve): lack of prerequisite skills
NP 2 = No progress (will **not** achieve): need more time
NP 3 = No progress (will **not** achieve): inadequate assessment
NP 4 = No progress (will **not** achieve): excessive absences/tardiness
NI = Not introduced
O = Other (specify)

*Indicates extent to which progress is sufficient to achieve goal by the end of the year

Figure 8.2. Sample individualized education program form. (*Key:* MLTU, mean length of T-unit; SLP, speech-language pathologist.) (*Source:* Connecticut State Department of Education, 2013.)

Modifications/adaptations in general education, including nonacademic and extracurricular activities and collaboration/supports for school personnel

Student: _____Sam Johnson_____   DOB: _____7/25/2004_____   Date: _____10/2/2012_____

Modification/adaptations in regular education, including nonacademic and extracurricular activities				Sites/activities where required and duration	Required supports for personnel and frequency and duration of supports**
Materials/books/equipment				*Writing lab times Tuesday–Thursday 1 h each*	*SLP will work in classroom with teacher on Tuesday. Teacher will provide support Thursday.*
☐ Alternative text	☐ Consumable workbook	☐ Modified worksheets	☒ Access to computer		
☐ Tape recorder	☐ Supplementary visuals	☐ Large print text	☐ Calculator		
☒ Assistive technology (specify) *Software with synthesized speech*					
Test/quizzes/time					
☐ Prior notice of tests	☐ Preview test procedures	☐ Test study guide	☐ Simplify test wording	☐ Oral testing	
☐ Limited multiple choice	☐ Student writes on test	☐ Shortened tasks	☐ Hands-on projects	☐ Reduced reading	
☐ Alternative tests	☐ Objective tests	☐ Extra credit options	☐ Extra time-written work		
☒ Extra time/tests	☐ Extra time/projects	☐ Extra response time	☐ Modified tests		
☐ Pace long-term projects	☐ Rephrase test questions/directions		☐ Other (specify)		
Grading				*Any formal graded activities*	
☒ No spelling penalty	☒ No handwriting penalty	☐ Grade effort + work	☐ Grade improvement	☐ Course credit	
☐ Base grade on IEP	☐ Base grade on ability	☐ Modified grades	☐ Pass/fail	☐ Audit course	
☒ Other (specify) *Provide feedback on spelling and keep data*					
Organization					
☒ Provide study outlines	☐ Desktop list of tasks	☐ List sequential steps	☐ Post routines	☐ Post assignments	
☐ Give one paper at a time	☐ Folders to hold work	☐ Pencil box for tools	☐ Pocket folder for work	☐ Assignment pad	
☐ Daily assignment list	☐ Daily homework list	☐ Worksheet formats	☐ Extra space for work	☐ Assign partner	
☐ Other (specify)					
Environment				*Any formal instruction*	
☐ Preferential seating	☐ Clear work area	☐ Study carrel	☐ Other (specify)		
Behavioral management					
☐ Daily feedback to student	☐ Chart progress	☐ Behavior contracts	☐ Parent/guardian sign homework		
☐ Positive reinforcement	☐ Collect baseline data	☐ Set/post class rules	☐ Parent/guardian sign behavioral chart		
☐ Cue expected behavior	☐ Structure transitions	☐ Break between tasks	☐ Time out from positive reinforcement		
☐ Proximity/touch control	☐ Contingency plan	☐ Other (specify)			
Teaching Strategies				*During writing lab times and any other times when general ed teacher deems appropriate*	*SLP will work in classroom with teacher on Tuesday during writing lab sessions.*
☒ Check work in progress	☐ Immediate feedback	☐ Preteach content	☒ Have student restate information		
☐ Extra drill/practice	☐ Review sessions	☐ Review directions	☐ Provide lecture notes/outline to student		
☐ Use manipulatives	☐ Modified content	☐ Assign study partner	☐ Computer-assisted instruction		
☐ Monitor assignments	☒ Provide models	☐ Repeat instructions	☐ Support auditory presentation with visuals		
☐ Multisensory approach	☐ Highlight key words	☐ Oral reminders	☐ Display key vocabulary		
☐ Visual reinforcement	☐ Pictures/charts	☐ Visual reminders	☐ Provide student with vocabulary word bank		
☐ Mimed clues/gestures	☐ Concrete examples	☐ Use mnemonics	☒ Personalized examples		
☐ Number line	☐ Other (specify)				

Figure 8.2. (continued)

IDEA reads as follows: "In determining whether a child has a specific learning disability, a local educational agency may use a process that determines if the child responds to scientific, research-based intervention as part of the evaluation process" (IDEA 20 U.S.C. § 1414(b)(6)(B)). Failure to respond to the intervention might be considered an indicator that a student has a specific learning disability that requires special education.

The option to use RTI as part of the evaluation process for learning disabilities was part of the changes in policy that made it permissible for school districts to spend up to 15% of their IDEA Part B funds on early intervention services in general education settings. Special education personnel and SLPs could now participate in preventive instructional activities with children not identified under IDEA as having a disability. These changes were made in response to research showing that early interventions might be more effective before young students' reading problems become "severe and intractable" (Yell & Walker, 2010, p. 126), thus avoiding the "wait-to-fail" elements of the discrepancy model.

The provision to allow RTI services has implications, however, that go beyond the identification of any one disability. Simonsen et al. (2010) described RTI as a schoolwide intervention model that is undergoing rapid development. A common interpretation conceptualizes RTI as a triangle with three tiers of services characterized by increasing intensity and individualization, with each tier required by smaller numbers of students. The expectation is that at the base of the triangle, 80%–90% of students will respond to high-quality general instruction, referred to as Tier 1; an additional 5%–10% will respond when they are provided targeted group interventions in Tier 2; and yet another 1%–5% may respond to the intensive individualized services at the top level of Tier 3. Some school districts define Tier 3 as special education; others view it as a more intensive form of general education. The RTI model has implications for speech-language pathologists beyond the identification of students with learning disabilities (Ehren & Nelson, 2005; Staskowski & Rivera, 2005). Case Example 1 provides an illustration of how a school-based SLP might contribute to decision making using an RTI model.

 CASE EXAMPLE 1

As an SLP who works in a school district, you are concerned about the district's long-standing policy that students with language delays are not eligible for services unless formal tests show a discrepancy between IQ scores and language quotient scores. Brian is a 6-year-old child in the first grade with a history of preschool language problems involving phonology and syntax, but he did not receive language intervention services in kindergarten and does not currently have a diagnosis of language impairment. As a first grader, Brian is struggling with phonemic awareness, reading decoding, and spoken and written language comprehension. Although Brian now sounds okay when he talks, his teacher is worried and his mother has expressed concerns about his language as well as his reading. Brian's mother has asked his teacher whether he should be tested, but she has learned that the school guidelines require Brian to participate in

RTI services before he can be tested for special education. His mother contacts you as the clinician who worked with Brian as a preschooler. You help her to understand that such guidelines were developed to guide general practice but that RTI approaches are not to be used to delay assessment in cases like Brian's. That is, if there is a concern that a child might have a disability, a parent has the right to request testing for possible special education services at any time. If Brian's mother presents such a request in writing, the clock will be started right away requiring timely comprehensive assessment under IDEA.

When you and the school psychologist test Brian, you find that he has cognitive skills in the low–mid range. Thus, even though his language skills are quite low for his age and he has been struggling in first grade, he does not meet the cognitive referencing criteria historically used by SLPs in the district. As the SLP, you participate in an IEP meeting in which the team decides that Brian should be eligible for language intervention services under an IEP because the research literature does not support cognitive referencing (see review by Nelson, 2010) and because changes in IDEA 2004 prohibit states from requiring a severe discrepancy between achievement and intellectual ability to identify specific learning disability, which you argue, should apply to identification of language impairment as well. Thus, Brian becomes part of your caseload, and you coordinate your efforts with the reading specialist who is providing early intervention reading supports, which Brian continues to receive as part of general education.

Section 504 of the Rehabilitation Act

Section 504 of the Rehabilitation Act of 1973 (PL 93-112) is civil rights legislation that makes it possible for children and adults facing a range of challenges to receive accommodations if they need them to participate in important life activities. It specifies that an otherwise qualified individual with a disability cannot be excluded from participation in, denied the benefits of, or subjected to discrimination under any program or activity receiving financial assistance from the federal government—including those in public elementary, secondary, and postsecondary schools. To qualify for accommodations under Section 504, individuals must be identified as having physical or mental impairments that substantially limit one or more of their major life activities.

Protection from discrimination in education agencies means that schools must make reasonable accommodations, such as structural alterations and modifications of classroom materials and procedures, to make it possible for individuals with disabilities to participate. Educational agencies must ensure that students with disabilities have access to nonacademic services as well. At the postsecondary level, this requirement might include providing students with disabilities access to housing that is comparable to housing for students without disabilities. Other modifications in academic programs might include extra time to complete assignments, adjustments in the length of assignments, the use of peer tutors, provision of visual aids, the ability to audio record lectures, or the use of specialized curricular materials. Modification of tests might include permission to receive testing orally or from an audio recording, extra time to complete tests, permission to dictate test answers, and use of an altered test format or a test printed in an enlarged type. Provision of auxiliary aids and devices might include sign language interpreters, frequency modulated amplification systems, and other forms of assistive technology.

In requiring schools to be accessible, Section 504 does not require every part of a school to be modified as long as the school's educational programs as a whole are accessible. Evaluations under Section 504 must be conducted with procedures that are 1) validated for the specific purpose for which they are used; 2) administered by trained personnel; 3) tailored to assess specific areas of educational need; and 4) selected to ensure that when a test is administered to a student with impaired sensory, manual, or speaking skills, the test results reflect the student's aptitude or achievement accurately rather than the student's impairment.

The Rehabilitation Act of 1973 (PL 93-112) also makes it possible for adults and children with disabilities to qualify for services under the Rehabilitation Services Administration, a branch of the Office of Special Education and Rehabilitative Services within the U.S. Department of Education. Qualification occurs when an individual with a disability applies to his or her state office of vocational rehabilitation for the purpose of identifying a plan to procure or enhance a work opportunity. In the case of an adult with new onset of traumatic brain injury or stroke, SLP services may be provided for the restoration of or compensation for the language or cognitive skills that would enhance the individual's chances of successfully attaining or returning to gainful employment.

Americans with Disabilities Act of 1990

The three basic purposes of the Americans with Disabilities Act (ADA) of 1990 (PL 101-336) are to ensure that individuals with disabilities have equal opportunity to 1) participate fully in society, 2) live independently, and 3) have access to economic self-sufficiency through the removal of barriers. The legislation is divided into five areas, called *titles*, addressing employment, public services, public accommodations operated by a private entity, telecommunications, and miscellaneous other issues.

Title I applies to *employment*. It requires employers with 15 or more employees, employment agencies, labor agencies, and labor–management committees to make accommodations for qualified employees. Qualified employees include individuals who have a disability in one or more area but who can still perform the essential functions of an employment position with or without reasonable accommodation. Title I prohibits discrimination in the following areas: job application procedures; hiring, advancement, or discharge of employees; employee compensation; job training; and other terms, conditions, or privileges of employment. An SLP may be consulted when determining reasonable accommodations. These may include restructuring of the job; modification of work schedules; acquisition or modification of equipment or assistive devices; adjustment or modification of examination materials, training materials, or policies; and provision of qualified readers or interpreters. Procedures for determining reasonable accommodations include analyzing the requirements of the job, identifying potential accommodations in consultation with the individual with the disability, and considering the preferences of the individual when deciding which options to pursue.

Title II applies to *public services* in entities such as schools, colleges, and universities. It ensures that policies are in place to protect the educational opportunities of individuals with disabilities and to guard against discrimination.

Title III applies to *public accommodations operated by a private entity.* It protects the rights of individuals with disabilities to gain access to places of lodging, exhibition or entertainment, recreation, and education; places where social services are offered; and stores, shopping centers, bars, and restaurants. For example, architectural accessibility modifications must be made to remove architectural and structural barriers in existing facilities when the modifications are readily achievable. If they are not readily achievable, the private entities must provide alternative methods for gaining access to the public accommodations. New buildings are required to comply fully with ADA accessibility requirements. Some strategies for removing architectural barriers include installing ramps, repositioning shelves, adding raised markings on elevator control buttons and lowering elevator control panels, designating parking spaces, installing accessible door hardware, widening doors and doorways, and installing grab bars in toilet stalls.

Title IV applies to *telecommunication services.* It requires the provision of technical support for persons with hearing and speech impairments. This title is responsible for making telephone systems with teletypewriter devices available to the public in places such as airports and restaurants.

Title V applies to *due process* provisions. It includes notice that states are not immune from the law's provisions. States, as well as other public or private entities, may be sued for noncompliance. Other provisions allow courts to award attorney's fees to prevailing parties and indicate that the law prohibits retaliation and coercion against people with disabilities who are seeking enforcement of the policy. Although the ADA is enforced through court actions, parties are encouraged to resolve disputes through methods other than litigation if possible.

Medicare, Medicaid, and the Balanced Budget Amendments

Prior to 1961, public policies aimed at assisting older adults consisted primarily of retirement supplements and benefits for individuals of low socioeconomic status. In 1961, President John F. Kennedy sponsored a "Conference on Aging" to build national awareness of issues important to older adults. This conference identified the problems ("want–get gaps") that were distressing to older adults, such as health and income maintenance; opportunity to retire with dignity; and issues pertaining to housing, transportation, and social isolation (Brown, 1996). This conference set the stage for the development of several key pieces of legislation, including the Older Americans Act of 1965 (PL 89-73), which was reauthorized in 2000 as the Older Americans Act Amendments (PL 106-501), as well as Medicare and Medicaid (Brown, 1996). The purpose of the Older Americans Act of 1965 was to help older individuals by providing funds to states for programs and services such as education about nutrition, hot meals, transportation, legal assistance, and materials to train service providers in the area of gerontology (Gelfand, 1999). Medicare and Medicaid policies later extended this legislation (Brown, 1996; Rigby & Kipping, 2000).

Medicare   The Social Security Act (SSA) of 1935 (PL 74-271), which was originally passed under the leadership of President Franklin D. Roosevelt, was designed to alleviate conditions of poverty. The Medicare program was established in 1965 as Title 18 to the SSA. It was an initial attempt by the government to assist individuals to meet the costs of adequate health care.

Medicare assistance is administered by a federal agency called the Centers for Medicare and Medicaid Services (CMS). Medicare is available to individuals who turn 65 years of age and those younger than 65 who have been diagnosed with amyotrophic lateral sclerosis or have a qualifying disability, or persons of any age who have end-stage renal disease (CMS, 2012a). Medicare has two parts that most commonly pertain to the provision of speech-language pathology or audiological services: *Part A* provides prepaid hospital insurance, and *Part B* offers additional optional medical insurance.

Part A finances hospital insurance through payroll tax. Consequently, people who are eligible for Medicare do not pay additional premiums for hospital insurance, which covers inpatient care in hospitals, skilled nursing facilities, and a limited number of days for hospice care in any benefit period. A *benefit period* includes the time a patient first enters a hospital up to and including the day of discharge. The longer the stay in the hospital, the more out-of-pocket costs are charged to the individual and fewer costs are covered by Medicare. For example, Medicare covers the first 60 days after the individual has paid a deductible ($1,184 in 2013). For days 61–90, the individual is responsible for a copayment ($296 in 2013) for each day of hospital stay, and after 90 days a copayment of $592 per day up to 60 days over a lifetime (http://www.medicare.gov).

Part A benefits also cover limited days in skilled nursing facilities. These facilities, previously known as *nursing homes,* are identified as such because they include a percentage of residents who require services from skilled professionals, such as nurses and rehabilitation specialists, including SLPs. For the first 20 days in a skilled nursing facility, Medicare pays 100% of the costs. For days 21–100 a copayment is required (e.g., Medicare pays 80% of costs and the individual pays 20%). After 100 days, the individual must have a payment source other than Medicare. Such sources include private pay, Medicaid, or supplemental insurance plans.

Part B of Medicare consists of medical insurance that is financed through a monthly premium paid by the individual. As of 2013, the Medicare Part B monthly premium was $104.90 (http://www.Medicare.gov). After an annual deductible of $149 is met, Part B pays 80% of "reasonable and necessary charges" for covered services. Part B covers such services as home health services, physician medical and surgical services, supplies (including drugs that cannot be self-administered), diagnostic services, physical therapy, home dialysis, x rays, surgical dressings, casts, orthopedic devices, oxygen tanks, wheelchairs, ambulance services, prosthetic devices (but not dentures), and immunizations. Part B does not cover hearing aids, but coverage was added for augmentative and alternative communication (AAC) services and technology in January 2001 for individuals with a documented severe expressive impairment that is not expected to improve (Augmentative and Alternative Communication–Rehabilitation Engineering Research Center, 2001). In order to qualify for funding as a form of medical durable equipment, the AAC device must be appropriate for the individual's cognitive and physical abilities. In addition, the sole purpose of the device must be for speech (i.e., laptops, personal digital assistants, electronic tablets and notebooks do not qualify). However, if any of these other devices is used as a speech generation device, the specific software or application could be covered under Medicare (see http://www.asha.org/slp/healthcare/sgd/checklist).

As part of the Middle Class Tax Relief and Jobs Creation Act of 2012 (Sec. 3005g), beginning in 2013, SLPs who treat patients under Medicare Part B must report patient outcomes via nonpayable G-codes on claims forms or risk rejection of reimbursement. The set of G-codes will usually have the GN modifier when used under an SLP's plan of care (West, 2012) and will refer to one of eight sets: 1) swallowing, 2) motor speech, 3) spoken language comprehension, 4) spoken language expression, 5) attention, 6) memory, 7) voice, or 8) other. The "other" must relate to the primary functional limitation being treated. According to West, the G-code set will contain the patient's current status, projected goal status, and discharge status. This requirement or change in policy is related to efforts by CMS to collect data for creation of a new reimbursement system for therapy services. Note that ASHA played a significant role by developing the National Outcomes Measurement System (NOMS), which Medicare used in creating the required G-codes (Satterfield, Swanson, & Kander, 2012).

Managed care organizations (MCOs) provide additional forms of supplemental insurance to Medicare recipients. These organizations manage or control health care expenditures by closely monitoring how service providers (e.g., hospitals, physicians) treat patients and by evaluating the necessity, appropriateness, and payment efficiency of the health services.

Health maintenance organizations (HMOs) are examples of MCOs that provide a range of care on a prepayment basis. Individuals continue to pay Part B premiums, and the HMO receives payment from the federal government for each HMO member equivalent to 95% of the average Medicare costs. These organizations may cover costs that are not covered by Medicare. For example, HMOs may contract with or employ service providers and pay for a minimum of 2 months or 60 visits (whichever is greater) per condition for a combination of speech-language pathology, occupational therapy, and physical therapy services. Some HMOs interpret these visits as the maximum rather than the minimum, however, resulting in inadequately provided services. Some SLPs also have experienced problems with HMOs when attempting to get approval for necessary services, as illustrated in Case Example 2.

 CASE EXAMPLE 2

Mrs. Robinson, an outpatient at Cedar Rehabilitation Services, was referred to you for voice therapy by an ear, nose, and throat specialist following a medical treatment for vocal nodules. For each of the next 6 months after receipt of the referral, however, the HMO refused to approve the voice therapy treatment. When the treatment was approved, it was for 3 visits only. Based on past records, you know that 3 visits are insufficient to serve Mrs. Robinson adequately. You provide the HMO with evidence that additional sessions are needed to retrain Mrs. Robinson's vocal behaviors so that the vocal nodules are less likely to recur. You also work with Mrs. Robinson to write to her legislators about problems in the health care financing system, showing how they are interfering with her access to adequate health care.

The Balanced Budget Act and Medicare Modernization Act   On August 1, 1997, President William J. Clinton signed into law the Balanced Budget Act (BBA) of 1997 (PL 105-33). The BBA, as its name implied, was designed to balance the national budget. Thus, it included provisions to reduce overall spending on Medicaid and to slow the growth of Medicare spending over 5 years. These reductions included limiting the funds designated for preventive benefits not previously covered, such as mammograms, self-management of diabetes, and prostate and colorectal cancer screening. Funding limits also were placed on spending under the BBA, which resulted in some programs receiving more funds and other programs receiving less, causing agencies and providers to compete for limited resources. This new competitiveness had the effect of denying Medicare funds to individuals who most needed them (ASHA, 2005).

The Balanced Budget Refinement Act (BBRA) of 1999 (PL 106-113) was signed into law on November 29, 1999, also by President Clinton, with a 2-year moratorium on the $1,500 cap on Medicare Part B services for combined outpatient speech-language pathology and physical therapy services from January 2000 through December 2001. Through this refined act, speech-language pathology service was reinstated as an independent service no longer linked with physical therapy, which made it possible for SLPs and physical therapists to be reimbursed separately. The BBRA was initiated through the actions of legislators and the advocacy of professional groups such as ASHA, the American Occupational Therapy Association, and the American Physical Therapy Association. Although the $1,500 cap limits were not in effect from 2000 through 2002, keeping it that way has required subsequent passages of moratoriums by Congress, including the Middle Class Tax Relief and Job Creation Act of 2012. Therapy caps remain a subject of controversy that requires constant vigilance and advocacy efforts on behalf of all individuals affected by the provision of rehabilitative speech-language pathology services.

Medicaid   Congress established **Medicaid** in 1965 under Title 19 of the Social Security Act (SSA). Funding for Medicaid comes from state, federal, and city taxes. Hence, it is a federal–state matching program because both the state and federal governments must contribute to it. Medicaid is run by state governments under guidelines from the federal government, resulting in variability in eligibility benefits from one state to the next.

Medicaid was created by Congress to pay medical bills for persons of low socioeconomic status who have no other financial means to pay for medical care. It is an entitlement program in that Congress has set eligibility criteria based on age, income, retirement, disability, or unemployment, which entitle those individuals who qualify to its benefits (Dye, 1998). Most Medicaid spending goes to older individuals and to individuals with disabilities. In addition, anyone receiving public assistance through Supplemental Security Income or Temporary Assistance for Needy Families is automatically eligible for Medicaid.

Medicaid covers such services as payment to hospitals, prenatal and delivery services for those with no other insurance, and services to families of low socioeconomic status who do not receive cash assistance. It is possible to obtain Medicaid coverage for rehabilitation for individuals of low socioeconomic status without insurance, but this requires an evaluation and the completion of the appropriate Medicaid Prior Approval form. The Medicaid Prior Approval form includes information on expected duration, short-term objectives, and projected outcome of treatment, but the form has a waiting period for approval. In a similar manner, coverage for AAC devices may be obtained if the appropriate codes are used (Higdon, 2003). Medicaid also covers long-term care in a skilled nursing facility, but only after beneficiaries have exhausted all other income and forms of payment. Most benefits are limited to long-term rehabilitative care.

The federal government does not mandate states to provide speech-language pathology and audiology services under Medicaid, but there is an exception for providing services to Medicaid-eligible children under the age of 21. These children are mandated to receive comprehensive benefits, including periodic screenings and wellness checks through the Early and Periodic Screening, Diagnostic, and Treatment Services (EPSDT). As part of the required medical screening, speech-language pathology and audiology services are included to identify and diagnose children with speech or language impairments, provide speech and language services, make referrals to other medical professionals as needed for rehabilitation, and offer counseling and guidance to parents and teachers. In addition, Medicaid can reimburse school districts for the provision of school-based speech-language pathology and audiology services required by Part B of IDEA in an IEP (ASHA, 2003). The services must be compliant with the Medicaid requirements for coverage of services, including frequency, duration, scope, comparability, medical necessity, prior authorization, and provider requirements.

The Patient Protection and Affordable Care Act   President Obama signed into law the Patient Protection and Affordable Care Act (ACA; PL 111-148) in March 2010. According to information available at http://www.healthcare.gov (June 2012), the ACA contains 10 Titles outlining four key features relating to individual rights and protections, insurance choices, insurance costs, individuals 65 and older, and employers. The primary intent is to ensure that all Americans have access to affordable quality health care. Provisions within the measure also aim to control rising health care costs and hold insurance companies accountable. Health insurance companies are required to use a uniform glossary of terms (Sec. 2715), such as *deductible* and *copayment*, and to give detailed coverage examples to make it easier to shop for and compare health care plans (http://www.healthcare.gov).

One part of the legislation (Sec. 2714) went into effect immediately upon its passage in 2010, extending the age limit to 26 years of age for individuals to remain on a parent's insurance plan even if they are married, not living with the parent, and not dependent on the parent financially. This has led to an increase in coverage for individuals in this age group, who due to their relative poverty and low access to employee-sponsored health insurance are at risk for being uninsured (Holahan & Kenney, 2008).

Another provision in the legislation with significant potential to affect clinical practice is the mandating of "essential health benefits" (Sec. 1302). Participating in the discussion to define the scope of these services to ensure that speech, language, and audiology services are included remains a major public policy agenda issue for ASHA (n.d.).

ADVOCACY

Professionals have responsibilities for understanding, implementing, and influencing public policy. Thinking of professional roles in **advocacy** may conjure up intimidating images of visits to Capitol Hill in Washington, D.C. This is one important avenue, which is not nearly as scary as it may seem at first, but active advocacy roles also may be assumed at other levels, including at the level of the individual client.

As discussed in this chapter, policies are in place to govern who is eligible for service and who will pay for it, as well as how services are to be delivered. Audiologists and SLPs are responsible for seeing that individuals receive services according to the policies written to address their needs. This means that professionals must know how to conduct assessments and write reports that maximize their ability to deliver high-quality services. For example, this includes the responsibility to advocate for individuals who at first might appear not to qualify for services because of overly strict interpretation of eligibility guidelines, as discussed in Case Example 1. It also refers to advocacy efforts in calling and writing to third-party payers on behalf of individual clients who have been denied funding for needed services. Advocacy at the individual client level also may include working with others to make policy implementation effective and to help clients and families learn how to advocate for themselves, as illustrated in Case Examples 3 and 4.

 CASE EXAMPLE 3

You have been working as an SLP for a year in an elementary school in which the students with disabilities traditionally have been served in separate classrooms or pulled out of general education classrooms for speech-language therapy. You are concerned that this approach is not meeting the students' needs and begin to work with the early and later elementary special education teachers to bring more aspects of the general education curriculum into the special education room and to explore more ways for the students with disabilities to participate actively with their peers in the general education classrooms by using a writing lab approach (Nelson, Bahr, & Van Meter, 2004) or enriched writers' workshop (Sturm, 2012).

CASE EXAMPLE 4

Mr. Rivers resided in a skilled nursing facility 2 years prior to having a stroke. Following the stroke, you conducted an assessment of his abilities and found that Mr. Rivers required dysphagia treatment. You recommended treatment for 5 days per week for 3 weeks. Mr. Rivers's HMO, however, approved treatment for only 5 days for 1 week. You provided this treatment and trained the nursing staff to feed and support Mr. Rivers during mealtimes. His records, however, show that the limited time approved for therapy was insufficient to establish and monitor a routine with the nursing staff charged with managing Mr. Rivers's care. Consequently, the staff frequently failed to assist Mr. Rivers during mealtimes. He experienced several episodes of aspiration and eventually reverted to his original swallowing problem. You continued to advocate with the HMO to justify more treatment sessions and communicated with Mr. Rivers's legislators about the dangers inherent in the current system, some of which were life threatening or could potentially require a costly readmission to an acute care hospital.

Advocacy Strategies

Grassroots advocacy involves efforts of individuals. Such efforts are particularly effective in gaining the attention of legislators because it is individuals who are eligible to vote for policy makers. Professional associations often guide the process, however, making it less daunting. Associations serve as a resource for clarifying issues, keeping individuals informed, employing lobbyists, and establishing opportunities to communicate with key policy makers (see http://www.asha.org/advocacy/grassroots). For example, according to ASHA's public policy agenda (2012b), ASHA continues to work on behalf of SLPs and audiologists at the federal level with regard to Medicare issues, as well as in other domains. The association encourages its members to contact federal representatives with respect to equitable reimbursement for beneficiaries of Medicare, to eliminate the reimbursement cap, to reform the rate formula for reimbursement under the Medicare Part B fee schedule, and to support Medicare coverage for audiologists performing diagnostic and rehabilitative services and to have the right to opt out of the Medicare program. At both the state and federal level, advocacy efforts also support the ability of SLPs and audiologists serving children in schools to provide quality services. In its public policy agenda, ASHA asks its members to advocate for reauthorizing ESEA and IDEA, including "funding of speech, language and hearing services and devices in all federal literacy legislation" (2012b), and to use common terminology in defining *highest qualified provider* in ESEA and IDEA.

In nearly all states, ASHA has key members appointed by state speech-language-hearing associations who advocate for improvements in health care coverage and for reasonable reimbursement. These proactive state advocates for reimbursement (STARs) form one of three groups creating a network linking ASHA's advocacy efforts to states (ASHA, n.d.). These STARs seek to communicate with policy decision makers, such as health care insurance executives, officials in public agencies, and local legislators. They also rely on colleagues to help actuate change. In addition, state speech-language-hearing associations may appoint representatives to ASHA's State Medicare Administrative Contractor Network (SMAC) to influence policy decisions as they pertain to Medicare coverage (ASHA, n.d.). Finally, state associations may appoint state education advocacy leaders (SEALS) to advocate on issues that affect the delivery of speech-language pathology and audiology services in education settings. The SEALS appointees then advocate for such issues as workload or caseload, salary, and clinical management skills (ASHA, n.d.). Collectively, these three groups seek to connect national association priorities to state-level efforts.

Understanding Current Policy and How to Change It   The steps for attempting to influence existing policy include 1) gaining access to the official wording of the policy (this can usually be done through Internet research), 2) identifying which government body or agency made the policy or rule, 3) determining whether the policy might have flexibility that was previously unnoticed, and 4) exploring whether the policy allows exceptions or variations that can overcome the immediate problem or concern without modifying the policy itself. If current policy still presents a problem, professionals may choose one of three options: They may

- *Study the rationale for the policy and decide to accept it.* In some cases, investigating the rationale for a policy may lead to greater understanding about why the policy was established, and professionals may decide there is no need to influence change.

- *Seek approval for a policy exception.* If a policy includes any room for negotiation or for exceptions, professionals may pursue such options. Obtaining permission for an exception to the rule may make it possible to gather additional data, which can then be used to make a case for more widespread change if it still seems desirable.

- *Work to change the official policy.* If a policy clearly needs changing, professionals have an obligation to work within official systems to advocate for change.

Communicating Directly with Policy Makers   The framing of a new bill requires direct involvement with legislators, particularly those on the committee where the bill will first be considered. Professional associations often employ legislative specialists, also called lobbyists, who are familiar with this complicated process and how to influence it. If the change needed is at the level of regulation rather than legislation, it may be more appropriate to start by communicating with the agency of the executive branch of government that is responsible for implementing the policy. One important question in such cases is whether the agency expects regulations for the policy to be opened for change any time soon.

When communicating directly with policy makers, it is important to note that most employers do not want their employees to write letters with political implications on agency stationery. Political advocacy messages should be conveyed as personal communication by individuals. This approach makes it clear that a constituent's views do not necessarily represent the official position of the

☐ **Short:** Is my letter one page or less in length?

☐ **Direct:** Is my letter to the point?

☐ **Client-based rationale:** Does my letter show how the proposed policy or change will influence the lives of constituents of the person to whom I am addressing the letter?

☐ **Data rather than emotions:** Does my letter provide information that will help the policy maker decide (rather than making an emotional plea)?

☐ **Ask for a specific action:** Does my letter make it clear what action I am requesting from the policy maker?

☐ **Responsive:** Does my letter indicate who I am and how I may be contacted for further information? (This also implies that I will follow up with the policy maker to express appreciation for considering my input and, if appropriate, to thank the policy maker for action consistent with my request.)

☐ **Personal:** Is my letter on my personal stationery unless I have obtained specific permission to use the stationery of the agency where I am employed?

Figure 8.3.   Checklist for advocacy letters.

individual's employer. In fact, personal communication coming from a constituent's home address to his or her legislative representative or senator (state or national) generally has the most meaning for policy makers. Figure 8.3. summarizes considerations for writing advocacy letters or composing e-mail messages.

Working within Professional Associations   Some of the most effective efforts occur when members of professional associations work together. Consider ASHA, for example, which keeps its members informed of policies and their implications through both its web site (http://www.asha.org) and its publications, particularly *The ASHA Leader*. The ASHA Government Relations and Public Policy Board is responsible for developing an annual public policy agenda to prioritize the advocacy activities of the association. The goal is to address issues that are of major concern to speech-language-hearing scientists, SLPs, audiologists, and the individuals whom they serve.

At a minimum, professionals who pay their dues to both state and national professional associations help to maintain professional organizations so that they can monitor public policy and communicate with their members, the public, and the policy makers at local and national levels. At a level of slightly greater involvement, professionals can make voluntary contributions to political action committees, which are in a position to lobby directly for change. At the most active level, professionals can become personally involved by writing letters, sending e-mail messages, and making telephone calls or personal visits to policy makers. State professional organizations often organize and facilitate these actions to communicate with state legislators. Individual SLPs and audiologists have played important roles in the development and modifications that have been made over the years in many of the key pieces of legislation discussed in this chapter.

CONCLUSION

Public policies guide many aspects of clinical decision making. It is the responsibility of professional practitioners to understand how public policies are generated, legislated, and regulated. Although professionals are expected to implement public policies, they also can question the wisdom of some policies, and when problems are evident, it is professionals' responsibility to advocate for change. Effective advocacy involves gathering and presenting data in a way that clearly communicates to policy makers a need at the level of the policy and the individuals affected by the policy.

STUDY QUESTIONS

1. List and discuss three reasons why it is important for SLPs and audiologists to know about public policies.

2. What are the key elements guaranteed by NCLB and IDEA? In what ways are the two laws compatible? In what ways are they distinct? In what ways might they exert conflicting requirements?

3. Contrast the important aspects of Section 504 of the Rehabilitation Act and the ADA.

4. Explain the influence of Medicare, Medicaid, and managed care organizations on speech-language pathology and audiology service provision in medical settings.

5. Describe levels of advocacy and discuss why it is important for audiologists and SLPs to take on advocacy roles.

REFERENCES

American Speech-Language-Hearing Association. (n.d.). *ASHA's state advocates for reimbursement (STARs): A state-based reimbursement network*. Retrieved from http://www.asha.org/practice/reimbursement/private-plans/reimbursement_network.htm

American Speech-Language-Hearing Association. (n.d.). *ASHA state education advocacy leaders* (SEALS). Retrieved from http://www.asha.org/advocacy/state/seals

American Speech-Language-Hearing Association. (n.d.). *The Patient Protection and Affordable Care Act (ACA): Essential health benefits*. Retrieved from http://www.asha.org/practice/Health-Care-Reform/Essential-Health-Benefits

American Speech-Language-Hearing Association. (2003). *Medicaid and third party payments in the schools*. Retrieved from http://www.asha.org/members/issues/reimbursement/medicaid/thirdparty-payment.htm

American Speech-Language-Hearing Association. (2012a). *Therapy cap advocacy center: Background on therapy cap*. Retrieved from http://www.asha.org/advocacy/federal/cap

American Speech-Language-Hearing Association. (2012b). *2013 Public Policy Agenda*. Retrieved from http://www.asha.org/2013-ASHA-Public-Policy-Agenda

Americans with Disabilities Act (ADA) of 1990, PL 101-336, 42 U.S.C. §§ 12101 *et seq.*

Annett, M.M. (2003, December 16). No Child Left Behind: A key focus of 2003 schools forum—ED officials address law, students with disabilities. *The ASHA Leader, 3*, 33.

Augmentative and Alternative Communication–Rehabilitation Engineering Research Center. (2001). Medicare. In *Medicare AAC device coverage guidance* (National Coverage Decision No. 50.1). Retrieved from http://aac-rerc.com/pages/Medicare/RMRP.htm#ncd

Ayres, K.M., Lowrey, K.A., Douglas, K.H., & Sievers, C. (2011). I can identify Saturn but I can't brush my teeth: What happens when the curricular focus for students with severe disabilities shifts. *Education and Training in Autism and Developmental Disabilities, 46*(1), 11–21.

Balanced Budget Act (BBA) of 1997, PL 105-33, 111 Stat. 251.

Balanced Budget Refinement Act (BBRA) of 1999, PL 106-113.

Blosser, J., Roth, F.P., Paul, D.R., Ehren, B.J., Nelson, N.W., & Sturm, J.M. (2012). Integrating the core. *The ASHA Leader, 17*(10), 12–15.

Brown, D.K. (1996). *Introduction to public policy: An aging perspective*. Lanham, MD: University Press of America.

Centers for Medicare and Medicaid Services (CMS). (2012a). Medicare program—General information. Retrieved from http://cms.gov/Medicare/Medicare-General-Information/MedicareGenInfo/index.html

Centers for Medicare and Medicaid Services (CMS). (2012b). *Therapy cap.* Retrieved from http://cms.gov/research-statistics-data-and-systems/monitoring-programs/medical-review/therapycap.html

Children's Health Act of 2000, PL 106-310,114 Stat. 1101, 42 U.S.C. §§ 201 *et seq.*

Connecticut State Department of Education. (2013). *IEP manual and forms.* Retrieved from http://www.sde.ct.gov/sde/lib/sde/PDF/DEPS/Special/IEPManual.pdf

Courtade, G., Spooner, F., Browder, D., & Jimenez, B. (2012). Seven reasons to promote standards-based instruction for students with severe disabilities: A reply to Ayres, Lowrey, Douglas, & Sievers (2011). *Education and Training in Autism and Developmental Disabilities, 47*(1), 3–13.

Dye, T.R. (1998). *Understanding public policy* (9th ed.). Upper Saddle River, NJ: Prentice Hall.

Early Hearing Detection and Intervention Act of 2010, PL 111-337.

Education for All Handicapped Children Act of 1975, PL 94-142, 20 U.S.C. §§ 1400 *et seq.*

Education of the Handicapped Act (EHA) of 1970, PL 91-230, 84 Stat. 121-154, 20 U.S.C. §§ 1400 *et seq.*

Ehren, B., & Nelson, N. (2005). The responsiveness to intervention approach and language impairment. *Topics in Language Disorders, 25*(2), 120–132.

Elementary and Secondary Education Act (ESEA) of 1965, PL 89-10, 20 U.S.C. §§ 241 *et seq.*

Etscheidt, S. (2012). Complacency with access and the aggregate? Affirming an individual determination of educational benefit under the Individuals with Disabilities Education Act. *Journal of Disability Policy Studies, 22*(4), 195–207.

Gelfand, D.E. (1999). *The aging network: Programs and services* (5th ed.). New York, NY: Springer-Verlag.

Higdon, C. (2003). CPT coding for AAC/SGDs. *The ASHA Leader* [Online publication]. Retrieved from http://www.asha.org/about/publications/leader-online/b-line/bl030527.htm

Holahan, J., & Kenney, G. (2008, June). *Health insurance coverage of young adults: Issues and broader considerations.* Published by Urban Institute: Timely Analysis of Intermediate Health Policy Issues. Available from the Urban Institute web site, http://www.urban.org/UploadedPDF/411691_young_adult_insurance.pdf

Individuals with Disabilities Education Act (IDEA) of 1990, PL 101-476, 20 U.S.C. §§ 1400 *et seq.*

Individuals with Disabilities Education Improvement Act of 2004, PL 108-446, 20 U.S.C. §§ 1400 *et seq.*

Metcalf, S. (2002, January 28). Reading between the lines. *The Nation.* Retrieved from http://www.thenation.com/doc.mhtml?i=20020128&s=metcalf

Meyer, L. (2004, May 27). No Child Left Behind fails to pass fairness test. *Albuquerque Journal.* Retrieved from http://ourworld.compuserve.com/homepages/JWCRAWFORD/AJ2.htm

Middle Class Tax Relief and Jobs Creation Act of 2012, PL 112-96, 26 U.S.C. §§ 3005 *et seq.*

Moore-Brown, B.J., & Montgomery, J.K. (2005). *Making a difference: In the era of accountability.* Eau Claire, WI: Thinking Publications.

Moores, D.F. (2011). Waist deep in the big muddy: The Individuals with Disabilities Education Act (IDEA) and No Child Left Behind (NCLB). *American Annals of the Deaf, 155*(5), 523–525.

National Center for Hearing Assessment and Management (NCHAM). (2012). *EHDI legislation: Overview.* Logan: Utah State University. Retrieved from http://www.infanthearing.org/legislation

National Governors Association Center for Best Practices, Council of Chief State School Officers. (2010). *Common core state standards.* Washington, DC: Author.

Nelson, N.W. (2010). *Language and literacy disorders: Infancy through adolescence.* Boston, MA: Allyn & Bacon.

Nelson, N.W., Bahr, C.M., & Van Meter, A.M. (2004). *The writing lab approach to language instruction and intervention.* Baltimore, MD: Paul H. Brookes Publishing Co.

Newborn and Infant Hearing Screening and Intervention Act of 1999, PL 93-406, 88 Stat. 829.

No Child Left Behind Act of 2001, PL 107-110, 115 Stat. 1425, 20 U.S.C. §§ 6301 *et seq.*

Older American Act Amendments of 2000, PL 106-501, Stat. 2226, 42 U.S.C §§ 3001 *et seq.*

Older Americans Act of 1965, PL 89-73, 42 U.S.C. §§ 3001 *et seq.*

Patient Protection and Affordable Care Act of 2010, PL 111-148, 42 U.S.C §§ 1302, 2714 & 2715 *et seq.*

Rehabilitation Act of 1973, PL 93-112, 87 Stat. 355.

Rigby, S., & Kipping, P. (2000). *The speech-language pathologist's guide to managing the new Medicare.* Austin, TX: PRO-ED.

Satterfield, L., Swanson, N., & Kander, M. (2012). SLPs must report Medicare outcomes in '13. *The ASHA Leader, 17*(15), 1, 10.

Simonsen, B., Shaw, S.F., Faggella-Luby, M., Sugai, G., Coyne, M.D., Rhein, B., ... Alfano, M. (2010). A schoolwide model for service delivery: Redefining special educators as interventionists. *Remedial and Special Education, 31*(1), 17–23.

Social Security Act of 1935, PL 74-271, 42 U.S.C. §§ 301 *et seq.*

Staskowski, M., & Rivera, E.A. (2005). Speech-language pathologists' involvement in responsiveness to intervention activities: A complement to curriculum-relevant practice. *Topics in Language Disorders, 25*(2), 132–147.

Sturm, J.M. (2012). An enriched writers' workshop for beginning writers with developmental disabilities. *Topics in Language Disorders, 32,* 335–360.

U.S. Department of Education. (2002). *No Child Left Behind: Overview.* Retrieved from http://www2.ed.gov/policy/elsec/leg/esea02/index.html

U.S. Department of Education. (2005). *Spellings announces new special education guidelines, details, workable "common-sense" policy to help states implement No Child Left Behind.* Retrieved from http://www.ed.gov/news/pressreleases/2005/05/05102005.html

West, P. (2012, December 12). *Preparing for therapy required functional reporting implementation in CY 2013.* Retrieved from Medicare Learning Network web site, http://cms.gov/site-search/search-results.html?q=preparing%20for%20therapy%20functional%20reporting

Yell, M.L., & Walker, D.W. (2010). The legal basis of response to intervention: Analysis and implications. *Exceptionality, 18*(3), 124–137.

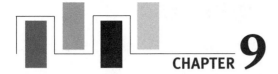

CHAPTER **9**

Clinical Service Delivery and Work Settings

Mary H. Purdy, Paul W. Cascella, and James J. Dempsey

CHAPTER OBJECTIVES

After reading this chapter, students will be able to

- Describe the role of the speech-language pathologist across medical and educational settings

- Identify the audiologist as an entry-level practitioner and identify multiple work settings for the qualified audiologist

Speech-language pathologists (SLPs) and audiologists provide a broad range of professional services aimed at assessing, treating, and preventing speech, language, voice, hearing, swallowing, and related communication disabilities. Estimates suggest that one out of every six Americans has a communication disorder and nearly 29 million Americans have a hearing impairment (American Speech-Language-Hearing Association [ASHA], 2008b). As audiologists and SLPs, we strive to create **service delivery models** that can accommodate the broad range of communication disabilities faced by our patients, while matching the particular needs of each individual. Service delivery models are the systems that are used to organize speech-language and hearing programs within employment settings. These models define our roles in the rehabilitation of persons with communication disorders.

This chapter introduces contemporary service delivery models and work settings within the field of communication disorders. Service delivery includes the formats by which services are rendered, including where, when, and with whom services are provided. To illustrate service delivery, this chapter highlights the typical and unique work settings that are included in professional preparation programs for audiologists and SLPs. A list of common service delivery terms and their acronyms is included in Table 9.1.

SERVICE DELIVERY FEATURES

It is important to become familiar with the core vocabulary that distinguishes one service delivery model from another. In service provision, particular features characterize each approach.

Table 9.1. Common acronyms related to service delivery

Affordable Care Act (ACA)
American Academy of Audiology (AAA)
Americans with Disabilities Act (ADA)
American Federation of Teachers (AFT)
American Occupational Therapy Association (AOTA)
American Physical Therapy Association (APTA)
American Speech-Language-Hearing Association (ASHA)
Auditory brainstem response (ABR)
Augmentative and alternative communication (AAC)
Birth-to-3 services (B–3)
Commission of the Accreditation of Rehabilitation Facilities (CARF)
Certificate of Clinical Competence (CCC)
Continuum of care (COC)
Certified occupational therapy assistant (COTA)
Committee on Special Education (CSE)
Comprehensive System of Personnel Development (CSPD)
Ear, nose, and throat doctor (ENT; otolaryngologist)
Electronystagmography (ENG)
Emergency department (ED)
Extended school year (ESY)
Free and appropriate education (FAPE)
Home health care (HHC)
Health maintenance organization (HMO)
Hard of hearing (HOH)
Health Care Financing Administration (HCFA)
Intermediate care facility/mental retardation (ICF/MR)
Intensive care unit (ICU)
Individualized education program (IEP)
Individualized family service plan (IFSP)
Individuals with Disabilities Education Act (IDEA)
Joint Commission on the Accreditation of Health Care Organizations (JCAHCO)
Local education agency (LEA)
Least restrictive environment (LRE)
National Education Association (NEA)
National Association for the Education of Young Children (NAEYC)
Neonatal intensive care unit (NICU)
Otoacoustic emissions (OAE)
Occupational therapy (OT)
Occupational therapist, registered (OTR)
Office of Special Education Programs (OSEP)
Office of Special Education and Rehabilitative Services (OSERS)
Planning and placement team (PPT)
Physical therapist (PT)
Physical therapy (PT)
Physical therapy assistant (PTA)
Residential care facility (RCF)
Registered nurse (RN)
State Education Agency (SEA)
Speech-language pathologist (SLP)
Speech-language pathology assistant (SLPA)
Skilled nursing facility (SNF)
Transitional living center (TLC)
University-affiliated program (UAP)
World Health Organization (WHO)
World Health Organization International Classification of Functioning, Disability and Health (WHO-ICF)

Direct and Indirect Services

Direct services occur when a clinician works in a face-to-face format with an individual patient or a group of patients. In the hospital setting, an SLP might provide direct swallowing rehabilitation with a patient at bedside. In an elementary school, a clinician might work directly with a small group of students with language delays who are learning the vocabulary associated with their first-grade math curriculum. **Indirect services** occur when the clinician does not have hands-on contact with the client but instead is likely to consult with the client's family members, teachers, and/or medical personnel about the client's communication needs. An example of this occurs when a classroom teacher follows the suggestion of a clinician and deliberately emphasizes the way particular sounds are pronounced by the students during a "letter of the week" activity in a kindergarten class. Another example is when the staff of a group home follow a clinician's suggestion and develops a picture board that helps an adult with a developmental disability communicate during community outings.

Clinical and Consultative Services

Direct services can include both clinical and consultative or collaborative services. In a clinical model, a school SLP typically takes children out of their classroom in order to provide intensive one-to-one or small-group instruction in a separate location. A clinical model is advantageous when trying to initially teach children particular speech-language skills and when standardized testing needs to be completed. A clinical model can also be utilized when a child needs a less distracting environment and when the intervention protocol warrants privacy. This may be necessary, for example, among children who stutter and need a safe place in which to talk about their feelings. The clinical model is also utilized within medical speech-language pathology, when, for example, an adult who has had a stroke leaves his or her home and comes to a university clinic to practice communication skills.

Consultative or collaborative services occur when members of an intervention team work together and share responsibility for client outcomes. In a school setting, the classroom teacher and the SLP can support each other's efforts to enhance students' academic success and communication skills. In one example, an SLP might work directly in a classroom and embed language objectives into small-group learning activities using materials from the academic curriculum. In another example, an SLP might work on literacy by leading phonological awareness activities during class reading time or might assist in monitoring progress in reading to determine students' responses to reading instruction and identify students who need additional help. By engaging in collaborative or consultative services, the SLP becomes better aware of the language demands within the academic curriculum and the social communication demands within the children's peer groups.

Another format for the consultative or collaborative approach occurs when an SLP works indirectly with a client by providing guidance to the client's family members and professional colleagues (i.e., general and special education teachers, preschool teachers, skilled nursing facility staff, birth-to-3 professionals, **psychologists**) who work more directly with the patient. This can occur when we teach parents how to provide home-based language models, when we help birth-to-3 professionals facilitate early feeding skills among infants with Down syndrome, or when we make recommendations to home health care staff about communication strategies for people with **Alzheimer's disease** after a speech-language evaluation.

Collaborative partnerships require that professionals from different disciplines work together in an effort to integrate patient goals, objectives, and intervention strategies. In these partnerships, participants bring their own field of expertise to their professional colleagues when they mutually design instructions, solve problems, and share teaching responsibilities. In both clinical and consultative or collaborative therapy services, there needs to be considerable scheduling coordination among team members. For example, when using a clinical model to address dysfluency in an elementary school student, SLPs need to work with teachers to schedule therapy sessions so they interfere as little as possible with the academic curriculum. In the consultative or collaborative model, SLPs need to work with teachers to determine how the SLP's collaboration in the classroom will be organized, whether as a "guest teacher," as the leader of a small group of students within the classroom using a response-to-intervention model, and so forth. School personnel must also have scheduling flexibility to meet to discuss the integration of speech-language goals into academic curricula. Often, a client's speech-language intervention plan calls for both clinical and collaborative or consultative services.

Individual and Group Services

Sometimes, the SLP will vary the number of clients in a therapy session. *Individual services* are intense and one-to-one in nature and are typically aimed at teaching the client a specific communication skill. An example of individual services occurs when Tom, an adult with apraxia of speech, works on speech production strategies during an individual intervention session at a rehabilitation center. *Group services* include two or more patients who are apt to be working on similar speech-language skills or who need to practice the generalization of learned skills to additional communication partners. For example, after Tom learns speech production strategies during individual services, he might participate in a group session in which he is expected to converse with other adults. Although individual services might focus on skill practice and strategies, a group session enables Tom to receive natural feedback from his peers. Another example of group services occurs in a **self-contained classroom** when the SLP is the primary educator providing both academic instruction and intensive speech-language remediation. This can occur, for example, when we run a class for preschoolers who need focused stimulation because they have severe speech sound disorders.

Multidisciplinary, Interdisciplinary, and Transdisciplinary Models

SLPs are often asked to work with their professional colleagues from the education, medical, and allied health (i.e., physical therapy, occupational therapy) fields in order to conjointly develop intervention plans that are unified and coordinated by content, objectives, and strategies (see Figure 9.1). There are currently three models that identify the relationships shared by team members in the facilitation of patient progress. The first two, multidisciplinary and interdisciplinary, are often interchanged depending on the work setting, and both are popular in medical settings and schools. In a *multidisciplinary model*, each individual discipline

	Birth to 3	School settings	Medical settings
Audiologist	X	X	X
Chaplain			X
Child care worker	X		
Dietitian			X
Neuropsychologist			X
Nurse	X	X	X
Nurse's aide			X
Occupational therapist	X	X	X
Pediatric developmental specialist	X	X	
Physical therapist	X	X	X
Physician	X	X	X
Psychologist	X	X	X
Recreational therapist			X
Rehabilitation paraprofessional	X	X	X
School counselor		X	
Social worker	X	X	X
Special education teacher	X	X	
Speech-language pathologist	X	X	X
Teacher (general education)	X	X	X

Figure 9.1. Service delivery professionals.

conducts its own assessment and develops discipline-specific goals with minimal integration of these goals across disciplines. Each discipline has its own plan for the patient, with goals reflecting only its own field of expertise.

In an *interdisciplinary model,* each discipline conducts its own particular assessment but also communicates with other disciplines about the results of these assessments. This communication fosters complementary goal development so that as each discipline creates its plan for the client, all disciplines incorporate elements of the goals and objectives of related fields into the plan. For example, when working with a patient with TBI, language sequencing may be one objective for the SLP. As part of the program, the SLP might have the patient write down the steps associated with daily tasks (e.g., turn off alarm, get out of bed, go to the bathroom, brush teeth). While writing, the patient can be given instructions about holding the pencil correctly and using eye–hand coordination, strategies that had been suggested to the SLP by the patient's occupational therapist. Conversely, during an occupational therapy session, the therapist can include verbal sequencing as part of therapeutic activities.

A *transdisciplinary model* is used when team members have an ongoing dialogue in which they share information, knowledge, and skills in order to develop and implement a single integrated service plan for the client. In this model, there is a single assessment of the client that is completed in unison by professionals from several disciplines. As a team, they review the assessment data and weave together objectives reflective of all the disciplines. The team typically authorizes one person who, along with the client's family members or caregivers, becomes responsible for carrying out the client's intervention plan. For example, a 17-year-old client with developmental disabilities who is making the transition to living and working independently is likely to have a job coach. This job coach is responsible

Table 9.2. Service delivery guidelines from the American Speech-Language-Hearing Association and the American Academy of Audiology

ASHA and AAA codes of ethics	Provide an ethical code governing clinician behaviors and actions
ASHA and AAA scope of practice guidelines offered by these professions	Describe the broad range of services and supports
ASHA preferred practice guidelines	Outline acceptable client care, clinical processes, and anticipated outcomes
ASHA practice guidelines and technical reports	Recommend clinical practice parameters in specific work settings
ASHA position statements	Describe policies in matters of professional practice

Key: AAA, American Academy of Audiology; ASHA, American Speech-Language-Hearing Association.

for teaching vocational skills by integrating several educational domains (i.e., academic, social, speech-language, activities of daily living) as the client learns job and communication skills and how to dress and socialize appropriately in the job setting. In this situation, the job coach can link together the educational plan, and the SLP can teach the job coach strategies to facilitate workplace communication skills.

PROFESSIONAL GUIDELINES FOR SERVICE DELIVERY

In both speech-language pathology and audiology, there are guidelines from ASHA and the American Academy of Audiology (AAA) that provide direction about clinical activities within service delivery and work settings. These guidelines (see Table 9.2) establish professional practice parameters for ethical practice, specific speech-language-hearing disorders, and typical clinical activities. For example, an ASHA technical report outlines the role of an audiologist in occupational hearing conservation and hearing loss prevention (ASHA, 2004a) and the role of an SLP in school-based preferred practice (ASHA, 2000), and an ASHA position statement identifies the role of an SLP who provides clinical services via telepractice (ASHA, 2005a). Two examples of guidelines from AAA are 1) AAA's standards of practice guidelines (AAA, 2012) and 2) the position statement on the audiologist's role in the monitoring of ototoxicity (AAA, 2009).

CONTEMPORARY ISSUES IN SERVICE DELIVERY

Historically, speech-language service delivery has concentrated on the one-to-one or small-group intervention approach in which skills are strengthened through a hierarchy of task demands and prompts. Service delivery has seen vast changes since the 1970s, and current service delivery models reflect evolving government agencies, health care management, educational philosophy, and human service principles. As service providers, we need to be aware of the many issues that influence service delivery approaches. Table 9.3 provides examples of contemporary issues that affect service delivery. For an extensive review of public policies that affect clinical practice, see Chapter 8.

EDUCATION WORK SETTINGS FOR THE SPEECH-LANGUAGE PATHOLOGIST

In the field of speech-language pathology, professionals work in a variety of educational settings for children from birth to age 21. Some of the programs you

Table 9.3.   Contemporary issues that influence service delivery

Issue	Speech-language pathologists challenged to
Functional communication	Develop protocols that relate to classroom curricula, independent living and vocational skills, and the natural situations in which their clients communicate
Assistive and instrumental technology	Increase their technical competence with alternative and augmentative communication (AAC), assistive technology, and medical technology (i.e., ventilators, tracheotomy tubes, nasendoscopy, videofluoroscopy)
Evidence-based practice	Investigate and verify that their assessment and treatment approaches are supported by clinical expertise, research evidence, and client values
Managed care	Develop effective and efficient service delivery programs
Affordable Care Act (ACA); Federal Health Care Reform	Ensure all Americans have access to quality health care that is affordable
Accountability	Justify the worth of their clinical services in terms of client progress, cost, and time
Inclusion	Ensure that communication supports assist children with special needs as they access the regular education curriculum
Collaboration	Coordinate speech-language services with other education and medical personnel
Educational standards	Support and document how speech-language intervention can enhance the academic achievement outcomes of students in public schools
Multicultural issues	Provide services that are culturally sensitive and applicable
Transition services	Help clients make life transition decisions (e.g., high school to work and reintegration to employment after adult onset disorders)
Regulations and accreditation	Stay familiar with the regulatory and accreditation guidelines governing service delivery
Self-advocacy, family involvement, and client rights	Respect clients and family members as integral participants in designing, implementing, and evaluating the effectiveness of treatment programs
Eligibility and exit criteria	Balance the opinions of clients, families, and regulatory bodies that may have different opinions about when services are warranted and/or when services are no longer needed
Speech-language pathology assistants and paraprofessionals	Understand the issues and guidelines surrounding the use of support personnel

are likely to participate in as part of your graduate clinical practica in speech-language pathology are introduced here.

Early Intervention Programs

Chapter 8 discusses the public policies that affect clinical practice, including public laws that govern early intervention services. Early intervention applies to children from birth to kindergarten. Two systems of early intervention exist, one for children age birth to 3 years and the second for preschoolers age 3 to kindergarten.

Birth-to-3 services emphasize that the family of the child with a disability is the recipient of services. This means that the SLP must understand family-guided practice that is both culturally sensitive and specific to each family's circumstance. In this model, family members are integral to the design, implementation, and evaluation of services, and they are considered partners with education and rehabilitation professionals in their child's developmental growth (Rini & Whitney, 1999; Chapter 12). Birth-to-3 service provision often operates using a transdisciplinary model by designing a single integrated individualized family service plan (IFSP). When speech-language objectives are recommended for the child, these are designed to coincide with objectives being addressed across other areas of development. The primary interventionist represents every discipline, and, for example, when we assume that role, we facilitate not only communication skills, but also any other goals on the child's IFSP (e.g., fine and gross motor skills, cognition, socialization, adaptive behavior, transition). In this model, service provision occurs in a variety of settings (e.g., the child's home, a child care center, a clinic, a segregated or inclusive playgroup) and our role may be direct or indirect, individual or group, and consultative or clinical.

A primary goal of many birth-to-3 programs is to mainstream young children with disabilities in order to provide rich peer language models and promote social development. In doing so, the interventionist becomes responsible for creating educational activities that adapt typical routines by training child care providers and promoting social skills with peers.

Preschool and School-Based Services

The 2003 ASHA omnibus survey indicated that a majority of SLPs work in educational settings (i.e., preschool and school-age). In fact, ASHA estimates that nearly 1.1 million school children ages 6–21 have a primary diagnosis of "speech-language impairment" (ASHA, 2008a), and school-based clinicians also provide services to children who have other educational disabilities that affect communication processes. Table 9.4 highlights some of the most frequent communication and educational diagnoses of school-age children and the percentage of school-based SLPs who report serving these children.

Among school-based SLPs, particular service delivery models seem to occur for particular communication disorders. A traditional clinical model is common, either alone or in conjunction with other approaches, for children with disorders of articulation or phonology, fluency, and voice. Classroom-based models are often utilized for children with augmentative and alternative communication needs, as

Table 9.4. Percentage of school-based clinicians serving communication and related educational disorders

Disorder	Percentage of school-based clinicians
Communication	
Articulation and phonology disorders	91.8%
Fluency disorder	67.5%
Specific language impairment	61.1%
Childhood apraxia	59.4%
Augmentative and alternative communication	50.8%
Hearing disorders	45.8%
Cognitive communicative disorders	43.6%
Voice and resonance disorders	33.8%
Dysphagia	13.8%
Related education	
Autism spectrum disorders	77.4%
Learning disability	72.4%
Intellectual and developmental disability	70.9%
Reading and/or writing disability	35.7%

Table 9.5. Individuals with Disabilities Education Improvement Act of 2004 requirements for school-based speech-language services

Identification	Students must be screened to determine whether they have speech-language concerns in need of further assessment.
Assessment	Students who are potentially eligible for speech-language services must participate in nonbiased assessment of their strengths, weaknesses, disorders, and/or delays.
Intervention	Students deemed eligible for services are entitled to receive free and appropriate speech-language intervention services in the least restrictive environment.
Consultation and counseling	Family members and educators who are primarily responsible for students with disabilities are entitled to ongoing discussion about the students' problems and remediation plans.
Referral	Students with communication disorders are entitled to the professional advice of related education and rehabilitation disciplines.

well as for children with language and literacy disorders, cognitive-communication needs, and autism spectrum disorders. Collaborative and consultative models occur most frequently for children with language concerns, autism spectrum disorders, and cognitive-communication needs. Children with related educational diagnoses often receive collaborative or consultation services.

As noted in Chapter 8, school-age children are eligible for speech-language services through the Individuals with Disabilities Education Improvement Act (IDEA) of 2004 (PL 108-446), the planning and placement team (PPT) process, and the individual education program (IEP). The 2004 legislation, IDEA 2004, is the mechanism typically used for providing special services to students with disabilities. Table 9.5 outlines IDEA 2004-mandated school speech-language pathology services. Preschool and school-based speech-language services require the child to be identified as having speech-language impairment or another educational diagnosis that will affect speech-language development and use (i.e., specific learning disability, autism spectrum disorder, intellectual disability, hearing impairment, attention-deficit/hyperactivity disorder).

Although school-based clinicians spend a majority of their time in direct intervention, they are likely to have other clinical tasks, including conducting diagnostic evaluations, screenings, and report writing; attending parent and staff meetings; completing paperwork; and supervising student clinicians and/or colleagues. Many SLPs are also involved on school literacy teams and have the responsibility for planning, delivering, and evaluating literacy instruction. In addition, with the adoption of Common Core State Standards across the country, many SLPs will take part in the planning and delivery of language-related services that advance curricular goals for struggling students. School clinicians are also often asked to take part in tasks shared by the entire teaching staff. These might include performing lunch and bus supervision duties, assisting with kindergarten registration, creating hallway bulletin boards, and helping with school plays and concerts. These additional duties may seem time consuming, given our large caseloads, travel between schools, and lack of planning time. Yet, these tasks provide opportunities to interact cooperatively with the other faculty members and enable us to observe and stimulate children out of the typical classroom and therapy context.

CASE EXAMPLE 1

Luis was born with a cleft palate. He received birth-to-3 services from the time he left the hospital with his mother. The services were aimed at helping his mother feed him and developing his early vocal and language skills. By the time he turned 3, he had had several surgeries to correct his lip and palate and was talking, although he was a bit hard to understand. He entered preschool and worked with the SLP there to improve speech intelligibility and was monitored closely by the audiologist to catch ear infections early and treat them to avoid any significant loss of hearing. When Luis entered kindergarten, his speech was fairly intelligible, but he failed a language screening and was given small-group language stimulation services in kindergarten. His first-grade class used a response-to-intervention (RTI) model for teaching reading, and the SLP worked often in the classroom with children who were having difficulty mastering early reading skills, monitoring children's progress, and providing small-group instruction for children who were not progressing adequately. Luis was found to need these services, and he worked with the SLP in a small group for 10 weeks during the school year. By the end of first grade, he was reading on grade level and had only residual speech errors on /s/ sounds.

MEDICAL WORK SETTINGS FOR THE SPEECH-LANGUAGE PATHOLOGIST

There are numerous medical conditions that may result in communication or swallowing disorders (see Table 9.6), and therefore approximately 35% of certified SLPs are employed in health care settings (ASHA, 2006). The most common work settings are general medical hospitals and skilled nursing facilities. Other medical settings include rehabilitation hospitals, outpatient clinics, home health agencies, or pediatric hospitals. In general hospitals and skilled nursing facilities, a large portion of your time as an SLP may be spent treating individuals with dysphagia. In both inpatient and outpatient rehabilitation centers, however, more time may be spent with remediation of **aphasia** or **cognitive-communication disorders** (ASHA, 2011; see Table 9.7). In each of these settings, our role typically includes assessment and **differential diagnosis,** development of an intervention plan, and patient and family education, although the proportion of these duties may vary depending on the setting.

ASHA has adopted the **World Health Organization's** (WHO) International Classification of Functioning, Disability, and Health (ICF) framework (WHO, 2001) for guiding assessment and intervention services to people with communication disorders (ASHA, 2004b). This framework considers the influence of body structure and function on the performance of daily activities and an individual's ability to participate in life functions. Participation may be further influenced by a variety of personal or environmental variables. For example, Rick was diagnosed with a brain tumor (health condition) and underwent surgery. As a result of the brain damage sustained from removal of the tumor, he demonstrated a cognitive-communication disorder (impairment in body structure and function). Rick now has difficulty remembering names and organizing his thoughts to express himself

Table 9.6. Medical conditions resulting in communication and/or swallowing disorders

Medical conditions	Communication and swallowing disorders
Stroke	Aphasia
Traumatic brain injury	Dysarthria
Progressive disease	Apraxia
Spinal cord injury	Cognitive-linguistic disorder
Head and neck tumors	Dysphonia
Brain tumors	Aphonia
Dementia	Speech-language delay or disorder
Vocal fold abnormalities	Dysphagia
Acquired immune deficiency syndrome	Velopharyngeal insufficiency
Respiratory disorders	
Congenital disorders	
Genetic disorders	
Premature birth	

Table 9.7. Percentage of time spent by medically based clinicians

Dysphagia	42%
Aphasia	20%
Cognitive communication	20%
Motor speech	10%
Voice	6%
Other	2%

clearly in conversation (activity limitation). In addition, he experienced difficulty returning to work at his law firm, where he was a partner, due to problems organizing his day and scheduling appointments (participation limitation). However, Rick is highly motivated to get back to work and eagerly follows through with all strategies you suggest (positive personal variable), and his law firm is willing to make adaptations to his schedule and provide additional support to facilitate Rick's return to work (positive contextual variable) (see Figure 9.2). Knowing the impact of the communication disorder on daily life functioning helps the SLP manage patients' care and facilitate transitions from one medical setting to another as the patients recover and the goals of rehabilitation change.

The transition through various settings is referred to as the **continuum of care** (COC) (see Figure 9.3). As part of the intervention team, SLPs participate in the decision to move patients through the continuum. Various regulatory bodies, however, also influence the placement of a patient in a specific type of facility. One of the major issues related to service delivery in medical settings is the concept of **managed care.** This is the collective term for approaches to the delivery of health care that attempt to control quality while containing costs. Third-party payers that cover the costs of rehabilitation (e.g., Medicare, private insurance) have a great influence in determining the number of sessions a patient may receive and may even influence how a patient progresses through the COC. In addition, the passing of the Patient Protection and Affordable Care Act (PL 111-148) in 2010 is likely to have a significant impact on how we deliver services to individuals in medical settings. The purpose of the legislation is to ensure that all Americans have access to quality health care that is affordable. However, the exact manner in which this health care reform will affect our practice is yet to be seen.

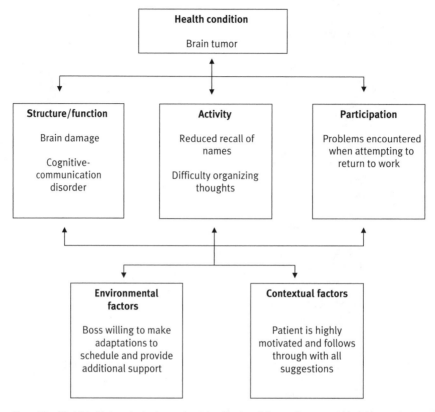

Figure 9.2. World Health Organization international classification of disease. (*Source:* World Health Organization, 2001.)

Other regulatory bodies that may influence service delivery are the accreditation commissions. The **Joint Commission on the Accreditation of Health Care Organizations** (JCAHCO) and the **Commission of the Accreditation of Rehabilitation Facilities** (CARF) both have regulations that must be met regarding documentation, amount of therapy provided, communication among team members, goal setting, and inclusion of the patient in the plan for his or her intervention. As service providers, SLPs must adhere to the guidelines imposed by both the insurance companies and the accrediting bodies.

General Medical Hospitals

Individuals are admitted to a general medical hospital due to needs for immediate medical management. Many patients are initially admitted through the emergency department, where very specific protocols are followed to manage a variety of illnesses and traumas. New regulations for stroke management require that these patients have their ability to swallow screened within a few hours of admission. The SLP may be called to the emergency department to perform a swallowing screen, or nursing staff who have been trained by the SLP may be qualified to perform the screen. If the patient is found to have problems with

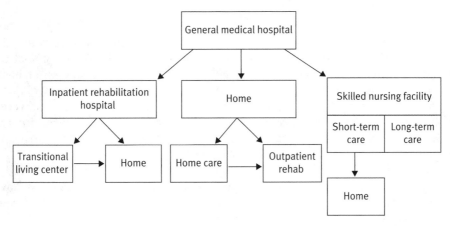

Figure 9.3. Continuum of care.

swallowing, the SLP may recommend a fiberoptic evaluation of swallowing (FEES) or a **videofluoroscopic swallowing study** (VFSS) to determine the specific swallowing problem and possible management approaches. A FEES may be performed at the patient's bedside, whereas a VFSS is conducted in the Radiology Department along with a **radiologist.** Following the evaluation, the SLP may recommend a **nasogastric tube** as an alternative method of feeding. To ensure the proper feeding plan is instituted, the SLP collaborates with nursing and dietary professionals.

Some individuals may be medically unstable and therefore placed in the **intensive care unit** (ICU), where they receive continuous medical monitoring. Many of these patients have tracheal tubes and are on ventilators to help them breathe. Because the placement of the tracheal tube prohibits air from reaching the vocal folds, these patients are unable to speak. Therefore, as the SLP you may receive a referral from the pulmonologist to see the patient to help with communication. You may recommend a one-way speaking valve or a communication board.

Some patients may be directly admitted to the main hospital. Because hospital stays are often brief, as SLPs we typically have the role of a consultant. We are responsible for evaluating the patient in order to determine the presence, type, and severity of the communication or swallowing disorder and have the task of educating the patient, family, and staff regarding the findings and recommendations of the evaluation. For example, we may receive a referral from an oncologist for a patient who will be undergoing a **laryngectomy.** We will see the patient prior to the surgery to educate him or her about the changes that will occur in communication and swallowing as a result of the laryngectomy. We will also provide some training with an intraoral electrolarynx to provide the patient with a means of communication immediately after surgery. Following the surgery, we will continue to train the patient to use the electrolarynx effectively and will educate the patient about other forms of communication that may be options at a later time, such as transcutaneous electrolarynx or esophageal speech.

Children's Hospitals

Some SLPs may work in a hospital that provides medical care specifically to children from infancy through late adolescence. Within many hospitals, premature infants or other infants with severe medical problems immediately after birth may be transferred to the **neonatal intensive care unit** (NICU). Many of these infants have feeding and swallowing problems. For example, an infant delivered at 32 weeks' gestation has numerous respiratory problems and an uncoordinated suck or swallow. The SLP may observe and evaluate the baby during feedings and provide suggestions to parents and nursing staff.

Some of these children may have communication or swallowing difficulties as a result of a birth defect such as **Möbius syndrome.** Other children may have an acquired communication or swallowing disorder resulting from a medical condition such as a brain tumor or traumatic brain injury. The role of the SLP in children's hospitals is largely the same as in the general medical setting: the SLP is responsible for evaluation, intervention, education, and discharge planning as part of the interdisciplinary team.

In addition, the SLP in a children's hospital may act as a consultant once a child is discharged. For example, as the hospital's SLP, you may meet with a child's elementary school teachers and school-based SLP following the child's discharge from the hospital following a traumatic brain injury in order to provide as smooth a transition as possible from the hospital to the school. Or, you may be part of a specialized medical team to provide continuous care for infants and children who require long-term follow-up. For example, a child with cleft lip and palate will need multiple surgeries to repair the cleft. As part of the craniofacial team, you as the SLP will assist with the development and remediation of speech and swallowing skills as the child grows.

Rehabilitation Units and Hospitals

Some hospitals have a dedicated rehabilitation unit, whereas other intensive rehabilitation programs are housed in specialized rehabilitation hospitals. Rehabilitation hospitals often have specific programs for acquired brain injury (e.g., stroke, traumatic brain injury), spinal cord injuries, degenerative diseases (e.g., **multiple sclerosis** or **Parkinson's disease**), or respiratory dysfunction. The SLP may be assigned to a single unit or required to work in all programs. Patients admitted to these programs are generally medically stable and are able to participate in several hours of therapy each day, which can be a combination of speech, occupational, physical, recreational, and/or psychosocial therapies. The SLP's first role is to assess the patient. At this stage, patients can tolerate longer sessions and the assessment can be more in depth than in the general hospital. When testing is completed, an appropriate intervention plan is developed given the specific diagnosis and needs of the patient. The SLP also functions as a member of a team. Depending on the philosophy of the rehabilitation program, the type of team may vary (multi-, inter-, transdisciplinary). In this setting, the SLP will likely provide a combination of individual and group therapy. In addition, the SLP may cotreat patients with professionals from other disciplines. For example, if a patient has executive function deficits that interfere with carrying out daily tasks, as the SLP you might conduct an intervention session with the occupational therapist in a kitchen, where you focus on assisting the patient with organization and sequencing skills required for the patient to prepare a meal and the occupational therapist addresses the patient's hand and arm control and trains the patient in the use of adaptive equipment. The primary goal of therapy is to enhance communicative and cognitive functioning and prepare the patient for discharge home. Regular team meetings are held to discuss the patient's progress, and, prior to discharge, a meeting is held with the patient and family to assist with the transition home.

Outpatient Rehabilitation Centers

Outpatient rehabilitation centers may be affiliated with a general medical hospital or a rehabilitation hospital, or they may be an independent center. Individuals participating in outpatient rehabilitation programs transport themselves from their homes to the center. The responsibilities of SLPs working in outpatient rehabilitation facilities are similar to those within inpatient programs: As SLPs, we evaluate the patient and set up an individualized intervention plan. The patient and his or her family are likely to have significant input into the goals of intervention. For example, a patient with dysphagia as a result of a hemiglossectomy for the management of tongue cancer may report, "I want to be able to eat by mouth and get rid of my feeding tube." Or, an elementary school teacher with dysphonia due to vocal nodules may communicate, "I want to learn to use my voice so that I don't get hoarse at the end of the day." Goals are typically geared toward maximizing communicative functioning in the home and the community or establishing and maintaining a safe and efficient swallow. The intensity of intervention may vary from daily to once a week, depending on the individual's specific needs, prognosis, or even insurance coverage. Individual and/or group interventions may be provided. Some interventions may even occur in the community. For example, as the outpatient rehabilitation center's SLP, you may take a patient to a fast food restaurant to practice using his or her verbal skills or augmentative communication system to order a meal. Increasingly, this kind of intervention is also being offered via telepractice.

Some patients may receive speech and language services through specialty clinics that are associated with specific disciplines or research programs. For example, as an SLP, you may work for an otolaryngologist who specializes in the evaluation and management of vocal fold dysfunction, and your day may be spent treating individuals who have voice problems. Or, you may be part of a team who follows individuals with neurodegenerative diseases, in which you develop augmentative communication systems for individuals. Perhaps you will work for a clinic that specializes in the diagnosis and treatment of swallowing disorders. As the scope of speech-language pathology practice expands and understanding of medically based communication and swallowing disorders increases, so do the opportunities for SLPs.

Transitional Living Centers

Transitional living centers are geared toward those individuals who want to return to an independent lifestyle. Most residents of this type of program are young and have sustained a traumatic brain injury (e.g., as a result of a vehicular accident).

The SLP works very closely with other rehabilitation staff and directs intervention toward self-management and community reentry skills. For example, as SLPs we may help the nursing staff develop a plan to teach the patient his or her medication schedule and how to compensate for memory problems, or we may address ways of managing the patient's finances. Therapy is often provided in a group setting led by the SLP or cofacilitated by the SLP and another team member, depending on the focus of the group.

Skilled Nursing Facilities

Individuals are admitted to a skilled nursing facility if they need ongoing nursing and medical care that cannot be managed by family members in the home. These facilities often have two distinct units: *short-term* (or *subacute*) *care* and *long-term care*. Individuals on the short-term units typically have the goal of returning home. They may be slower to recover from an illness or injury and therefore do not qualify for intensive rehabilitation programs. For example, as SLPs we may see a patient on the short-term unit with speech and swallowing problems due to multiple sclerosis who was admitted to regulate his or her medications and to improve his or her endurance, self-care, speech intelligibility, and safety while swallowing. The goal for intervention may be to train the patient and the patient's family members and caregivers to use strategies to make swallowing easier and to recognize any signs of difficulty when the patient returns home. In contrast with patients in short-term care, individuals in long-term care are likely to remain in the facility for the rest of their lives. These patients may have a progressive neurological disease such as Alzheimer's disease. These individuals may be seen in a group setting for general cognitive stimulation. In addition, education and training may be provided to caregivers regarding supportive communication techniques. Because Alzheimer's disease is progressive, the goal of intervention would not be to improve the patients' memory and communication but, rather, to facilitate and maintain communication as long as possible to improve quality of life. Medicare regulations have greatly influenced the provision of speech therapy and other rehabilitation services within these facilities. Strict guidelines must be followed regarding the amount and type of therapy provided.

Home Health Care

Individuals may be eligible to receive therapy in the home if they are considered "homebound"; that is, they have medical and/or physical problems that make it difficult for them to leave their homes. They may be transported by family members or other caregivers to their doctor appointments, but they do not leave the home for any other purpose. These individuals often require the services of a registered nurse and a home health aide. The SLP may, for example, be seeing an **oncology** patient who had his or her larynx removed and can no longer speak. The patient is still very weak and cannot drive. The patient has had difficulty maintaining weight due to side effects of medications and needs supplemental tube feedings. A nurse may help the patient manage the tube feedings, and a home health aide may assist the patient with bathing, dressing, and household chores. The SLP's role is to help the patient learn to communicate with an electrolarynx and to educate the patient and the caregivers regarding techniques that help facilitate communication.

Palliative Care

Another area in which the medical SLP has become involved is that of terminal care. The stark reality is that some of the patients we see as SLPs will not survive their diseases. We may be consulted to see these patients through palliative services. We have several roles to play with these individuals, including providing consultation and strategies to patients, family, and caregivers to optimize function related to communication and swallowing, to support the patient's role in decision making with the family and hospice team, and to improve overall comfort and satisfaction (Pollens, 2004).

CASE EXAMPLE 2

Bob is a 58-year-old man admitted to a **general medical hospital** with the diagnosis of a stroke. The SLP has completed an evaluation and has diagnosed a moderate aphasia. The physical therapist and the occupational therapist have determined that Bob has a paralysis of his right side and is unable to complete basic activities of daily living (e.g., dressing, bathing, cooking). Given Bob's age, motivation, and potential for good progress, the rehabilitation team has recommended that he be discharged to an **inpatient rehabilitation hospital.**

At the inpatient rehabilitation program, the SLP begins intensive intervention. Bob is scheduled for 1 hour of individual speech therapy per day. He makes progress in his ability to understand directions and questions, express some basic thoughts and ideas, and read sentences. Progress is also made in his physical therapy and occupational therapy, though Bob continued to need moderate assistance to complete his activities of daily living. After 3 weeks, the rehabilitation team determines that Bob's wife could manage him at home. After some education and training for his family members, Bob is discharged.

Once at home, Bob receives occupational, physical, and speech therapy through **home care services.** Rapid progress is made with his mobility and ability to perform his daily tasks. The SLP continues to work with him on his language skills. After 4 weeks, Bob has made significant progress in all language areas. Physically, he can now get around the house and in and out of the car, so the physical therapist discharges him. A referral to outpatient therapy is recommended for continued speech therapy.

Bob begins therapy at an **outpatient facility.** His speech and language program is geared toward return to work. He participates in individual and group therapy, as well as some activities in the community. After 8 weeks, Bob is ready to return to work on a part-time basis.

OTHER WORK SETTINGS FOR SPEECH-LANGUAGE PATHOLOGISTS

Private Practice

Running an independent private practice is similar to running any other small business. The challenges and risks, both financial and emotional, of such an endeavor are greater than in other professional settings. The rewards of a successful private practice, however, are equally great. The SLPs who work in a private practice have a lot of flexibility in choosing the setting in which they may work. Some may see individuals in a private office; some may contract with various facilities such as hospitals, rehabilitation agencies, schools, or group homes; and some may act primarily as consultants. In private practice, the SLP can specify the types of communication disorders he or she may treat and accept only those referrals. Depending on the setting and type of client seen in a private practice, these SLPs may work completely independently or be part of a team. For example, one SLP may specialize in the management of communication disorders in children with autism spectrum disorders. He or she may contract with several school systems and be called to evaluate a child, provide specific intervention recommendations, and train the teachers in management of the child's intervention. Another SLP may be hired by parents of children with communication disorders to provide therapy outside of school. Or, an SLP may have contracts with several nursing homes or hospitals, which would contact the SLP when a client needs to be evaluated and requires an intervention plan set up. This SLP may also be hired privately by a family to provide therapy in the home.

A growing area of private practice is corporate speech-language pathology. This involves consulting with specific companies, their employees, or their customers. In that position, you offer assessment and training in many aspects of communication, such as articulation, fluency, voice, and language and hearing education, as well as other services uniquely needed by the business world. These include presentation skills, foreign and regional accent modification, professional diction and grammar, interviewing skills, business writing, and business communication etiquette. You may even help clients communicate more effectively with their customers by training customer representatives to work with their clients with hearing loss (Christensen, 2006).

Colleges and Universities

Some SLPs may function as professors or clinical supervisors in a college or university setting. Here, they may provide direct services to their clients, but their main role as SLPs is to provide undergraduate and graduate education and supervise graduate student clinicians who are training to become SLPs themselves. Services may be provided at a university-based clinic or in a variety of educational or medical settings with whom the university has a contract. When SLPs function as clinical instructors, their role is to provide a foundation in the principles of diagnosis and intervention and expose students to a wide variety of communication disorders encountered in children and adults. In this college or university setting, SLPs may act as consultants to provide a second opinion to school- or hospital-based SLPs.

Psychiatric Centers

Some SLPs work in a psychiatric facility among individuals who present with severe behavioral disabilities secondary to psychiatric illness, mental health concerns, and/or social-emotional maladjustment. For this population, the SLP needs an understanding of behavior management and the potential communicative function of aberrant or challenging behavior. In psychiatric centers, SLPs work with **psychiatrists,** behavior modification specialists, and psychiatric social workers.

Group Home and Employment Settings for People with Developmental Disabilities

Since the mid-1970s, small, local community group homes have gradually replaced large state institutions for people with developmental disabilities, autism spectrum disorder, and/or intellectual disability (i.e., mental retardation). Service provision to these individuals is often indirect and consultative. Assessment includes documenting the skills of the individual, and determining whether the individual is provided opportunities to actualize communication skills during daily routines. Intervention strategies focus on functional communication within everyday routines and community recreational events (Cascella & McNamara, 2004; ASHA, 2005b). For high-functioning individuals with autism spectrum disorder, SLPs may work with clients to function within the higher education setting, providing social and organizational skills support.

WORK SETTINGS FOR AUDIOLOGISTS

Audiologists practice their profession in a variety of settings. The majority of audiologists practice in some type of health care setting and/or private practice. A smaller number of audiologists practice in school systems, universities, and industrial environments.

Current graduate programs in audiology lead to a clinical doctoral degree, most being the doctor of audiology (Au.D.). All such programs require the completion of a full-time clinical externship in the final year of study. This externship is designed to provide audiology externs with opportunities to develop clinical skills, knowledge, and professional judgment. The AAA maintains an externship registry to help students and university programs determine placements for this final-year experience.

Scope of Practice

In defining the scope of practice for the field of audiology, it is important to realize that audiologists are autonomous professionals. This means that they have earned the right to function independently. Patients who seek the services of an audiologist can do so directly, without the referral of a physician. In order to maintain this autonomy, it is important that the audiologist provide services that fall under the true mission of the profession.

Audiologists are involved in activities that identify, assess, diagnose, manage in a nonmedical fashion, and interpret test results related to disorders of human hearing, balance, and other neural systems (AAA, 2004; ASHA, 2004c). These activities would include traditional **behavioral audiological tests** of hearing sensitivity (i.e., air and bone conduction thresholds) as well as **electrophysiological tests** (i.e., **auditory brainstem response** [ABR]). Audiologists are uniquely qualified to assess the hearing sensitivity of children and adults. In addition to assessing peripheral hearing sensitivity, audiologists are also involved in the evaluation and management of children and adults with auditory processing disorders.

Audiologists often serve in a consultative capacity. When dealing with school-age children, audiologists may be called upon to consult with an educational team regarding the educational implications of a hearing loss, educational programming, classroom acoustics, and large-area amplification systems for children with hearing impairments. Audiologists may also serve as consultants with regard to compliance with the Americans with Disabilities Act (ADA) of 1990 (PL 101-336). In this capacity, the audiologist may be called on to determine accessibility for persons with hearing loss in public and private buildings and facilities. Many audiologists serve as expert witnesses for legal interpretations of audiological findings and the general effects of hearing loss. Consulting with industrial businesses regarding the prevention of noise-induced hearing loss and implementing **hearing conservation** techniques has been a staple of the audiological profession for many years. More recently, many audiologists have gotten involved in consultation and provision of rehabilitation to persons with balance disorders through habituation, exercise therapy, and balance retraining.

The scope of practice for the audiologist has been rapidly expanding in recent years. One area in which audiologists have become involved is in the use of **otoscopic** examination and external ear canal management for removal of **cerumen.** In the past, cerumen management was a function performed exclusively by physicians or nurses. An ear canal that is clear of excessive cerumen is critical to obtaining an accurate audiological evaluation and impression of the external ear. In an attempt to expedite the diagnostic evaluation process, many audiologists have become involved in cerumen management.

Technological advances have led to additional activities becoming part of the audiological scope of practice. Many audiologists who are familiar with electrophysiological equipment now find themselves working in the operating room side-by-side with surgeons. In these instances, the audiologist is providing neurophysiologic **intraoperative monitoring** and cranial nerve assessment. The purpose of intraoperative monitoring is to try to alert the surgeon to possible nerve damage during surgery in an attempt to maintain complete nerve function.

Another technological advancement that has broadened the scope of practice of the audiologist is the **cochlear implant.** Audiologists are involved in determining candidacy for cochlear implants as well as fitting, programming, or mapping the device. Audiologists also provide rehabilitative services to optimize the benefits derived from the cochlear implant.

Although audiologists have been involved in newborn hearing screening programs for many years, legislation in many states during the 1990s has increased the need for involvement in this area. Many states now have mandated universal hearing screening for all newborns. The development of the otoacoustic emission test battery has provided one tool by which these universal screening programs can be carried out. The ABR also continues to be used for this purpose.

Audiologists are also involved in **tinnitus** assessment and management. New developments in nonmedical management of tinnitus using biofeedback, masking, hearing aids, education, and counseling have led to an increase of work in this area by many audiologists.

The reduction of communication disorders is a primary theme that runs through the activities of the audiologist. Audiologists screen for obvious speech-language

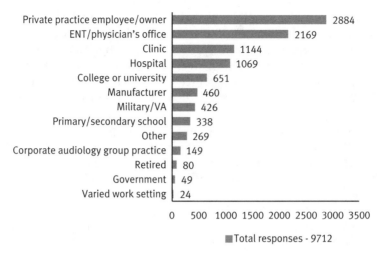

Figure 9.4. Primary settings in which audiologists practice. (*Source:* American Academy of Audiology, 2013.)

disorders, are involved in the use of sign language, and provide rehabilitative services including speech, reading, and communication management strategies.

Practice Settings

Audiologists work in a wide variety of settings (AAA, 2013). Figure 9.4 contains a breakdown of the primary settings in which audiologists practice.

Schools Those individuals who work in the school systems are referred to as educational audiologists. Their role will be mainly rehabilitative in nature. Educational audiologists work in a collaborative fashion with educators as a member of an interdisciplinary team. Educational audiologists provide input about amplification issues as well as communication management, educational implications of hearing loss, educational programming, and classroom acoustics.

An example of a common scenario faced by an educational audiologist would be the case of a 10-year-old girl with a moderate to severe hearing loss who has recently moved into the school district. The educational audiologist in this setting would be called upon to provide input to the child's educational team regarding use of a **frequency modulation** (FM) **amplification system** in the classroom. The audiologist would also provide information regarding the expected influence of the hearing loss on the educational performance of this child.

Hospitals or Medical Centers Approximately 20% of audiologists work in a hospital or medical center. In this setting the audiologist is almost always an employee of the hospital. The hospital setting provides a broad array of duties for audiologists. Diagnostic procedures will include in-depth electrophysiological and behavioral assessments of inpatients and outpatients of all ages. If the hospital is a birthing hospital, audiologists will likely be involved in a universal neonatal hearing screening program. Audiologists may also be involved in hearing screenings and diagnostic evaluations of babies who spend time in the NICU.

In many hospital settings, audiologists will have the opportunity to be involved in intraoperative monitoring in order to measure the integrity of various nerves during surgical procedures. The hospital setting is the environment in which audiologists are most likely to be involved in working with cochlear implants. It is also in the hospital or medical center where audiologists are most likely to be called upon to assess the possible **ototoxic** effects of various types of drug therapies.

One example of a clinical scenario in the hospital setting would be the case of the 20-year-old man with **cystic fibrosis.** This patient's team of doctors has recently prescribed the drug Amikin to help him with his breathing. This particular drug is known to have possible ototoxic side effects. The other team members have asked the hospital audiologist to perform repeated serial audiograms in order to monitor the patient's hearing sensitivity very closely. Ototoxic effects are usually first evident as shifts in hearing sensitivity in the very high frequencies. Under these circumstances, audiologists may choose to perform a combination of repeated high-frequency audiograms as well as repeated otoacoustic emission tests.

Medical Practices Approximately 25% of audiologists work in a medical practice. In this setting, audiologists are most often an employee of the corporation that is usually managed by a physician or a group of physicians. The medical specialty of the physicians who hire audiologists is almost always **otolaryngology.**

The duties of audiologists in this setting will usually have a diagnostic emphasis. In addition to routine behavioral diagnostic measures of hearing sensitivity, audiologists will often be called to perform electrophysiological tests such as the ABR and **electronystagmography** (ENG) to assist the physician in making diagnoses regarding hearing and balance disorders.

An example of a common clinical scenario in a medical private practice could be seen in the case of a 62-year-old man who has been seen by the otolaryngologist with a complaint of episodes of dizziness. The physician has referred the patient to the audiologist for an audiological evaluation to measure hearing sensitivity and an ENG to evaluate the vestibular (balance) system. The audiologist's responsibility is to perform the requested tests and provide the results to the physician. The audiologist's role in this case is primarily diagnostic in nature, and interpretation of test results will usually be left up to the otolaryngologist.

Private Practices The practice setting that has grown most dramatically in the past few years and is most likely to continue to grow is the independent private practice. Approximately 30% of audiologists currently work in this setting. One obvious reason for the growth in this area is related to a change in the official scope of practice guidelines for the profession (AAA, 2004; ASHA, 2004b). In the 1970s, dispensing hearing aids was not considered to be in the audiologist's scope of practice. At present, dispensing hearing aids is an integral part of the audiologist's duties and has provided the main source of income for many who are maintaining an independent private practice. Although diagnostic evaluations are an important part of most private practices, the emphasis is usually on the rehabilitative services of dispensing and fitting hearing aids. Most private practitioners state that they experience a tremendous feeling of satisfaction in running their own business. In addition, the potential for financial benefit is great as well. Median earnings for a successful independent private practice are estimated to be between 33% and 100% higher than the salary of other audiologists (Stach, 1998).

An example of a common clinical scenario in an independent private practice is illustrated by the case of a 72-year-old woman who has recently noticed a decrease in her hearing sensitivity. This client has sought the advice of her family physician regarding her increase in communication difficulties. The physician has provided medical clearance for amplification to her and has referred her to the audiologist's private practice. Audiologists in private practice are responsible for assessment of the client's hearing sensitivity as well as the selection and fitting of appropriate hearing aids. In addition to the formal test protocols that may be used, a good deal of the audiologist's efforts will be rehabilitative in nature. The audiologist will spend significant time counseling the client regarding proper use of the instruments and establishing realistic expectations concerning aided performance.

Industry Audiologists who work in industry are referred to as industrial audiologists or as environmental audiologists. Industrial audiologists are involved in the prevention of hearing loss to a greater extent than are audiologists in other professional settings. A primary role of industrial audiologists is to be a manager of an effective hearing conservation program.

An industrial hearing conservation program includes assessing the levels of noise exposure experienced by workers, performing baseline and annual audiometric evaluations, and providing recommendations for utilizing hearing protection devices. An important part of an effective hearing conservation program is providing education to workers and supervisory personnel regarding noise-induced hearing loss. In addition, many industrial audiologists will be called on to make suggestions for engineering and administrative controls that will reduce the levels of noise exposure to employees.

Colleges and Universities Some audiologists work at colleges and universities as professors or clinical instructors. Although these professionals may be involved in clinical activities, their main role is to provide graduate-level education and training to audiology students. It is common for audiologists in these settings to divide their time between lecturing to graduate students regarding diagnostic and rehabilitative procedures and providing actual services to a clinical population.

Hearing Aid Manufacturers Companies that manufacture hearing aids employ some audiologists. In this setting, the audiologist will be responsible for bringing ideas to the company regarding the design of instruments and communicative needs of hearing-impaired individuals. Audiologists working for hearing aid companies will often serve as in-house consultants to practicing audiologists regarding specific instruments produced by their company. These audiologists are available to provide hearing aid fitting suggestions over the telephone to other audiologists. On occasion, audiologists working in this capacity will travel to various facilities as a product representative for their particular company.

CONCLUSION

In conclusion, SLPs and audiologists have myriad opportunities to match their personal interests and styles to a work setting. All settings in which speech-language and hearing professionals practice make high levels of demand in terms of productivity, accountability, and technical competence. All settings also provide the personal satisfaction that is unique to our profession, knowing that we are helping clients to engage in one of the most important human functions: communication.

STUDY QUESTIONS

1. Describe some of the service delivery features that influence the role of the SLP. What are the relative strengths and weaknesses of these service delivery features?

2. Contrast multi-, inter-, and transdisciplinary service provision.

3. Describe some of the contemporary factors affecting speech-language service provision in birth-to-3, public schools, and medical settings.

4. How is the work setting of the SLP in birth-to-3 services uniquely different from that of the school-based clinician?

5. Describe the parameters that contribute to a patient's progression through the continuum of care.

6. Compare and contrast the role of an SLP in a medical setting with that of an SLP in a school setting.

7. Describe three different settings in which audiologists may practice. Which one of these appeals to you the most and why?

8. How have recent technological developments broadened the scope of practice of the audiologist?

REFERENCES

American Academy of Audiology. (2004). *Scope of practice*. McLean, VA: Author.

American Academy of Audiology. (2009). *Position statement and clinical practice guidelines: ototoxicity monitoring*. Retrieved from http://www.audiology.org/professional/positions/ototoxicity

American Academy of Audiology. (2012). *Standards of practice for audiology*. McLean, VA: Author.

American Academy of Audiology. (2013). *Membership demographics* [Unpublished]. McLean, VA: Author.

American Speech-Language-Hearing Association. (2000). *Guidelines for the roles and responsibilities of school-based speech-language pathologist*. Rockville, MD: Author.

American Speech-Language-Hearing Association. (2003). *2003 omnibus survey: Practice trends in audiology*. Rockville, MD: Author.

American Speech-Language-Hearing Association. (2004a). The audiologist's role in occupational hearing conservation and hearing loss prevention programs: Technical report. *ASHA Suppl. 24*. Rockville, MD: Author.

American Speech-Language-Hearing Association. (2008a). *Communication facts: Incidence and prevalence of communication disorders and hearing loss in children.* Retrieved from http://www.asha.org/research/reports/children.htm

American Speech-Language-Hearing Association. (2008b). *Incidence and prevalence of hearing loss and hearing aid use in the United States.* Retrieved from http://www.asha.org/research/reports/hearing.htm

American Speech-Language-Hearing Association. (2004b). *Preferred practice patterns for the profession of speech-language pathology.* Rockville, MD: Author.

American Speech-Language-Hearing Association. (2004c). Scope of practice in audiology. *ASHA Suppl. 24.* Rockville, MD: Author.

American Speech-Language-Hearing Association. (2005a). *Roles and responsibilities of speech-language pathologists serving persons with mental retardation/developmental disabilities.* Retrieved from http://www.asha.org/policy/GL2005-00061.htm

American Speech-Language-Hearing Association. (2005b). Speech-language pathologists providing clinical services via telepractice: Position statement. *ASHA Suppl. 25.*

Americans with Disabilities Act (ADA) of 1990, PL 101-336, 42 U.S.C. §§ 12101 *et seq.*

Cascella, P.W., & McNamara, K.M. (2004). Practical communication services for high school students with severe disabilities: Collaboration during the transition to adult services. *The ASHA Leader, 9*(9), 6–7, 18–19.

Individuals with Disabilities Education Improvement Act of 2004, PL 108-446, 20 U.S.C. §§ 1400 *et seq.*

Rini, D.L., & Whitney, G.C. (1999). Family centered practice for children with communication disorders. *Child and Adolescent Psychiatric Clinics of North America, 8*(1), 153–174.

Stach, B. (1998). *Clinical audiology: An introduction.* San Diego, CA: Singular Publishing Group.

World Health Organization. (2001). *International Classification of Functioning, Disability and Health* (ICFDH). Geneva: Author.

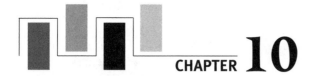

CHAPTER 10

Issues of Cultural and Linguistic Diversity

Brian A. Goldstein and Aquiles Iglesias

CHAPTER OBJECTIVES

After reading this chapter, students will be able to

- Define cultural and linguistic diversity
- Outline the effects of culture on communication
- Understand issues of bilingualism and dialects
- Apply principles of least biased assessment and intervention

Nina is a 4-year-old girl of Latino descent who was referred by her classroom teacher to the speech-language pathologist (SLP) at her preschool because she was communicating in short sentences and was difficult to understand at times. Nina lives at home with her mother, father, and older sister, who is in the first grade. The family speaks both English and Spanish at home and in the community. The family reports that Nina uses more Spanish with them but more English with her older sister, Ana. Nina is increasingly using English at home and sometimes refuses to use Spanish. Nina's mother indicates that she can understand what Nina is trying to say.

Not every SLP will have access to individuals who can provide cultural and linguistic information about clients or will have been enrolled in a training program with a major focus on providing appropriate clinical management skills to individuals such as Nina from culturally and linguistically diverse populations. It should be noted, however, that the American Speech-Language-Hearing Association (ASHA) mandates academic and clinical education that prepares students in accredited programs to practice in a multicultural society (ASHA, 2004). This chapter provides a road map to the linguistic and cultural differences found in the United States today and shows how those differences influence the field of speech-language pathology. The overarching goal of this chapter is to better prepare and equip you, as clinicians, for situations in which you provide clinical services to individuals who do not share your cultural and/or linguistic experiences.

CULTURALLY AND LINGUISTICALLY DIVERSE DEFINED

What individuals are considered *culturally and linguistically diverse*? For the most part, normative information about speech and language development and disorders comes from English-speaking, European American, middle-class individuals. That is, from a historical perspective, clinicians have tended to base their diagnostic and intervention approaches on one group. In a sense, everyone except those who make up that group falls into the category of culturally and linguistically diverse, and those are the individuals with whom we are concerning ourselves.

DEMOGRAPHICS

Historically, the United States has been called a "melting pot" because individuals from many countries came representing diverse races, ethnic groups, religions, languages, and so forth, and then were thought to assimilate into mainstream American culture, however *mainstream* is defined. The obvious disadvantage to assimilation was the loss of cultural and linguistic identities. In the early 21st century, the term *mosaic* is more commonly used to represent how individuals new to the United States help form the fabric of the country. Individuals retain some or all of their historical identities while creating a new and different picture of the United States. In the future, that picture will continue to change. Table 10.1 represents U.S. population statistics from 2010 and projected for the year 2050 (U.S. Bureau of the Census, 2010a).

By the year 2050, it is predicted that the percentage of culturally and linguistically diverse individuals will increase as the percentage of individuals of European descent declines. The percentage of individuals of Asian descent will double, and the percentage of individuals of Hispanic descent will increase by 6%. The percentage of African Americans/Blacks[1] in the U.S. population will increase by 3%; the percentage of Native Americans will increase to just above 1%. The percentage of Whites (i.e., European Americans) will decrease, forming slightly over half the population.

There is a misperception that individuals from culturally and linguistically diverse populations exist mainly in large, urban areas such as Chicago, New York, Philadelphia, and Los Angeles; however, that is clearly not the case. For example, there are large Spanish-speaking communities in Arkansas, Georgia, Nebraska, and Oregon. The highest percentage increase in Hispanics in the United States from 2000 to 2010 was in South Carolina, at 148% (U.S. Bureau of the Census, 2010b). There are Native Americans in North Carolina and Minnesota. There are sizable Hmong (Southeast Asian) communities in Massachusetts, Minnesota, and California. This linguistic diversity extends to speakers of English **dialects** as well. For example, Washington and Craig (1994) indicated that the number of children speaking African American English is increasing and will continue to do so in the foreseeable future. Thus, children from culturally and linguistically diverse populations are well represented in U.S. school systems. In 2008, approximately 49 million children were enrolled in elementary and secondary schools in the United States, 45% of whom were from culturally and linguistically diverse

---

[1]Terms are those used by the U.S. Department of Commerce, Bureau of the Census (2010a, 2010b).

Table 10.1. United States population statistics, 2010 and 2050

Group	Number[a] (2010)	Percentage[b] (2010)	Percentage[b] (2050)
African American	38.9	12.7	15.7
Asian American	14.7	4.8	10.3
Hispanic	50.5	16.6	22.5
Native American	2.9	0.9	1.1
White	197.0	64.8	52.5
Total	**304.0**	**99.8**[c]	**102.1**

Source: U.S. Bureau of the Census (2010a).

[a]In millions.

[b]Represents percentage of total U.S. population (http://www.census.gov/population/www/pop-profile/natproj.html).

[c]Not 100% due to rounding.

populations (U.S. Department of Education, 2008). In addition, there were more than 11 million English language learners (ELLs; i.e., children who are in the process of acquiring a second language and who lack sufficient mastery of English to successfully achieve in an English-language classroom without additional support) in public schools during the 2009–2010 academic year, an increase from 9.8 million students in 2000 (U.S. Department of Education, 2009). This diversity influences school-based SLPs directly. Roseberry-McKibbin, Brice, and O'Hanlon (2005) surveyed school-based SLPs on a number of issues concerning students from culturally and linguistically diverse backgrounds, particularly ELLs. The authors found that 11.3% of all the children on SLPs' caseloads were ELLs. The most commonly reported issues that SLPs faced in working with ELLs included 1) inability to speak the language of the child, 2) lack of least biased assessments, 3) lack of support personnel who speak the child's language, and 4) lack of information on developmental norms in the student's home language. In a national survey of SLPs, Roseberry-McKibbin and Eicholtz (1994) found that 78% of SLPs had on their caseloads 0–3 students with limited English proficiency, 11% had 4–7 students, 4% had 7–10 students, and 6% had more than 10 students. The majority of SLPs were working with children of Latino descent, although they were also working with children of Chinese, Filipino, Hmong, Korean, European, Middle Eastern, Portuguese, and Vietnamese descent.

COMMUNICATION AND CULTURE

Anderson and Fenichal define *culture* as "the totality of socially transmitted behavior patterns, arts, beliefs, institutions, and all other products of human work and thought. . . . The predominating attitudes and behavior that characterize the functioning of a group or organization ... the cultural framework must be viewed as a set of tendencies of possibilities from which to choose" (1989, p. 8). The way in which we communicate reflects, among many things, the culture in which we were raised. Parents socialize their children to be "good" (i.e., appropriate) communicators within their own community. Given the diversity that exists in the United States, SLPs may find that the ways in which parents interact with their children vary greatly. That variation might be reflected in the responses to the tasks we ask families to perform during the clinical management process. For example, during Nina's evaluation, a student clinician asked Sra. Flores, Nina's mother, to go into the diagnostic room and "play with your child as you do at home." Nina and Sra. Flores entered the playroom, which was full of toys and games appropriate for Nina's age. After entering the room, Nina promptly went to the kitchen area and began playing with the pots and pans. Sra. Flores sat nearby and observed Nina as she played. Every once in a while, Sra. Flores would ask Nina in Spanish to bring her something to drink or eat. Nina complied with all requests that were repeated more than twice. Nina's verbal utterances were limited in quantity and quality. The student clinicians in the observation room were dismayed because they felt Nina and Sra. Flores's interaction was stilted and the language sample was not rich. They wondered why Sra. Flores did not ask questions, make comments or statements, or engage with her daughter in play. The student clinicians began to wonder whether Nina's low verbal output and possible language delay was due in part to Sra. Flores's interaction style.

The clinical supervisor then asked one of the student clinicians to go into the playroom with a rather complex puzzle. The student was instructed to ask Sra. Flores to explain to Nina how to put the puzzle together. After hearing the instructions, Sra. Flores asked Nina to sit in a chair next to her. She began asking Nina questions and making commands using a large number of nonspecific words (e.g., "Where do you put this one?" "Put that one next to that thing"). Nina's expressive language was more complex and receptively she appeared to understand all of Sra. Flores's utterances. The language output, however, was still less than one would expect of a 4-year-old child, and the student clinicians were almost positive that Nina had a language delay. Finally, Nina's 6-year-old sister, Ana, was brought into the room, and the two were allowed to play together. Ana informed Nina that they were going to play school, pulled out a book, and proceeded to play the role of the teacher. She asked such questions as "What is the girl's name?" "What happened when she sat in the Papa Bear chair?" and "What happened next?" Nina's verbal output in this situation amazed the evaluation participants. She used language for a variety of purposes, her sentences were complex, and her vocabulary was diverse. The student clinicians were not prepared for the fact that there are cross-cultural differences in parent–child interaction and communication that vary by context (Iglesias & Quinn, 1997). For example, parents do not necessarily engage in cooperative play with their children. Parents may see their role as being that of a caregiver, and in a situation in which language is contextualized, parents may use a high degree of nonspecific vocabulary (Scheffner Hammer, Miccio, & Rodriguez, 2004).

It is necessary to gather cultural and linguistic information to provide appropriate services to individuals who come from cultures other than your own or speak languages other than yours. You might read and study about various cultural groups, talk to and work with individuals from a variety of cultures, participate in the life of someone from another culture, and/or learn another language (Lynch, 2011). There are a number of specific **sociolinguistic factors** (both verbal and nonverbal) that might influence your interaction with a client and his or her family (Damico & Hamayan, 1992; Kayser, 1993; Lynch, 2011; Roseberry-McKibbin, 1994, 2002; Terrell & Terrell, 1993; Wyatt, 2002). First, child socialization practices and children's play characteristics should be considered. For example, children who typically utilize peers as conversational partners might be less comfortable interacting in play situations with adults. In terms of the assessment process, the SLP would want to use peers (or perhaps siblings) to interact with the client in order to obtain a language sample. Second, family characteristics also need to be taken into account (e.g., Westby, 2000). These include factors such as country of birth, degree of acculturation into American society, knowledge of the U.S. education system, family attitude toward English and English speakers, family attitude toward disabilities, family structure, geographic location (e.g., urban, rural), religious beliefs, social status, and socioeconomic status. For example, adults from some cultures may be more comfortable interacting with female clinicians rather than male clinicians (Roseberry-McKibbin, 2002). Third, in assessing clients from culturally and linguistically diverse populations, SLPs must also consider individual differences. For example, not all African Americans speak African American English, and speakers of African American English are all not African Americans (Wolfram & Schilling-Estes, 1998).

BILINGUALISM AND DIALECTS

In providing assessment and intervention services to individuals from culturally and linguistically diverse populations, as SLPs you will undoubtedly encounter individuals who either speak more than one language (e.g., are bilingual) or speak a dialect of English (here, we focus on dialects of English, although all languages have dialects). In this chapter, we first discuss bilingualism and then turn our attention to dialects.

Bilingualism

Speaking only one language is the exception to the norm if we take a world perspective. According to the Linguistic Society of America (1996), the majority of the world's countries are at least bilingual and many are multilingual. For example, the European Union has more official languages than does the United Nations, and nearly 60% of Europeans have learned a second language (Sollors, 1998). The United States, though officially not bilingual, is home to approximately 57.1 million speakers of languages other than English (U.S. Bureau of the Census, 2010a). In addition, of those 57 million, 24 million speak English less than "very well." According to the U.S. Bureau of the Census (2009), there are 37 languages spoken in the United States and more than 100,000 speakers, ranging from Scandinavian languages, with 126,000 speakers, to Spanish, with more than 35 million speakers. In addition to Spanish, there are over 1 million speakers of German, Vietnamese, French, Tagalog, and Chinese (the variation of which is not specified).

Historically, bilinguals have been placed in one of two categories, simultaneous or sequential (Paradis, Genesee, & Crago, 2011). Traditionally defined, *simultaneous learners* were individuals who acquired both languages from birth (*bilingual first-language acquisition* is a term also used for this group; see De Houwer, 2009), and *sequential learners* were those who acquired one language after the other (e.g., the second language typically being acquired on entrance into the school system). As Baker said, however, "defining who is or is not bilingual is essentially elusive and ultimately impossible. Some categorization is often necessary and helpful to make sense of the world" (1996, p. 13). Thus, bilingualism should be viewed on a continuum with changing levels of input, output, use, and proficiency over time. At the two extremes of the continuum are monolingual individuals raised and living in monolingual environments (e.g., Spanish-speaking children raised and living in remote areas of Mexico). Bilingual individuals fall between those ends of the continuum and will differ from monolingual speakers of each language across phonological, semantic, morphosyntactic, and pragmatic areas (e.g., Goldstein, 2012; Paradis, Genesee, & Crago, 2011). The degree of bilingualism achieved by an individual will be dependent on linguistic, social, emotional, political, demographic, and cultural factors (e.g., Baker, 1996; Hakuta, 1986; Pease-Alvarez, 1993). In addition, studies in bilingualism suggest that the degree of bilingualism depends on such factors as generational level, age, occupation, opportunity for contact with speakers of English, exposure to English media, and the nature of interactions with members of their community (Romaine, 1995, 1999).

Bilingual speakers demonstrate various degrees of proficiency in either language depending on the situation, topic, interactants, and context. Many bilingual individuals appear indistinguishable in normal social interactions, what Cummins (1984) referred to as possessing basic interpersonal communication skills (BICS). Differences, however, are evident in cognitively demanding, decontextualized interactions—what Cummins refers to as having cognitive academic language proficiency (CALP).

For an illustration of that difference, we return to the example of Nina's evaluation for a possible language delay. In the first interaction between Sra. Flores and Nina, they both were speaking in Spanish, although in the second interaction Sra. Flores used English and Spanish. The interaction between Nina and Ana was all in English. The first interaction could be classified as one in which Nina was relying heavily on her BICS to communicate with her mother. The second interaction was more demanding and required Nina to understand and use more cognitively demanding language. To facilitate the linguistic experience in this interaction, Sra. Flores used contextual cues (using modeling behaviors) and also used both languages to facilitate the conversation. Sra. Flores's use of both languages is typical of that seen when both speakers are bilingual. The interaction of Nina and Ana was all in English and required Nina to further use more cognitively and academically demanding language. As a result of the situations, the speakers, and the topics, Nina demonstrated different proficiencies in the two languages.

Although there are many specific definitions of bilingualism, most people accept Grosjean's "holistic" view of bilingualism (1989, 1992, 1997). This view posits that the languages of bilinguals are an integrated whole that cannot be easily separated into the component languages. According to Grosjean, bilinguals have one linguistic system that results in different surface structures. This interdependence between the two languages allows for the transfer of skills across languages. From the standpoint of an SLP, adopting this view of bilingualism means that the communication assessment of bilinguals, both children and adults, will necessitate 1) studying bilinguals as a whole without comparison to monolinguals, 2) examining both of the bilingual's languages, and 3) investigating how bilinguals organize and use both languages (cf. Goldstein, 2012).

Dialects

There are many dialects spoken in the United States, including those such as Southern White Standard, Appalachian English, Caribbean English, African

American English, and General American English. A *dialect* is a rule-governed variety of a language characterized by social, ethnic, and geographical differences in its speakers (e.g., Oetting & McDonald, 2002). Dialects are mutually intelligible forms of a language associated with a particular region, social class, or ethnic group. Dialects may differ across all areas of language—phonology, syntax, morphology, lexicon, and pragmatics. In fact, every person has his or her own unique way of speaking, termed an **idiolect.** Varieties of a language that depend on the context and conversational participants are called **registers,** which change depending on the participants, setting, and topic. For example, an individual usually uses one register when talking to a potential employer and another variety when speaking to friends. The terms *dialect* and **accent** are often (erroneously) used interchangeably. The term *dialect* refers to all aspects of a language, and *accent* refers only to the pronunciation of a language variety. Accent does not take into account lexical, syntactic, morphological, and pragmatic aspects of the language variety.

No dialect of any language is superior to any other dialect (Green, 2004). This is not to say that all varieties of a language are equally prestigious. Some varieties of a language, specifically those used by the "dominant" groups in any socially stratified society, will be considered to have higher prestige (Wolfram, 1986), to be preferred in the educational system (Adler, 1984), and to be valued by the private sector of the society (Terrell & Terrell, 1983). General American English is considered the prestige dialect in the United States and is preferred in the educational system. Because of mass media saturation, there have been some decreased differences between dialects and greater acceptance of others. There has also been, however, increasing difference between dialects because of the isolation of some groups, especially those in the lower socioeconomic status in society (Wolfram & Schilling-Estes, 1998). The increased immigration and ethnic isolation that has occurred among some subgroups has further increased the number of ethnic dialects. At least in terms of dialects, the "melting pot" hypothesis appears to be a myth for certain segments of our society.

COMPLETING MOST APPROPRIATE ASSESSMENTS

To complete reliable and valid assessments, SLPs will need to use information on communication and culture, bilingualism, and dialects. The goal of an assessment with an individual from a culturally and linguistically diverse population is to conduct a least biased assessment. This means that you understand the individual's culture and language (and/or dialect) and understand how the factors cited previously might influence the diagnostic process. The result of a least biased assessment is to differentiate individuals developing typically who may have a **language difference** (i.e., expected community variations in syntax, semantics, phonology, pragmatics, lexicon) from those with **language disorders** (i.e., communication that deviates significantly from the norms of the community; see Taylor & Payne, 1994).

So why is it necessary to make adjustments in the way that individuals from culturally and linguistically diverse populations are assessed? Historically, individuals from culturally and linguistically diverse populations have not been assessed appropriately (Goldstein & Horton-Ikard, 2010). For example, bilingual adults with aphasia have only been assessed in one language (i.e., English) because of the lack of a bilingual SLP or trained support personnel. In the case of school-age children, this lack has resulted in an overreferral to and enrollment in special education for children from culturally and linguistically diverse populations despite recognition of cultural differences and their influence on linguistic development. That is, many children from culturally and linguistically diverse backgrounds were placed in special education because of a language difference, not a language disorder. It has also meant, in some cases, an underidentification of language disorders due to the assumption that any variation from what is expected is attributable to cultural and linguistic differences.

Many laws have been passed and lawsuits have been brought to help ensure that children are placed appropriately into special education. For example, public laws such as the Individuals with Disabilities Education Improvement Act (IDEA) of 2004 (PL 108-446) mandate that a child's native language must be used in all direct contact with the child. Thus, SLPs must find means to conduct assessments employing the language the child uses in the home or learning environment. Lawsuits such as *Larry P. v. Riles* (1979) nullified the use of standardized IQ tests in California to place African American children in special education. Thus, society-at-large and the courts have acknowledged the rights of linguistic minority populations. This acceptance has resulted in greater acceptance of the variety of dialects that are spoken in the United States. Although General American English is the most common and dominant language variety spoken in the United States, there has been a realization that other varieties have a right to exist in the linguistically pluralistic society. These laws have a definite influence on conducting least biased assessments.

To diagnose individuals who truly have a communication disorder, communicative standards of one group cannot be imposed on another. Operationally, a *communication disorder* is defined as communication that differs from the norm. It is imperative that the norm be, among other things, culturally based (Taylor & Clarke, 1994). To be certain that least biased assessments take place, you should take into account factors that may influence the assessment process (e.g., Goldstein, 2000; Iglesias, 2001; Kayser, 1993, 1995a; Langdon, 2008; Roseberry-McKibbin, 2002; Seymour & Pearson, 2004; Terrell & Terrell, 1993).

Clinician Factors

Prior to conducting an assessment, clinicians must assess their cultural and linguistic competence. Our attitudes, knowledge, and actions have an influence on the quality of the services we provide. To respond optimally to the individuals we serve, we must have 1) a positive attitude toward the families' values and beliefs, even if they are significantly different from our own; and 2) an understanding of typical and atypical language development, including an understanding of what is considered to be a disorder across different groups. As we gain a better understanding and an appreciation of the families we serve, our intervention goals and approaches will be congruent with those of the families.

We must also assess the extent to which our linguistic skills in a language other than English are sufficient to evaluate our assessment tools and carry out an assessment. Although some working knowledge of a language is helpful, clinicians should be aware that less-than-native or near-native proficiency in a language is not sufficient to carry out a proper assessment. In the case of a bilingual child, the clinician not only must be proficient in both languages but also should able to create an environment where the child can freely code-switch or mix, thus using his or her full linguistic repertoire. In preparing to complete a least biased assessment, you should conduct a self-assessment (i.e., know your own culture and worldview), have a solid understanding of variations across and within cultural-linguistic groups, and determine whether you have the language skills and training to provide assessment and intervention for bilingual individuals. According to ASHA (1989), an SLP or audiologist may be considered bilingual if he or she speaks one native language and speaks a second language with native or near-native proficiency in lexicon, semantics, phonology, morphology, and pragmatics. To provide bilingual clinical services in the child's language, the bilingual SLP should

- Be able to describe typical speech and language development using contemporary data and theory

- Possess knowledge of dialects in the child's home language

- Use least biased evaluation tools to gauge speech and language skills

- Administer and interpret formal and informal evaluation tools

- Apply intervention strategies in the child's language

- Recognize cultural factors that affect assessment and intervention

- Be able to aid parents and other professionals in understanding the diagnosis, assessment results, and intervention options and approaches

General Assessment Factors

During the assessment process, there are ways in which you can increase the likelihood of an appropriate diagnosis. First, use an assessment framework, such as the one outlined by Gillam and Hoffman (2001). Although the framework was designed for children, it has implications for adults as well and can be adapted for that purpose, especially as it relates to assessing the client across multiple contexts with multiple interlocutors. They suggest that assessment should take place in four domains: 1) functions and activities (e.g., interviews, language samples, dynamic assessment), 2) participation (e.g., portfolios with homework, class assignments, tests, writing samples) and naturalistic observation in the home and at school, 3) contextual areas (e.g., curriculum measures, reading miscues; see Laing, 2002), and 4) decontextual settings (e.g., standardized tests). Using such a framework will increase the likelihood of a least biased assessment. Second, administer several formal (i.e., standardized) and informal (i.e., nonstandardized) measures. Using both types of measures will allow for a more representative sample of the individual's abilities. Third, assess skills in all languages or dialects. It is quite common for individuals to exhibit some skills in one language or dialect and other skills in the other language or dialect. For example, Nina first learned the names of colors in English because her English-speaking teacher produced the names of colors in English. If she were tested in Spanish only, she might not label colors in Spanish, leading the SLP to mistakenly believe that she did not know color names. Bilingual adults with aphasia may recover some language skills in the one language but other skills in the other language (Paradis, 2001). Clinicians should also observe whether the language disorder exists in all languages or dialects; it should. Fourth, recognize that different modes of communication may be in effect and that performance may vary because of those factors rather than the client's abilities. A mismatch of communicative styles between the family and the SLP is always possible.

Assessment Tool Factors

Most SLPs administer formal (i.e., standardized) assessment tools to their clients. Not all formal assessments will, however, be appropriate for all clients. In administering formal assessments to your clients, you should take into account the following issues (e.g., Goldstein, 2000; Kayser, 1993, 1995a; Langdon, 2008; Roseberry-McKibbin, 2002; Wyatt, 2002):

- Examine each item before administering the test to determine whether the client may have had prior access to the information and if failure should be considered indicative of a disorder.

- Determine whether modification of specific test items can reduce bias.

- Consider first administering a child's test to an adult in order to get information on the appropriateness of test items and the likely responses from a child.

- Have families complete case history information, permission forms, and release-of-information documents in person.

- Make an effort to identify in the normative sample those measures that include individuals from culturally and linguistically diverse populations.

- Observe *code-switching*, or alternations between languages at the word, phrase, or sentence levels (e.g., an individual may start a sentence in one language and finish it in another; see Mattes & Omark, 1991), and **language interference,** or the influence of one language on another (e.g., a native speaker of Japanese may pronounce English with a Japanese accent; see Roseberry-McKibbin, 2002).

- Report all modifications of standardized administration procedures.

- Report norms only if they are valid for the population being assessed.

- Select a test that examines those aspects of language that need to be assessed.

- Use a variety of elicitation procedures.

ALTERNATIVE METHODS OF ASSESSMENT

Just as you would, as clinician, alter the assessment process for evaluating someone with a language disorder versus someone with a voice disorder, you also need to tailor the assessment of individuals from culturally and linguistically diverse populations to their specific language and culture. That is, you design your assessment to fit the specific needs of the client. Alternative methods of assessment also need to be used in order to make a proper differential diagnosis. Without using such modifications, there is a chance for either **overdiagnosis** or **underdiagnosis.** Overdiagnosis might occur when an individual is labeled with a communication disorder because his or her abilities were assessed using a test standardized based on a sample from which the client does not come. For example, Nina might be overdiagnosed using a standardized test that did not include bilingual children in the norming sample. Underdiagnosis might occur because the examiner assumes that all "errors" produced are due to dialect or second-language acquisition. For example, in the assessment of a 5-year-old child who speaks African American English, the SLP may find a language sample and note some anomalies in form (e.g., "He eated the doughnut") that were initially erroneously labeled as a dialect feature (i.e., "eated" is not grammatically correct in African American English). Further, Nina's production errors might be misinterpreted as second-language acquisition or dialectal and thus not considered true errors.

A number of suggestions in completing alternative methods of assessment have been suggested by many researchers (compiled from Cheng, 1993; Erickson & Iglesias, 1986; Goldstein, 2000; Goldstein & Horton-Ikard, 2010; Kayser, 1989, 1993, 1995a; Langdon, 1992, 2008; Norris, Juarez, & Perkins, 1989; Roseberry-McKibbin, 1994, 2002; Taylor & Payne, 1983; Terrell & Terrell, 1993; Toliver Weddington, 1981; Van Keulen, Weddington, & DeBose, 1998; Vaughn-Cooke, 1986; Wyatt, 2002). Utilizing such alternative strategies increases the likelihood that children such as Nina will undergo a least biased assessment. These suggestions include solutions such as developing new tests, standardizing existing tests on individuals from culturally and linguistically diverse backgrounds, and administering standardized tests in nonstandardized ways. No matter which route you choose, if a standardized test does not include individuals from culturally and linguistically diverse populations in the standardization sample, you should question the test's validity. Because many standardized assessments must still be developed with these populations in mind, clinicians frequently use tests already in existence and administer them to their clients in alternative ways. If you use an alternative format when assessing a client, your assessment report must detail how the test was modified and the report must indicate the underlying motivation of the modifications. For example, you might alter a test by allowing an individual to go back to revise his or her test responses, repeating and/or rewording instructions, providing additional time for an individual to respond, testing beyond the ceiling of the assessment, adding practice items, and asking an individual to explain his or her answers. If modifying existing tests will not yield helpful information, another option is to restandardize the existing tests by developing **local norms.** You can do this by administering the test to individuals without language disorders in the community in which you are working, note the scores they receive and the quality of their responses, and use their test results as the standard to which the client's test scores can be compared.

Because it can be difficult and time consuming to restandardize existing tests or develop new tests, it is also recommended that clinicians use alternative testing formats (i.e., measures other than standardized tests). Alternative testing formats might include these:

- *Criterion-referenced tests:* These are tests that specify the linguistic behaviors to be tested, establish criteria for acceptable responses, and do not compare the client's responses against some other standard. One disadvantage is that the criteria used to develop these tests often come from standardized assessments.

- *Dynamic assessment* (e.g., Kapantzoglu, Restrepo, & Thompson, 2012; Peña, 1996; Peña, Iglesias, & Lidz, 2001): Performance is gauged by examining **modifiability** (i.e., change through mediation or teaching). Examiners can determine how a client learns, what is needed for a client to learn, and how a client generalizes a task to new situations. Modifiability is composed of three factors: 1) client responsiveness (i.e., how a client responds to and uses new information), 2) examiner effort (i.e., the quantity and quality of effort needed to make a change), and 3) transfer (i.e., the generalization of new skills).

- *Portfolio assessment:* This is a procedure in which you collect a client's work over time representing a variety of tasks and assignments; assignments might include writing samples, observations from teachers, parents, and so forth; language samples; and tapes of performance.

- *Ethnographic assessment* (Heath, 1982, 1983; Westby, 2000): This is a procedure in which you observe the client in many contexts with many conversational partners. You ask family members about their own culture, their attitudes about the host culture (i.e., the new culture in which they are living), and their communication in the home. You interact with clients, being sensitive to their culture, their frame of reference, and what they see as important. In addition, you describe clients' communicative abilities during genuine communication in a naturalistic environment.

- *Probe techniques:* This assessment technique assesses a small amount of information over a short period of time (e.g., weekly, biweekly) to gauge rate and amount of learning.

If a school-age child is being evaluated, the SLP might obtain academic information from teachers and school records in addition to utilizing the alternative testing formats described above. Damico (1993) and Gillam and Hoffman (2001) suggested that clinicians obtain information by observing in the classroom, analyzing academic tasks and the curriculum, and assessing the child's test-taking abilities during structured activities.

As an SLP, you should also follow some testing guidelines to decrease the possibility of misdiagnosis (Kayser, 1993; Langdon, 2008; Roseberry-McKibbin, 1995).

1. Do not use norm-referenced tests only.

2. Do not use only a language sample to qualify someone for services.

3. Do not use multiple assessments in order to get low scores so that someone will be qualified for services.

4. Do not use translations of tests (Roseberry-McKibbin, 1994). First, there are differences in structure and content in each language. The same translated item may differ in structure and difficulty across the two languages.

Second, using such tests mistakenly implies that children acquiring English proficiency and English-speaking children receive similar socialization, life experiences, language input, academic instruction, and so forth. Third, differences in the frequency of target words vary from one language to the next. Fourth, grammatical forms may not be equivalent between the languages. Fifth, translated tests do not tap an individual's ability to acquire language.

5. Do not use only one elicitation technique.

6. Do not use tests administered in English-only if the individual is bilingual.

7. Do not assume that features of a second language or a dialect of English are characteristics of a disorder.

8. Do not assume that support personnel are automatically trained to aid in the diagnostic process.

RESPONSIBILITIES AND ROLES OF THE MONOLINGUAL SPEECH-LANGUAGE PATHOLOGIST

Given the demographic changes occurring in the United States and the fact that most SLPs are monolingual and English speaking, ASHA has developed guidelines regarding the responsibilities of monolingual SLPs to individuals who are bilingual. These guidelines should be followed in evaluating a child such as Nina. According to ASHA (1998; see also ASHA, 2004), monolingual SLPs may test in English, perform the oral-peripheral exam, conduct hearing screenings, complete nonverbal assessments, and conduct the family interview (with appropriate support personnel) in English. In preparing to assess an individual whose language they do not speak, monolingual SLPs should research the culture, language, and dialect of the person they are going to assess and use least biased assessment tools. They should also be prepared to ask for help if necessary, be an advocate for the individual, and be willing to refer the individual to another clinician if necessary.

Monolingual SLPs might also consider some other alternatives (ASHA, 1998):

1. Establishing contacts and hiring bilingual SLPs as consultants or diagnosticians to provide clinical services

2. Establishing cooperative groups in which a group of school districts or programs might hire an itinerant bilingual SLP

3. Establishing networks such as forging links between university settings and work settings to help recruit bilingual speakers into the workforce

4. Establishing clinical fellowship year and graduate student practica sites

5. Establishing interdisciplinary teams in which monolingual SLPs are teamed with bilingual professionals from other fields

6. Training support personnel such as bilingual aides, students, family members, or members of the community (Paul & Norbury, 2012, p. 164)

You should be aware that there is a limit as to the types of tasks that support personnel can complete (ASHA, 1996). Support personnel can conduct speech-language screenings, follow intervention plans or protocols, document client progress, and assist during assessment, but there are also other tasks that support personnel should not complete. These tasks include performing standardized or nonstandardized diagnostic tests; interpreting test results; participating in parent conferences, case conferences, or any interdisciplinary team without the supervising SLP present; and writing, developing, or modifying a client's individualized intervention plan.

INTERVENTION

Intervention is a process by which a clinician deliberately sets out to systematically change the course of an ongoing behavior. This process always involves an expert who has an awareness of what is appropriate behavior (i.e., intervention goal) and what to do to achieve this goal (i.e., intervention approach). The specific goals and approaches selected are driven by the clinician's values, beliefs, and knowledge. As clinicians, it is our ethical responsibility to examine how our own biases and the limits of our knowledge base influence the direction and outcome of our intervention. To achieve this, we must identify and overcome our biases and engage in activities that expand our conceptual perspective of sociocultural and linguistic factors that have an influence on intervention. We must be aware that in many cases we will be implementing interventions based on limited empirical research. The majority of our intervention programs will be based on this limited knowledge coupled with logic and experience. Ongoing evaluation of our goals, intervention approaches, and outcomes should be a source for our ongoing decision-making process.

Let us return to our example of Nina being evaluated for a language disorder. Based on the results of the evaluation, the supervising clinician decided that Nina needed to receive intervention to facilitate her language acquisition and that one of the goals of the intervention should be to increase Nina's use of questions, commands, and statements. The SLP reasoned that greater use of these communicative functions would increase Nina's academic communication skills. Unfortunately, Nina's parents were excluded from the decision-making process. Although on the surface the goal appears to be appropriate, the clinician should have noted that this goal required a shift in Sra. Flores's child-rearing practices; now Nina is to view her parent as an equal partner instead of as a caregiver. The clinician did not consider whether this shift would create new adjustment problems for the family. Sra. Flores returned to the clinician 3 weeks later to complain about Nina's new, disrespectful behavior toward adults. Another intervention strategy may have worked better while still assuming the same goals. For example, the clinician could have discussed with the Sra. Flores the need to achieve these goals and asked her advice on optional ways to attain them. Perhaps Sra. Flores would have suggested that the SLP explicitly state that this type of communication be used only in Nina's classroom or that the intervention should be carried out in a group situation where Nina would be interacting with her peers. There is even the possibility that once the SLP thoroughly explained the intervention strategy, Sra. Flores would have agreed to change her own rules regarding what behaviors of Nina's are appropriate. Any or all of these strategies could have avoided the negative side effects of

Nina's intervention. Providing appropriate intervention services to individuals from culturally and linguistically diverse populations has often proved to be difficult. There is a severe lack of research into effective intervention strategies. We have, however, provided you with general intervention guidelines to apply when treating individuals with communication disorders who hail from culturally and linguistically diverse populations (compiled from Beaumont, 1992; Cheng, 1989, 1996; Damico & Hamayan, 1992; Damico, Smith, & Augustine, 1996; Goldstein, 2000; Kayser, 1995b; Kohnert, Yim, Nett, Kan, & Duran, 2005; Langdon, 2008; Seymour, 1986).

General Considerations

There are a number of general guidelines you should follow when providing intervention services to individuals from culturally and linguistically diverse populations. First, assess the individual continuously. Each session should be a miniassessment that will help you plan for the next session. Complete comprehensive reevaluations of the individual's intervention needs periodically (e.g., every 3–6 months). Second, set up opportunities for language to be used in natural interactions, utilize natural language-learning activities, and interrelate activities. The activities, and the materials used in them, should be meaningful and interesting. We acquire new knowledge in situations that require us to use multiple bases of knowledge. Third, consider a holistic strategies approach by encouraging clients to 1) explain new information in their own words, 2) abstract information, 3) generalize information to new contexts, and 4) analyze new information (Roseberry-McKibbin, 2002). Keep in mind that SLPs should focus on language meaning as well as language structure; have clients relate new information to previously learned information; teach strategies for learning and remembering new content; and use an intervention strategy that teaches the "whole" of a concept, breaks the concept down into its "parts," and then reconstructs it into a "whole" again (Roseberry-McKibbin, 2002). Fourth, allow clients to think, discuss options, make decisions, establish accountability, and show knowledge both verbally and nonverbally. If the use of printed material is emphasized during the intervention, SLPs will need to build a literacy-rich environment for clients, which will help empower individuals as learners. Fifth, use a variety of social organizations (e.g., large-group projects, small-group projects, peer–peer projects) and use individual, peer–peer, and group work. Sixth, if appropriate, use a bidialectal and/or bilingual approach. That is, incorporate clients' home language and/or dialect into the intervention process. Research has shown that language skills in the second language can be predicted, in part, by skills in the first language (e.g., Cobo-Lewis, Eilers, Pearson, & Umbel, 2002; Lopez & Greenfield, 2004; Perozzi & Sanchez, 1992). For example, because Nina uses both Spanish and English at school and in the community, intervention will need to take place in both languages and not only in English. As Kohnert (2008) indicates, a disorder in bilinguals is not caused by bilingualism or cured by monolingualism. Finally, use all resources available to you (e.g., if you are working in a school, get help from English-as-a-second-language teachers, general classroom teachers, and so forth; if you are employed in a health care setting, utilize a cross-disciplinary approach).

Family-Centered Intervention

It is likely that the people who will know your client best are his or her family members. Therefore, it is imperative to involve your client's family in the intervention process (Lynch & Hanson, 2011). Family members' involvement, however, must be at a level at which they are most comfortable. Some families may be comfortable actually participating in the intervention by being in the room with you, whereas other families may wish to observe the intervention sessions and ask questions following the intervention.

There are some specific ways in which you ought to work with families like Nina's in the intervention process. First, educate the family about the purpose of the sessions and who will be present in them. Second, attempt to involve the family in the decision making, if appropriate. Third, match your client's goals to the family's concerns and needs. Fourth, allow time for the family to ask questions but also be prepared to answer the same question posed by different members. Fifth, utilize practices that are culturally appropriate. These strategies include checking often for comprehension, emphasizing key words continually, reviewing previously learned material on a daily basis, including literacy activities, rephrasing information, teaching concepts in naturalistic situations, teaching the client to monitor his or her own learning activities, using all modalities, and using stories and narratives. These strategies have been shown to be effective for individuals from culturally and linguistically diverse populations (Roseberry-McKibbin, 2002).

CONCLUSION

Providing appropriate assessment and intervention services to individuals from culturally and linguistically diverse populations is challenging. Before the assessment even takes place, you will probably have to gather information on your client's language, dialectal variety, verbal and nonverbal communication styles, and so forth. This information will have to be applied to the specific person you are evaluating. It may be necessary for you to employ support personnel to aid in the clinical management process, particularly if you do not speak the client's language. You may also have to alter your typical assessment protocol in order to ensure that you are making a valid diagnosis. Accurate diagnosis will lead to intervention approaches and techniques that are suited to your particular client.

STUDY QUESTIONS

1. Describe your own culture, language, and dialect. How have aspects of each one changed since high school? How does your culture, language, and dialect compare to the group you think is most different from you? How might your culture, language, and dialect influence assessment and intervention of an individual from a different cultural and/or linguistic group?

2. How do culture and communication relate? Consider three ways in your own experience that culture and communication are interrelated.

3. Describe four alternative methods of assessment in the diagnosis of communication disorders of individuals from culturally and linguistically diverse populations.

4. What is the relationship between child socialization practices and language development? In an assessment, how might you determine that a child's linguistic performance was due to socialization and not the result of a communication disorder?

5. Gather different definitions of bilingualism. How might monolingual SLPs assess and treat bilingual individuals?

6. Do you think immigrants to the United States should maintain their home language? Provide a rationale for your response. How would their maintenance or loss of their home language influence your selection of an intervention approach and intervention goals?

7. Using data from the U.S. Census Bureau (http://www.census.gov), determine the racial or ethnic composition of your community.

8. Go to the grocery store, department store, or airport (or anywhere diverse groups of individuals congregate) and describe the different ways that individuals interact with one another. You might compare how adults interact with other adults, how adults interact with children, and how children interact with other children.

9. An idiolect is

   a. Each person's unique way of speaking
   b. A variety of a language dependent on context
   c. A rule-governed variant of a language
   d. The way individuals pronounce their words

10. Which of the following is an alternative testing format?

    a. Back translation
    b. Accent modification
    c. Probe technique
    d. Dialect density

11. A "holistic" view of bilingualism means that

    a. Every bilingual person has his or her own way of speaking
    b. The languages of bilinguals are an integrated whole
    c. Bilinguals speak in the same way as monolinguals
    d. Bilinguals have difficulty organizing their thoughts

12. The possibility of misdiagnosing an individual from a culturally and linguistically diverse population can be decreased by

    a. Using one test
    b. Assuming that support personnel are trained

    c. Using a variety of testing formats

    d. Using translated tests

13. Monolingual SLPs should

    a. Complete assessments in both languages for bilinguals

    b. Train support personnel

    c. Always refer bilinguals to bilingual SLPs

    d. Have tests translated into the bilingual's non-English language

FURTHER READING

American Speech-Language-Hearing Association. (2005). Cultural competence. *ASHA* Suppl. 25.

Bedore, L., & Peña, E. (2008). Assessment of bilingual children for identification of language impairment: Current findings and implications for practice. *International Journal of Bilingual Education and Bilingualism, 11*(1), 1–29.

Goldstein, B. (2006). Clinical implications of research on language development and disorders in bilingual children. *Topics in Language Disorders, 26,* 318–334.

Jackson, J., & Pearson, B. (2010). Variable use of features associated with African American English by typically developing children. *Topics in Language Disorders, 30,* 135–144.

Shatz, M., & Wilkinson, L. (Eds.). (2010). *The education of English language learners.* New York, NY: Guilford Press.

Stockman, I. (2010). A review of developmental and applied language research on African American children: From a deficit to difference perspective on dialect differences. *Language, Speech and Hearing Services in Schools, 41,* 23–38.

Texas Speech-Language-Hearing Association. (2013). *Resources & information.* Retrieved from http://www.txsha.org/diversity_issues/diversity_issues.aspx

REFERENCES

Adler, S. (1984). *Cultural language differences: Their educational and clinical-professional implications.* Springfield, IL: Charles C. Thomas.

American Speech-Language-Hearing Association. (1998). *Provision of instruction in English as a second language by speech-language pathologists in school settings* [Position Statement]. Retrieved from www.asha.org/policy

American Speech-Language-Hearing Association. (1989). Definition: Bilingual speech-language pathologists and audiologists. *ASHA, 31,* 93.

American Speech-Language-Hearing Association. (1996, Spring). Guidelines for the training, credentialing, use, and supervision of speech-language pathology assistants. *ASHA, 38*(Suppl. 16), 21–34.

American Speech-Language-Hearing Association. (2004). *Accreditation manual: Council on Academic Accreditation in Audiology and Speech-Language Pathology.* Rockville, MD: Author.

Anderson, P., & Fenichal, E. (1989). *Serving culturally diverse families of infants and toddlers with disabilities.* Washington, DC: National Center for Clinical Infant Programs.

Baker, I. (1996). *Foundations of bilingual education and bilingualism* (2nd ed.). Clevedon, England: Multilingual Matters.

Beaumont, C. (1992). Language intervention strategies for Hispanic LLD students. In H. Langdon (Ed.), *Hispanic children and adults with communication disorders: Assessment and intervention* (pp. 272–333). New York, NY: Aspen Publishers.

Cheng, L.R.L. (1989). Intervention strategies: A multicultural approach. *Topics in Language Disorders, 9,* 84–91.

Cheng, L.R.L. (1993). Asian-American cultures. In D. Battle (Ed.), *Communication disorders in multicultural populations* (pp. 38–77). Boston, MA: Andover Medical Publishers.

Cheng, L.R.L. (1996). Enhancing communication: Toward optimal language learning for limited English proficient students. *Language, Speech, and Hearing Services in the Schools, 27,* 347–354.

Cobo-Lewis, A., Eilers, R., Pearson, B., & Umbel, V. (2002). Interdependence of Spanish and English knowledge in language and literacy among bilingual children. In D.K. Oller & R.E. Eilers (Eds.), *Language and literacy in bilingual children* (pp. 118–134). Clevedon, England: Multilingual Matters.

Cummins, J. (1984). *Bilingualism and special education: Issues in assessment and pedagogy.* San Diego, CA: College-Hill Press.

Damico, J. (1993, October). Appropriate speech and language assessment for bilingual children. Seminar presented at *Bilingualism: What every clinician needs to know.* Symposium sponsored by the American Speech-Language-Hearing Association, Alexandria, VA.

Damico, J., & Hamayan, E. (1992). *Multicultural language intervention.* Buffalo, NY: Educom Associates.

Damico, J., Smith, M., & Augustine, L. (1996). Multicultural populations and language disorders. In M. Smith & J. Damico (Eds.), *Childhood language disorders* (pp. 272–299). New York, NY: Thieme

De Houwer, A. (2009). *An introduction to bilingual development.* Bristol, England: Multilingual Matters.

Erickson, J., & Iglesias, A. (1986). Assessment of communication disorders in non-English proficient children. In O. Taylor (Ed.), *Nature of communication disorders in culturally and linguistically diverse populations* (pp. 181–217). San Diego, CA: College-Hill Press.

Gillam, R., & Hoffman, L. (2001). Language assessment during childhood. In D. Ruscello (Ed.), *Tests and measurements in speech-language pathology* (pp. 77–117). Boston, MA: Butterworth-Heinemann.

Goldstein, B. (2000). *Cultural and linguistic diversity resource guide for speech-language pathology.* San Diego, CA: Singular Publishing Group.

Goldstein, B.A. (Ed.). (2012). *Bilingual language development and disorders in Spanish-English speakers* (2nd ed.). Baltimore, MD: Paul H. Brookes Publishing Co.

Goldstein, B., & Horton-Ikard., R. (2010). Diversity considerations in speech and language disorders (pp. 38–56). In J. Damico,

N. Müller, & M. Ball (Eds.), *Handbook of language and speech disorders* (pp. 38–56). Malden, MA: Wiley-Blackwell.

Green, L. (2004). Research on African American English since 1998: Origins, description, theory, and practice. *Journal of English Linguistics, 32,* 210–229.

Grosjean, F. (1989). Neurolinguists, beware! The bilingual is not two monolinguals in one person. *Brain and Language, 36,* 3–15.

Grosjean, F. (1992). Another view of bilingualism. In R. Harris (Ed.), *Cognitive processing in bilinguals* (pp. 51–62). New York, NY: Elsevier.

Grosjean, F. (1997). Processing mixed languages: Issues, findings, and models. In A. de Groot & J. Kroll (Eds.), *Tutorials in bilingualism: Psycholinguistic perspectives* (pp. 225–254). Mahwah, NJ: Lawrence Erlbaum Associates.

Hakuta, K. (1986). *Mirror of language: The debate on bilingualism.* New York, NY: Basic Books.

Heath, S. (1982). What no bedtime story means: Narrative skills at home and school. *Language in Society, 11,* 49–76.

Heath, S. (1983). *Ways with words: Life and work in communities and classrooms.* New York, NY: Cambridge University Press.

Iglesias, A. (2001). What test should I use? *Seminars in Speech and Language, 22,* 3–16.

Iglesias, A., & Quinn, R. (1997). Culture as a context for early intervention. In S.K. Thurman, J.R. Cornwell, & S.R. Gottwald (Eds.), *Contexts for early intervention: Systems and settings* (pp. 55–71). Baltimore, MD: Paul H. Brookes Publishing Co.

Individuals with Disabilities Education Improvement Act (IDEA) of 2004, PL 108-446, 20 U.S.C. §§ 1400 *et seq.*

Kapantzoglu, M., Restrepo, M.A., & Thompson, M. (2012). Dynamic assessment of word learning skills: Identifying language impairment in bilingual children. *Language, Speech and Hearing Services in Schools, 43,* 81–96.

Kayser, H. (1989). Speech and language assessment of Spanish-English speaking children. *Language, Speech, and Hearing Services in the Schools, 20,* 226–244.

Kayser, H. (1993). Hispanic cultures. In D. Battle (Ed.), *Communication disorders in multicultural populations* (pp. 114–157). Boston, MA: Andover Medical Publishers.

Kayser, H. (1995a). Assessment of speech and language impairments in bilingual children. In H. Kayser (Ed.), *Bilingual speech-language pathology: An Hispanic focus* (pp. 243–264). San Diego, CA: Singular Publishing Group.

Kayser, H. (1995b). Intervention with children from linguistically and culturally diverse backgrounds. In M.E. Fey, J. Windsor, & S.F. Warren (Eds.). *Language intervention: Preschool through the elementary years* (pp. 315–331). Baltimore, MD: Paul H. Brookes Publishing Co.

Kohnert, K. (2008). *Language disorders in bilingual children and adults.* San Diego, CA: Plural Publishing.

Kohnert, K., Yim, D., Nett, K., Kan, P.F., & Duran, L. (2005). Intervention with linguistically diverse preschool children: A focus on developing home language(s). *Language, Speech and Hearing Services in the Schools, 36,* 251–263.

Laing, S. (2002). Reading miscues in school-age children. *American Journal of Speech-Language Pathology, 11,* 407–416.

Langdon, H. (1992). Speech and language assessment of LEP/bilingual Hispanic students. In H. Langdon (Ed.), *Hispanic children and adults with communication disorders: Assessment and intervention* (pp. 201–271). New York, NY: Aspen Publishers.

Langdon, H. (2008). *Assessment and intervention for communication disorders in culturally and linguistically diverse populations.* Clifton Park, NY: Thomson Delmar.

Larry P. v. Riles. (1979). C-71-2270, FRP. Dis. Ct.

Linguistic Society of America. (1996). *Statement on language rights.* Washington, DC: Author.

Lopez, L., & Greenfield, D. (2004). The cross-linguistic transfer of phonological skills of Hispanic Head Start children. *Bilingual Research Journal, 28,* 1–18.

Lynch, E.W. (2011). Developing cross-cultural competence. In E.W. Lynch & M.J. Hanson (Eds.), *Developing cross-cultural competence: A guide for working with children and their families* (4th ed.). Baltimore, MD: Paul H. Brookes Publishing Co.

Lynch, E.W., & Hanson, M.J. (2011). Steps in the right direction: Implications for service providers. In E.W. Lynch & M.J. Hanson (Eds.), *Developing cross-cultural competence: A guide for working with children and their families* (4th ed.) Baltimore, MD: Paul H. Brookes Publishing Co.

Mattes, L., & Omark, D. (1991). *Speech and language assessment for the bilingual handicapped* (2nd ed.). Oceanside, CA: Academic Communication Associates.

Norris, M., Juarez, M., & Perkins, M. (1989). Adaptation of a screening test for bilingual and bidialectal populations. *Language, Speech, and Hearing Services in the Schools, 20,* 381–389.

Oetting, J.B., & McDonald, J.L. (2002). Methods for characterizing participants' nonmainstream dialect use in child language research. *Journal of Speech, Language, and Hearing Research, 45,* 508–518.

Paradis, M. (2001). Bilingual and polyglot aphasia. In H. Goodglass & A.R. Damasio (Eds.), *Handbook of neuropsychology* (2nd ed., pp. 69–91). New York, NY: Elsevier Science.

Paradis, J., Genesee, F., & Crago, M. (2011). *Dual language development and disorders: A handbook on bilingualism & second language learning* (2nd ed.). Baltimore, MD: Paul H. Brookes Publishing Co.

Paul, R., & Norbury, C. (2012). *Language disorders from infancy through adolescence: Listening, speaking, reading, writing, and communicating* (4th ed.). St. Louis, MO: Mosby.

Pease-Alvarez, L. (1993). *Moving in and out of bilingualism: Investigating native language maintenance and shift in Mexican-descent children.* Santa Cruz, CA: National Center for Research on Cultural Diversity and Second Language Learning.

Peña, E.D. (1996). Dynamic assessment: The model and its language applications. In K.N. Cole, P.S. Dale, & D.J. Thal (Eds.), *Communication and Language Intervention Series: Vol. 6. Assessment of communication and language* (pp. 281–307). Baltimore, MD: Paul H. Brookes Publishing Co.

Peña, E., Iglesias, A., & Lidz, C.S. (2001). Reducing test bias through dynamic assessment of children's word learning ability. *American Journal of Speech-Language Pathology, 10,* 138–154.

Perozzi, J., & Sanchez, M. (1992). The effect of instruction in L1 on receptive acquisition of L2 for bilingual students with language delay. *Language, Speech, and Hearing Services in the Schools, 23,* 348–352.

Romaine, S. (1995). *Bilingualism* (2nd ed.). Oxford, England: Blackwell Publishing.

Romaine, S. (1999). Bilingual language development. In M. Barrett (Ed.), *The development of language* (pp. 251–275). East Essex, England: Psychology Press.

Roseberry-McKibbin, C. (1994). Assessment and intervention for children with limited English proficiency and language disorders. *American Journal of Speech-Language Pathology, 3,* 77–88.

Roseberry-McKibbin, C. (1995). *Multicultural students with special language needs.* Oceanside, CA: Academic Communication Associates.

Roseberry-McKibbin, C. (2002). *Multicultural students with special language needs* (2nd ed.). Oceanside, CA: Academic Communication Associates.

Roseberry-McKibbin, C., Brice, A., & O'Hanlon, L. (2005). Serving English language learners in public school settings: A national survey. *Language, Speech, and Hearing Services in the Schools, 36,* 48–61.

Roseberry-McKibbin, C., & Eicholtz, G. (1994). Serving children with limited English proficiency in the schools: A national survey. *Language, Speech, and Hearing Services in the Schools, 25,* 156–164.

Scheffner Hammer, C., Miccio, A.W., & Rodriguez, B.L. (2004). Bilingual language acquisition and the child socialization process. In B.A. Goldstein (Ed.), *Bilingual language development and disorders in Spanish-English speakers* (pp. 21–50). Baltimore, MD: Paul H. Brookes Publishing Co.

Seymour, H. (1986). Clinical principles for language intervention among nonstandard speakers of English. In O. Taylor (Ed.), *Treatment of communication disorders in culturally and linguistically diverse populations* (pp. 115–133). San Diego, CA: College-Hill Press.

Seymour, H.N., & Pearson, B.Z. (Eds.). (2004). Steps in designing and implementing an innovative assessment instrument. *Seminars in Speech and Language, 25,* 27–32.

Sollors, W. (1998). Introduction: After the culture wars; or, from "English only" to "English plus." In W. Sollors (Ed.), *Multilingual America: Transitionalism, ethnicity, and the languages of American literature* pp. 1–13). New York, NY: New York University Press.

Taylor, O., & Clarke, M. (1994). Communication disorders and cultural diversity: A theoretical framework. *Seminars in Speech and Language, 15,* 103–113.

Taylor, O., & Payne, K. (1983). Culturally valid testing: A proactive approach. *Topics in Language Disorders, 3,* 8–20.

Taylor, O., & Payne, K. (1994). Language and communication differences. In G. Shames, E. Wiig, & W. Secord (Eds.), *Human communication disorders: An introduction* (4th ed., pp. 136–173). New York, NY: Merrill.

Terrell, S., & Terrell, F. (1983). Effects of speaking Black English upon employment opportunities. *ASHA, 25,* 27–29.

Terrell, S., & Terrell, F. (1993). African-American cultures. In D. Battle (Ed.), *Communication disorders in multicultural populations* (pp. 3–37). Boston, MA: Andover Medical Publishers.

Toliver Weddington, G. (1981). *Valid assessment of children.* San Jose, CA: San Jose State University.

U.S. Bureau of the Census. (2010a). *Statistical abstract of the United States, 2010.* Washington, DC: U.S. Department of Commerce.

U.S. Bureau of the Census. (2010b). *The Hispanic population, 2010.* Retrieved from http://www.census.gov/prod/cen2010/briefs/c2010br-04.pdf

U.S. Department of Education. (2008). *Percentage distribution of enrollment in public elementary and secondary schools, by race/ethnicity and state or jurisdiction.* Retrieved from http://nces.ed.gov/programs/digest/d10/tables/dt10_036.asp

U.S. Department of Education. (2009). *Number and percentage of children ages 5–17 who spoke a language other than English at home, 2009.* Washington, DC: National Center for Education Statistics. Retrieved from http://nces.ed.gov/programs/coe/tables/table-lsm-2.asp

Van Keulen, J., Weddington, G., & DeBose, C. (1998). *Speech, language, learning and the African American child.* Boston, MA: Allyn & Bacon.

Vaughn-Cooke, F. (1986). The challenge of assessing the language of nonmainstream speakers. In O. Taylor (Ed.), *Treatment of communication disorders in culturally and linguistically diverse populations* (pp. 23–48). San Diego, CA: College-Hill Press.

Washington, J., & Craig, H. (1994). Dialect forms during discourse of poor, urban African American preschoolers. *Journal of Speech and Hearing Research, 37,* 816–823.

Westby, C. (2000). Multicultural issues in speech and language assessment. In. J.B. Tomblin, H. Morris, & D.C. Spriestersbach (Eds.), *Diagnosis in speech-language pathology* (2nd ed., pp. 35–62) San Diego, CA: Singular Publishing Group.

Wolfram, W. (1986). Language variation in the United States. In O. Taylor (Ed.),

Treatment of communication disorders in cul-turally and linguistically diverse populations (pp. 73–116). San Diego, CA: College-Hill Press.

Wolfram, W., & Schilling-Estes, N. (1998). *American English: Dialects and variation.* Oxford, England: Blackwell Publishing.

Wyatt, T. (2002). Assessing the communicative abilities of clients from diverse cultural and language backgrounds. In D. Battle (Ed.), *Communication disorders in multicultural populations* (pp. 415–459). Boston, MA: Butterworth-Heinemann.

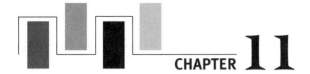

CHAPTER 11

Technology and Communication Disorders

Elizabeth S. Simmons, Donald A. Vogel, and Gladys Millman

After reading this chapter, students will be able to

- Define assistive technology
- Describe how technology is utilized in clinical practice
- Discuss how evidence-based decision making is implemented when using technology
- List commonly used technology for verbal expression and assistive listening
- Discuss the issues related to the use of mobile technology

Most of us use technology to make daily tasks a bit easier. Tracking your appointments with a calendar program on your computer or setting an alarm on your iPhone to ensure you do not miss an important meeting are both examples of ways most of us use technology to simplify our lives. For those individuals with **complex communication needs** (CCN), technology becomes more critical to support independence and promote quality of life.

As defined by the Technology-Related Assistance for Individuals with Disabilities Act (Tech Act) of 1988 (PL 100-407), **assistive technology** (AT) is any "item, piece of equipment, or system, whether acquired commercially, modified, or customized, that is commonly used to increase, maintain, or improve functional capabilities of individuals with disabilities." This definition encompasses a range of devices, including those used for improving the communication skills of individuals with CCN, but also those devices that assist with activities of daily living (e.g., a wheelchair for individuals with impairments in mobility). The use of technologies to improve both expressive and receptive communication skills in populations with communication impairment is the focus of this chapter.

Both audiologists and speech-language pathologists (SLPs) assess and treat a diverse population of individuals with equally diverse communication needs. Therefore, clinicians need to be knowledgeable about who might benefit from AT. There is a significant body of literature that discusses the use of AT with young

children as well as school-age students (e.g., see Campbell, Milbourne, Dugan, &
Wilcox, 2006; Johnston, Beard, & Carpenter, 2007; Sadao & Robinson, 2010).
Children and adults with developmental disabilities, such as autism or Down syndrome, may benefit from AT. Individuals with acquired impairments, including
those from traumatic brain injury or cerebrovascular accidents, may also benefit
from AT (de Joode, van Heugten, Verhey, & van Boxel, 2010; LoPresti, Mihailidis, &
Kirsch, 2004; Sohlberg, 2011). Individuals with hearing loss of varying etiology
are also candidates for AT, more specifically hearing aids and assistive listening
devices (Bess, Dodd-Murphy, & Parker, 1998; Lesner, 2003).

Historically, AT has been used to improve independent functioning of people with disabilities. Clinicians will likely encounter these individuals, including
those with CCN, hearing impairment, and cognitive impairments, on their caseload. Some individuals might use technology as a primary means of communication. For example, a child with Down syndrome might carry an electronic device
that when activated speaks a preprogrammed message. Others might use technology to aid cognition after a stroke by setting an alarm on their iPod reminding
them to take a medication at given intervals. Still others will use assistive listening devices to improve receptive language skills for learning in a classroom setting. It is our role as clinicians to identify those clients who might benefit from
technology, as well as the type of technology that might be useful. Part of this
process includes comprehensive assessment of the potential user of the technology, including the individual's strengths and areas of need. Another part includes
training caregivers, educators, and other staff on the technology. Continued education, monitoring, and adjustment of the technology are typically required as the
users' needs change over time.

EVIDENCE-BASED DECISION MAKING FOR TECHNOLOGY

The American Speech-Language Hearing Association's (ASHA) definition of evidence-based decision making includes the use of 1) clinical expertise, 2) external scientific evidence, and 3) client values. Despite the fundamental challenges
inherent in AT research, including the variability of users (e.g., type of disability,
severity of disability), the context in which the technology is applied (Peterson-
Karlan & Parette, 2007), and newness of technology (e.g., tablets, MP3 players,
cellular devices), it is possible to make informed decisions regarding these new
technologies using the guidelines set forth by ASHA. As described by Hill (2004),
application of evidence-based practice (EBP) includes characterizing the user, asking relevant questions, reviewing the literature for evidence of efficacy, and then
implementing intervention. In addition, clinicians are responsible for measuring
the changes in their client's behavior and evaluating these results. A detailed discussion of evidence-based practice and evidence-based decision making can be
found in Chapter 3.

One methodology that guides evidence-based decision making around AT is
referred to as SETT (Zabala, 1995). The SETT framework provides the clinician
with a means to organize the pertinent information as part of the AT decision-
making process. Although the SETT framework was initially designed as a tool
for school use, it has been successfully implemented with other populations (e.g.,
adults) and in other environments (e.g., outpatient rehabilitation facilities).

Table 11.1.   Student (Self), Environments, Tasks, Tools framework

	Considerations
Student/self	How does the student currently communicate?
	What are the student's communication needs?
	What are the expectations and concerns regarding the student's communication?
Environment	How will the environment be arranged to support the student's use of technology (e.g., physical support, instructional support)?
	Will there be access issues that need to be addressed?
	What are the ideas and expectations held by those who care for the student related to the use of the technology?
Tasks	What tasks does the technology support for participation in daily activities?
Tools	What devices will be useful for helping the student achieve greater independence?

From Zabala, J. (2005). *SETT*. Retrieved from http://www.joyzabala.com; adapted by permission.

SETT is an acronym for Student (Self), Environments, Tasks, Tools. Within each of these categories, a group of questions and suggestions that the clinician can use to help guide the AT decision-making process is supplied. *Student* (or Self) is the user of the technology. When selecting an AT device, it is important to have a knowledge of the user's communication skills, including areas of strength and areas of difficulty. *Environment* provides detailed descriptions of the various places where the AT device will be used (e.g., only at school, skilled nursing facility, home). *Tasks* are the demands that occur in the environment that the device can help accomplish. Last, *Tools* are the various supports and services needed by the student and others for the student to be successful (e.g., AT devices, training, teaching methodologies, strategies used to implement, and other accommodations). See Table 11.1 for an outline of the SETT framework.

Given that many AT users will be those with CCN, it is advisable to seek out and collaborate with other professionals who work with these individuals. Many SLPs are part of an AT team that includes others who have a role in making technology decisions. Obtaining the views, values, and ideas of many people through this team process increases the likelihood of successful device implementation, especially in school-based settings. The most common members of an AT team, in a school-based setting, are teachers, SLPs, and occupational therapists. Other individuals might be included (e.g., paraprofessionals, physical therapists) as needed (DeCoste, Reed, & Kaplan, 2005). The SLP may need to collaborate with the occupational therapist and physical therapist, who can provide consultation regarding device access. Device access, or how the user interfaces with the technology, can include direct activation by touching the device or might require specialized hardware. An individual with amyotrophic lateral sclerosis, for example, might require a large button or switch to access the communication device. Therefore, it would be imperative that the SLP collaborate with the occupational therapist and physical therapist to determine appropriate switch placement. Similarly, the SLP might need to consult with the client's caregiver to help choose vocabulary words that will be most functional for a new communication device.

A new category of equipment, **mobile technology** designed for daily use by the mainstream consumers, has emerged to function as AT that can be used both to teach a range of skills to those with disabilities (Bouck et al., 2012; Jones, Grogg, Anschutz, & Fierman, 2008) and to serve as **augmentative and**

alternative communication (AAC). Despite the limited empirical evidence to support their use, these technologies can still be incorporated by applying evidence-based decision making. Some of the most popular mobile technology devices are Apple's iPad, iPod Touch, and iPhone (from here on referred to as iOS devices) and Android-based technology. These devices and their applications (apps) have become increasingly popular for therapeutic use. Moreover, these devices and specialized apps are beginning to take the place of more traditional dedicated communication systems. Wakefield and Schaber (2012) provide an outline for choosing apps using an EBP approach. Their five-step model includes these activities for clinicians:

- *Frame your clinical question.* Your clinical question could be, "Will my client with autism use an iPad app to make a selection between a preferred and non-preferred food choice during snack?"

- *Search for evidence.* Wakefield and Schaber suggest setting a time limit of 30 minutes to complete an Internet search using high-yield databases. For our clinical question above, there is research suggesting that children with autism can make choices using paper-based picture systems (Bondy & Frost, 2001; Charlop-Christy, Carpenter, Le, LeBlance, & Kellet, 2002).

- *Assess the evidence.* What research did you find that supports your clinical question? Were these large, controlled trials or single-subject designs? Again, for our clinical question, we know that the research by Charlop-Christy and colleagues (2002) demonstrates some efficacy of using pictures for communication.

- *Search for an app in the App Store.* There might be many apps in the store that claim to do what you need them to do. If this occurs, compare and contrast the apps (e.g., features, costs, evidence).

- *Choose the app.* To make your app selection, you must go back to your clinical question and integrate the research and evidence. You must also use it with your client and assess his or her reaction to the app. This step is imperative because it integrates the student's values.

Although the foregoing example is geared toward selecting an app for a young child with autism, the same steps could be implemented with an adult client or when choosing an app for teaching new skills (e.g., language forms, turn taking, memory strategies).

ASSESSMENT OF NEED FOR ASSISTIVE TECHNOLOGY

Whereas there are many widely available standardized assessment tools to evaluate speech, language, and communication skills, there are limited formal assessment instruments available for evaluating an individual's ability to use technology. This is due in part to the heterogeneity of AT users; many of these individuals have unique communication, motor, and cognitive profiles. Despite the limited number of formal assessment tools, it is imperative to complete a comprehensive assessment in order both to evaluate client strengths and needs and to foster device acceptance and integration (Copley & Ziviani, 2005). The assessing clinician should utilize a range of assessment methodologies for collecting information regarding the client's AT requirements (Beigel, 2000; Copley & Ziviani, 2007). Johnston et al. (2007) suggest gathering information in a variety of environments, utilizing a range of tools, and incorporating caregivers into the process. Below is an outline of the steps suggested by Johnston and colleagues (2007) to be included as part of determining the assessment of need for AT.

As part of preparation for the AT assessment, clinicians conduct a comprehensive record review that includes information from a variety of sources, among them educational records (e.g., Individualized Education Program), medical records (e.g., hospitalizations, medications) and any previous evaluations (e.g., previous AT evaluations, occupational therapist evaluations, physical therapist evaluations). Gathering this background information is likely to help SLPs make decisions regarding the tools chosen for the subsequent portions of the technology assessment. It is also helpful to speak with other professionals working with the client, since they can provide invaluable information that might not be easily ascertained through written records.

During direct observation(s) of the client, the clinician collects information on cognitive functioning, sensory skills (e.g., audition, vision), motor functioning, and current communication modalities. Does the client communicate through nonverbal means such as gestures and eye contact? Does he or she use vocalizations? Is the client already using an AT device? These observations should take place where the client spends time and would likely use the technology. These environments may include school, home, community, or workplace. If possible, observations should be conducted at different times throughout the day because functioning can change based on both environmental and biological factors (e.g., fatigue).

Interviewing parents, teachers, caregivers, friends, and the individual who will use the technology can provide information not easily obtained using other assessment methods. Many clinicians will draft their own interview questions to yield client-specific information. Information that can be gleaned from an interview can include family and caregiver concerns regarding implementation of technology. It can also address expectations regarding the client's use of technology. Additional information such as the individual's ideas and preferences regarding the technology can also be obtained during the interview process. Finally, any additional information that might not have been readily available during the record review can be collected during the interview process.

Formal assessment of the individual's present level of functioning will need to be completed. This will likely be conducted by a range of professionals, including occupational therapists, physical therapists, special educators, and psychologists. As audiologists and SLPs, it is our responsibility to assess listening, speech, language, and nonverbal communication. One of the main purposes of formal assessment is to determine how the individual currently communicates and to determine the effectiveness of the current modality. Since many candidates for AT have CCN, the clinician will likely need to be creative when choosing appropriate assessment measures. These might include subtests from standardized tools that are administered in a nonstandard way. **Criterion-referenced tests** conducted in important environments may also be used (e.g., How does Ethan ask for help during centers at his preschool?).

Once the information is collected, the clinician is responsible for synthesizing the data collected into a cohesive unit to be presented to other professionals and family members. In the academic setting, this type of assessment will typically result in a lengthy written report documenting the student's current communication skills, areas of communicative competence, and needs. Documentation will differ from facility to facility, but some form of written documentation will usually be required, especially if the cost of the device is to be reimbursed by private health insurance, Medicaid, or Medicare.

ASSISTIVE TECHNOLOGY INTERVENTIONS

A range of AT tools have been used clinically to improve the communication and listening skills of individuals with disabilities. An increasingly popular subset of AT devices, mobile technology is included in this discussion of AT interventions. Along with the discussion of these popular devices is a discussion of their costs and benefits.

Listening Technology

Commonly used by schools for the deaf after the mid-20th century, assistive listening devices (ALDs), which amplify the teacher's voice above background noise levels, helped educators improve the educational achievement of students with significant disabilities. In the 1980s, ALDs were discovered to add value not only to severely hearing-impaired individuals but also to individuals with mild to moderate hearing loss. In the late 20th century, clinicians began to appreciate the value of ALDs for clients who could be classified as having a "minimal hearing loss" diagnosis (American Academy of Audiology, 2003; Bess et al., 1998). Current best practice suggests that the use of ALDs can provide children with all levels of hearing disorder an optimal listening environment in the classroom, treatment room, or social setting (Lewis, 1994).

Improving the **signal-to-noise ratio** (SNR) is a basic goal of all listeners, whether achieved subconsciously by leaning forward to hear someone better or consciously by assessing the environment and utilizing tools and strategies in an attempt to improve understanding of the speaker. The SNR is defined as the relationship between the sound levels of a message (signal) as it competes with background chatter (noise). The louder the signal relative to the noise, the greater the likelihood that the message will be received by the listener (Good & Gilkey, 1996; Welzl-Muller & Sattler, 1984).

The SNR is expressed as positive or negative sound pressure level. For example, +6 SNR indicates that the message is 6 dB louder than the background chatter. Conversely, an SNR of −3 SNR indicates that background noise is 3 dB less than than the message signal. If the intensities of both the background noise and the desired message are equal, SNR is 0. Improvements in listening occur when the positivity of the SNR value increases. The higher that number, the better the chances that the message will be understood. Clinicians need to be aware of environmental elements, such as ambient noise (i.e., background noise) and environmental acoustics, that contribute to listening situations and may decrease SNR.

Due to developments in mobile technology, clinicians have a variety of tools with which they can quickly assess the ambient noise of the environment. Reliable sound-level meter applications are available for free or at minimal cost on most smartphones and tablets. Reviewing the online ratings of such applications can help in selecting an appropriate tool for monitoring of noise in the environment.

Selection of an ALD requires basic knowledge of hearing loss. Consultation with an audiologist who can identify the degree, type, and site of hearing loss will assist the clinician working with hearing-impaired clients. Human hearing is sensitive to a range of frequencies between 20 Hz and 20,000 Hz (cycles per second). It is measured by an audiologist with **pure tone audiometers,** which are frequently calibrated to maintain their accuracy, in sound-treated suites. Hearing is commonly tested for frequencies between 250 Hz and 8,000 Hz. Although these frequencies represent only a portion of the range of human hearing, the sounds of speech are produced within this frequency range. Results of hearing testing are graphed onto a chart, known as an **audiogram** (see Figure 11.1), which displays the intensity needed to detect each of the frequencies tested for individual being assessed. Intensity is measured from −10 dB to 120 dB, calculated on a logarithmic scale of sound pressure.

Hearing impairments can be caused by both conductive and sensorineural losses. A **conductive hearing loss** occurs when there is decreased sensitivity stemming from an interruption in the normal conduit of sound into the ear via

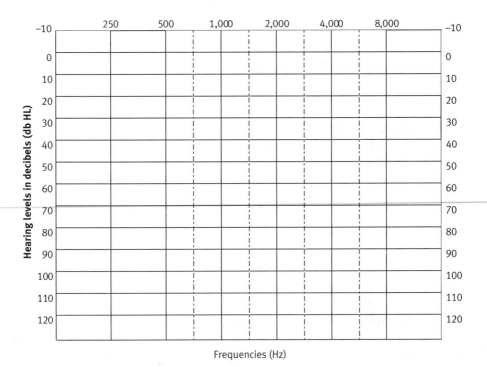

Figure 11.1 Results from a hearing test are graphed on this chart, called an audiogram. (*Source*: American Speech-Language-Hearing Association, 2013.)

the outer ear, tympanic membrane, and the middle ear. A conductive hearing loss can occur in one or both ears. Common etiologies of a conductive hearing loss include impacted cerumen (earwax), tympanic membrane (eardrum) perforation, and otitis media (middle-ear infection). Less common contributors to conductive hearing loss are diseases or malformations of the middle ear, including microtia, ossicular disarticulation, otosclerosis, cholesteatoma, and some hereditary disorders involving bone formation. Medical intervention by an otologist typically offers complete success in treating these disorders. A conductive hearing loss can dampen sound by as many as 60 dB (Feldman, 1963).

The cochlea, or inner ear, which is the end organ of the peripheral auditory system, transforms sound energy into usable information, and transmits it to the auditory nerves, which carry the message to the brain. **Sensorineural hearing loss** occurs when information processing in the cochlea is interrupted due to such issues as malformation or outer hair cell destruction, which often occurs with aging. Involvement of the auditory nerve contributes to the neural component. An audiologist can distinguish between a sensorineural hearing loss and a conductive hearing loss through commonly used clinical tools, including comparing air conduction to bone conduction test results and otoacoustic emissions assessment, which evaluates the integrity of the outer hair cells of the cochlea. Etiologies of sensorineural hearing loss may include diseases, such as meningitis, rubella, high fevers, and diabetes. Other contributors to sensorineural hearing loss may be genetic or syndromic factors, ototoxic medications, noise exposure, and aging.

A mixed hearing loss occurs when both conductive and sensorineural components are present. Although not as common as conductive or sensorineural hearing losses, the mixed hearing loss generates unique challenges to the audiologist in its identification. Few etiologies directly cause a mixed hearing loss. Instead, the additive effect of two different etiologies—creating one conductive component and another generating a sensorineural issue—are usually involved.

Although an audiologist will be the lead professional in quantifying the degree and type of hearing loss, collaboration with an SLP will help in determining candidacy for AT and in selecting and implementing interventions across environments such as school, workplace, and home.

When selecting the appropriate device, it is important to consider which of the available mechanical elements will offer optimal performance to the user. The selection of these components may include the types of volume control, power supply, telephone access, and ability to attach to an amplifier. The fitting of an ALD can be verified by an audiologist in a manner similar that used for amplification via probe-microphone measurement. This procedure helps to confirm that the electroacoustic profile of the instrument is in fact attaining its promised target in the client's ear. Both subjective reports from the client and instrumental measurements help to ensure that use of the instrument delivers benefit to the client.

There are three basic mechanical components to the majority of ALDs: microphone, transmitter, and receiver. The microphone picks up signals from the sound source. The transmitter converts the energy of sound picked up by the microphone to a usable form and then delivers it via the modality that is characteristic of the component (e.g., frequency modulated, hard wired, infrared).

Table 11.2. Types of assistive listening devices

Assistive listening device system	Description	Benefits	Disadvantages
Frequency modulation (FM)	Voice is captured via a microphone and transmitted through FM signals to a receiver worn by the individual.	Good sound quality Inexpensive installation	Interference from external sources such as low-frequency radio bands Limited range
Infrared	Voice is captured via a microphone and transmitted through infrared light to a receiver worn by the individual.	Good sound quality Inexpensive installation	Poor operation in low light or presence of large objects (e.g., room columns or dividers)
Induction loop	Voice is captured via a microphone that is hardwired to a magnetic coil that is placed around the room. The signal is received by the telecoil switch on the user's hearing aid.	Excellent sound quality Limited components that could be damaged	Expensive installation Typically requires a permanent installation

Source: Gelfand (2001).

Last, the receiver delivers the information at ear level to the client typically via headset or personal system. Table 11.2 provides an outline of the most widely used commercially available ALDs. The challenges of effectively and consistently wearing ALDs include client motivation, caregiver attention, teacher cooperation, and financial burden. For some populations, such as the elderly, ALDs may be the preferred alternative to hearing aids (Priutt, 1990). These devices are not limited to use in classrooms or other public venues such as churches or lecture halls. Some devices are designed to be used in the home; among these are infrared television amplifiers, vibrating alarms for the pillow, and flashing lights for doorbells.

Technology for Expression

For individuals who have not acquired functional spoken language or have lost language due to neurological insult, AAC can make an enormous difference in the client's quality of life. Traditional AAC systems span a continuum of technological complexity and specificity of usage. Specificity ranges from devices designed as dedicated tools, which serve only to function for augmenting communication, to mainstream consumer electronic devices, such as computers, tablets, and smartphones, that provide access to apps developed for AAC but serve many other functions. Complexity ranges from low- to mid- to high-tech systems. The level of complexity selected will be dictated by the user's communication needs, cognitive functioning, and motor skills. No-tech and low-tech strategies do not use any electronic devices. No-tech strategies make use of the human body in the form of gesture, body language, vocal intonation, and the like. Low-tech strategies involve nontech options such as common objects and a variety of visual supports such as pictures or photographs. Sign language is used by some nonverbal communicators and is considered a no-tech AAC system. The Picture Exchange Communication

System (PECS; Bondy & Frost, 2001) is an example of a low-tech strategy for communication. A PECS user is given a card with a picture of a preferred item (e.g., a line drawing of a cup of juice) and taught to exchange the picture with an adult for the item pictured. Although low-tech strategies may not always make use of assistive devices, many of these low-tech systems are being presented on technology platforms such as an iOS device to increase their mobility and convenience as well as to heighten a client's motivation to use them.

Mid-tech AAC devices include **speech-generating devices** with static or **fixed displays.** These devices are most commonly referred to as **voice output communication aides.** They can be as simple as a large button that plays a single prerecorded word or phrase when pressed. More sophisticated switches allow the user to program two, four, or many more messages. **Digitized speech** is usually used in mid-tech devices, which allow clinicians, educators, and caregivers to record in their own voice messages that are then stored in digitized form. Mid-tech devices typically have *static* or *fixed displays*, meaning the symbols, pictures, or real items used are affixed to a particular location on the device.

High-technology devices are those that primarily use **synthesized speech** and **dynamic displays,** although some may offer the added benefit of digitized speech. Computers, tablets, and devices with computer-like screens are classified as high-tech AAC. For these devices, synthesized speech is generated by software built into a device, like the text-to-speech function on an iPhone that translates typed text into phonemes and words. Synthesized speech capability allows users with a computer screen or dynamic display to generate novel language by typing or selecting letters that are then translated to speech by the software. There are two types of dynamic displays (Beukelman & Mirenda, 2013). The first employs a computer screen with symbols that represent messages. When the symbol is activated, a new set of symbols appears, allowing a greater number of messages to be generated. In the second type of display, the symbols are fixed; when the user activates the symbol, a prediction tool suggests the next possible symbols that user might need. Figure 11.2 illustrates the different types of AAC devices, from low- to high-technolgy options.

Users can activate these AAC devices or select items on them in a number of different ways. The two categories used to describe item selection or device activation are known as **direct selection** and **scanning** (Beukelman & Mirenda, 2013). Direct selection occurs when the user directly chooses or activates the device. This can occur through pressing a button or pointing to a given item on a communication board or tablet computer. These selection techniques are appropriate for individuals with motor functioning that includes pointing or with enough movement to be able to indicate a choice with some tool attached to the body, such as a head-mounted light or stick held in the mouth.

For users with severe motor impairment, scanning is sometimes a better selection vehicle. The purpose of scanning is to move through unwanted items displayed in sequence on a communication device until the target item is reached. Once the target is reached, the user indicates this as the choice. Scanning can be accomplished in one of two ways. Another person can act as a facilitator by removing the unwanted items, pictures, or choices. Once the desired item is reached, the user produces a predetermined behavior—perhaps an eye blink,

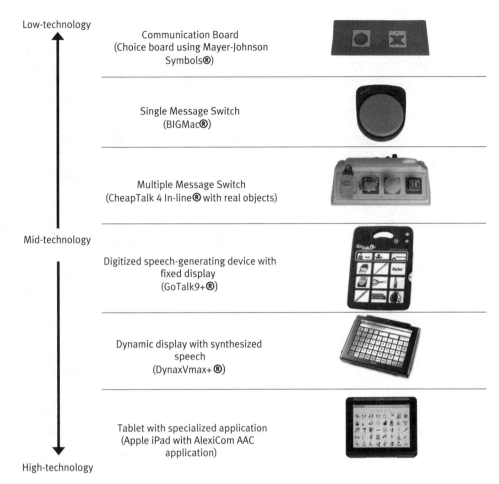

Low-technology

Communication Board
(Choice board using Mayer-Johnson
Symbols®)

Single Message Switch
(BIGMac®)

Multiple Message Switch
(CheapTalk 4 In-line® with real objects)

Mid-technology

Digitized speech-generating device with
fixed display
(GoTalk9+®)

Dynamic display with synthesized
speech
(DynaxVmax+ ®)

Tablet with specialized application
(Apple iPad with AlexiCom AAC
application)

High-technology

Figure 11.2 Continuum of augmentative and alternative communication technology.

for example—to select the item. Scanning can also be accomplished without a facilitator by using high-tech devices. Many of these devices include specialized software that scans independently. For example, when the scanning feature is activated, each button is highlighted until the desired button is reached. The user then activates this button via some form of switch access. For example, the user may activate a switch by moving his or her head to hit a switch mounted close by on the user's wheelchair, or the user employs a "sip and puff" device held in the mouth to allow sucking or puffing on the tube when the desired choice is highlighted. The tube is connected to an activating mechanism that is in turn connected to the computer display.

Dedicated communication devices such as the ones described above will continue to be appropriate choices for some individuals with CCN because they are sturdy, offer flexible access, and are covered by health insurance mandates as durable medical equipment. However, with the development of mobile technologies, devices that once functioned to play your favorite song or to answer a phone call are now being adapted to perform many of the functions previously performed by dedicated devices.

Mobile Technology for Communication

Android and iOS platforms have revolutionized many of the ways we communicate, including communication modalities for people with communication disorders. According to Melhuish and Falloon (2010), iOS devices offer "five distinct affordances for education" (p. 4) that other types of technologies do not necessarily provide. These affordances are as follows:

- Portability: diminutively sized, can easily be moved from one location to the next

- Affordability and accessibility: limited cost with continuous web access

- Frequent learning opportunities: user can process information anytime and anywhere

- Connectivity: enables user to connect with other people and devices

- Individualization: can be customized to the needs of the user

Given their limited expense and portability, these devices have found their way to the treatment of individuals with disabilities. Although there is limited research regarding the efficacy of these devices, their advantages in convenience, familiarity, and price have led to a boom in their use for educational purposes both with typically developing populations and those with special needs. Moreover, given their place in popular culture, the iOS devices are less stigmatizing and more socially acceptable compared to other more traditional, dedicated AAC systems, and their use by people with CCN helps them achieve greater social integration and acceptance.

Mobile technology can be implemented for two distinct purposes: as a therapeutic tool to teach a new skill or as dedicated functioning AAC communication device. There are many resources available to clinicians who are looking for information regarding choosing appropriate applications to teach a specific speech and language skill. *The ASHA Leader* has a published series on the utilization of iOS applications for therapeutic purposes (e.g., Sutton, 2012; Sweeney, 2012; Wakefield & Schaber, 2012). Because of the wealth of resources in this area, and also because the available apps change so rapidly, this chapter focuses on using new mobile technology as an AAC device through the use of specialized apps. Although you may be approached by caregivers or parents who have purchased an iPad to use with their loved one, it is important for you as a clinician to apply the same rules of evidence when making a determination on the use of a mobile device for AAC as you would for a more traditional piece of equipment. As suggested by Gosnell, Costello, and Shane (2011), hype surrounding iOS technology—including from well-meaning caregivers, parents, and the media—might lead professionals to abandon important clinical decision points when choosing an appropriate communication device for a client. Although mobile technology and apps for communication are relatively new to our field, practitioners can use the same clinical decision-making processes when deciding between an iPad and app or a dedicated communication device.

Gosnell and colleagues (2011) have outlined a framework of specific clinical questions to ask when determining an appropriate communication app for

Table 11.3. Feature matching process for selection of augmentative and alternative communication applications

Clinical feature	Description
Purpose	What is the application's intended function?
Output	Does the application provide speech output? If so, what type?
Speech settings	Does the application allow for customized speech settings, including changes to volume, pitch, and rate?
Symbols	Does the application include icons or symbols? Can you import your own symbols?
Display	Does the application allow for customization of display features? Can you change the layout, size of buttons, fonts, colors?
Feedback	Does the application provide visual or tactile feedback upon button activation?
Rate enhancement	Does the application provide rate enhancement features (e.g., word and grammar prediction) to increase the speed and accuracy of communication output?
Access	Does the application require the user to use direct selection? Are there other access options (e.g., switch access, scanning)?
Support	Does the application provide users with technical support if the need arises?
Miscellaneous	Does the application offer any other special features that might be useful?

Source: Gosnell, Costello, and Shane. (2011). From Alliano, A., Herriger, K., Koutsoftas, A., & Bartolotta, T. (2012). A review of 21 iPad applications for augmentative and alternative communication purposes. *Perspectives on Augmentative and Alternative Communication, 21*, 60–71; adapted by permission.

an iPad (or other mobile technology) to be used as a communication device (see Table 11.3). This framework is similar to that developed for traditional AAC practice (Schlosser, Koul, & Costello, 2007). The first relevant clinical question concerns feature matching. This is a process by which the clinician determines whether the features of a given device fit with the user's skills and communication needs (Beukelman & Mirenda, 2013; Quist & Lloyd, 1997). This process is completed by asking clinically relevant questions, observing the individual, and conducting clinical interviews. If the outcome of the feature match process supports the use of an iPad or other mobile technology, the next question to ask pertains to the type of app that would be most beneficial. It is important to stress that the intended outcome of the feature match process is not to fit a preexisting device to the user's needs but to find a new device that maps onto the needs of the user.

Gosnell et al. (2011) stress the importance of remaining knowledgeable about the latest technology trends. Doing so is extremely challenging when new apps are coming on to the market weekly. The number of commercially available apps that function as AAC tools, especially for iOS, is climbing steadily. As of March 2013, for example, there were 269 of these apps compared to just 133 in June 2011 ("Apps for AAC," 2013). With this ever-changing app landscape, it is difficult to know where to turn for comprehensive information. At this juncture, there are a range of web resources that can provide clinicians with information on AAC apps. Table 11.4 provides a list of resources for information on AAC apps for iOS devices.

CONSUMER-RELATED ISSUES: MOBILE TECHNOLOGY

With its high value in mainstream culture, impressive price point, and seemingly endless apps, mobile technology is a tempting modality. Still, it is important that clinicians be well-informed consumers of this technology and aware of both the benefits and the possible downfalls of this new and popular technology.

Table 11.4. Web-based augmentative and alternative communication application resources

Web address	Proprietor	Content
appsforaac.net	Will Wade, occupational therapist	Apps are categorized based on feature, including speech-output, symbols, and operating platform Provides a compare/contrast feature
aactechconnect.com	Debbie McBride, speech-language pathologist	AAC apps assistant available for a monthly/annual fee Provides in-depth information on available AAC apps Compares product features
spectronicsinoz.com	Jane Farrell, technology specialist	List of AAC apps and user ratings Brief written descriptions Continually updated with a list of dates and titles of new applications
atcoalition.org	Center for Accessible Technology	List of applications with a brief description of their features, including cost Categorized by age (e.g., appropriateness for children vs. appropriateness for adults) Alphabetized
bridgingapps.org	Volunteer community, including parents, clinicians, and teachers	Database of AAC apps searchable by developmental skill level

Key: AAC, augmentative and alternative communication.

Unlike traditional AAC devices, mobile technology is not covered by Medicare or Medicaid, even if it is used as a speech-generating device. The reason for the lack of coverage by these agencies is that, according to Goldman (2011), neither Medicare nor Medicaid considers an iPod or iPad **durable medical equipment**. Although at one time laptop computers, desktop computers, and personal digital assistants were also denied coverage because they did not meet the criteria for durable medical equipment, Medicare amended this rule to include these devices if they function as dedicated, AAC machines (Social Security Amendments, 2001). That is, if a computer solely operates AAC software, it can be covered by Medicare and Medicaid. Given the popularity and the limited expense of mobile devices, it is possible that these funding agencies will provide reimbursement for these technologies in the future. Until that time comes, clinicians must take this limitation into account when providing AAC recommendations to clients. However, whereas Medicare and Medicaid are currently not providing reimbursement for these devices, some third-party payers (e.g., insurance companies, school districts, health savings accounts) are willing to pay for an iPad or tablet (Goldman, 2011); this is so because these devices are much less expensive than other high-tech speech-generating devices, which can cost upward of $10,000. An iPad loaded with a speech-generating app and durable case costs less than $1,000. Given prices like this, it is more likely that the individual or family is able to pay for these devices, even out-of-pocket.

Another drawback of using mobile technology with individuals with disabilities is a problem of durability. For example, will the glass screen of an iPad shatter or crack when dropped repeatedly by a child with autism? Or will poor saliva management cause functionality issues when using an iPod? Answers to these questions are not yet fully known, and the challenges will differ from client to client. What is known is that these consumer electronics are more fragile than traditional AAC devices. This is one of the reasons that insurance companies and other funding agencies are hesitant to cover mobile technology devices. There are hundreds of cases available for tablets, MP3 players, and other mobile devices. These are designed to protect the device from mishaps of users without disabilities. Although some cases and accessories have been designed for use with individuals with disabilities, such items are limited and not well tested. The manufacturer of Apple products offers AppleProtection plans for a nominal fee; however, this plan does not cover "damage caused by accident, misuse, abuse, liquid contact," and so forth (Apple, 2011, p. 2). As mobile technology continues to gain popularity, it is possible that new accessories geared toward individuals with disabilities will be designed and tested to make these devices more usable for a wider range of populations.

An additional hurdle to new technology is available support. A large number of AAC companies provide extensive technical support as needed. What happens when the app you are using closes each time you access it? Or when a voice output app freezes when your client is using it to communicate a message? Who is responsible for troubleshooting this technology? Is it the programmer of the app? Is it the manufacturer of the device that is running the app? The clinician needs to be mindful of these unknowns and have a plan in place to tackle such issues. Some clinicians work in facilities that provide technology support, but many do not. Whereas Apple as well as other manufacturers will provide support related to hardware issues or preloaded software issues, they typically do not provide support for third-party-designed applications. If an iPad with a speech-generating app is the client's sole means of communication and the app crashes, what contingency plan will be in place if it takes days or weeks to fix the problem? Similarly, if a client requires switch access or other special accessories that must interface smoothly with a hardware device, support in troubleshooting problems with these accessories could also be needed. Raising such issues is meant not to dissuade clinicians from using new technologies but to guide the decision-making process. For example, when choosing a tablet for a client, it might be useful know that Apple has a high customer support satisfaction rating; it was ranked number one for customer satisfaction compared to other computing companies (Shah, 2012). However, if the app you want to try is available only for the Android operating system, support issues have to be factored into the decision. It is for these reasons that clinicians must be savvy and careful consumers.

A paper released by the AAC division of the Rehabilitation Engineering Research Center (AAC-RERC; 2011) provides clinicians with a way to think about who might benefit from mobile technologies and how benefits and costs can be weighed. The AAA division suggests that mobile technologies and associated applications might

- Be utilized for a primary communication system that meets the majority of the user's communication needs

- Be utilized as a backup communication system when the user's dedicated device is not available

- Be used in a habilitative or rehabilitative fashion to teach language (or other skills) as part of the user's intervention

- Not be a viable option for addressing the user's communication needs but be used for reasons other than communication (e.g., organization, memory support)

- Not be a viable option due to issues with device access, durability, cost, or user's preference

Another important issue raised by this group is related to service delivery. In times past, it was the primary responsibility of the clinician to make decisions regarding AT. However, these days, clinicians must often negotiate between evidence-based, empirically validated practices and a visit from a parent who says, "I bought an iPad for my child, and I want you to teach him how to use it to communicate." Although many new consumer electronics show promise, a sort of ecological validity, there remains limited objective, empirical information related to their efficacy in practice.

CONCLUSIONS

The use of AT for individuals with CCN is growing in popularity and accessibility as the sophistication and scope of consumer technology increases. In fact, AT can be implemented for a wide range of individuals, for those with mild hearing impairment to individuals with developmental disabilities to those with acquired neurological injury.

The ever-changing landscape of technology will require clinicians to remain vigilant and up-to-date regarding the newest assistive hardware and software that might be beneficial for their clientele. With mobile technology now providing clinicians and individuals with CCN with new treatment options, it is important to use the same evidence-based decision-making processes when making a technology recommendation for a client as would be applied to any other form of intervention.

STUDY QUESTIONS

1. Describe how a speech-language pathologist and audiologist might use assistive technology as part of their clinical practice.

2. Explain how evidence-based decision making is used to inform decisions when choosing technology for a client.

3. Discuss the components of a comprehensive assistive technology assessment.

4. Describe the groups of individuals who might benefit from assistive listening devices.

5. Compare and contrast the features of low-tech, mid-tech, and high-tech AAC devices.

6. Explain how mobile technology has changed the way people with and without communication disorders communicate with one another.

7. Describe the issues related to the use of mobile technology in populations with communication disorders.

REFERENCES

Alliano, A., Herriger, K., Koutsoftas, A., & Bartolotta, T. (2012). A review of 21 iPad applications for augmentative and alternative communication purposes. *Perspectives on Augmentative and Alternative Communication, 21*, 60–71.

American Academy of Audiology. (2003). *Pediatric amplification protocol.* Retrieved from http://www.audiology.org/resources/documentlibrary/Documents/pedamp.pdf

American Speech-Language-Hearing Association. (2013). *The audiogram.* Retrieved from http://www.asha.org/public/hearing/Audiogram

Apple. (2011, December 20). *AppleCare protection plan for iPad: Terms and conditions.* Retrieved from http://www.apple.com/legal/applecare/appforipad.html

Apps for AAC. (2013). Retrieved from http://www.appsforaac.net

Beigel, A. (2000). Assistive technology assessment: More than the device. *Intervention in School and Clinic, 35*, 237–243.

Bess, F.H., Dodd-Murphy, J., & Parker, R.A. (1998). Children with minimal sensorineural hearing loss: Prevalence, educational performance, and functional status. *Ear & Hearing, 9*, 339–354.

Beukelman, B., & Mirenda, P. (2013). *Augmentative and alternative communication: Supporting children and adults with complex communication needs* (4th ed.). Baltimore, MD: Paul H. Brookes Publishing Co.

Bondy, A., & Frost, L. (2001). The Picture Exchange Communication System. *Behavior Modification, 25*, 725–744.

Bouck, E.C., Shurr, J.C., Kinsey, T., Jasper, A.D., Bassette, L., Miller, B., & Flanagan, S.M. (2012). Fix it with TAPE: Repurposing technology as assistive technology for individuals with high-incidence disabilities. *Preventing School Failure: Alternative Education of Children and Youth, 56*, 121–128.

Campbell, P., Milbourne, S., Dugan, L., & Wilcox, M. (2006). A review of evidence on practices for teaching young children to use assistive technology devices. *Topics in Early Childhood Special Education, 26*, 3–13.

Charlop-Christy, M., Carpenter, M., Le, L., LeBlanc, L.A., & Kellet, K. (2002). Using the Picture Exchange Communication System (PECS) with children with autism: Assessment of PECS acquisition, speech, social-communicative behavior, and problem behavior. *Journal of Applied Behavior Analysis, 35*, 213–231.

Copley, J., & Ziviani, J. (2005). Barriers to utilization of assistive technology with children who have multiple disabilities. *Occupation Therapy International, 11*, 229–243.

Copley, J., & Ziviani, J. (2007). Use of a team-based approach to assistive technology assessment and planning for children with multiple disabilities: A pilot study. *Assistive Technology, 19*, 109–125.

de Joode, E., van Heugten, C., Verhey, F., & van Boxel, M. (2010). Efficacy and usability of assistive technology for patients with cognitive deficits: A systematic review. *Clinical Rehabilitation, 24*, 701–714.

DeCoste, D., Reed, P., & Kaplan, M. (2005). *Assistive technology teams: Many ways to do it well.* National Assistive Technology In Education (NATE) Network [Monograph series]. Roseburg, OR.

Feldman, A.S. (1963). Maximum air-conduction hearing loss. *Journal of Speech, Language and Hearing Research, 6*, 157–163.

Gelfand, S. (2001). *Essentials of audiology* (2nd ed.). New York, NY: Thieme Medical Publishers.

Goldman, A. (2011). Mobile information and communication technologies (ICT)—New tools for the SLP. *ASHAsphere.* Retrieved from http://www.asha.org

Good, M., & Gilkey, R. (1996). Sound localization in noise: The effect of signal-to-noise ratio. *Journal of the Acoustical Society of America, 99*, 1108–1117.

Gosnell, J., Costello, J., & Shane, H. (2011). Using a clinical approach to answer "What communication apps should we use?" *Perspectives on Augmentative and Alternative Communication, 20*, 87–96.

Hill, K. (2004). Augmentative and alternative communication and language: Evidence-based practice and language activity monitoring. *Topics in Language Disorders, 24*, 18–30.

Johnston, L., Beard, L., & Carpenter, L. (2007). *Assistive technology: Access for all students.* Upper Saddle River, NJ: Pearson.

Jones, M., Grogg, K., Anschutz, J., & Fierman, R. (2008). A sip-and-puff wireless remote control for the Apple iPod. *Assistive Technology, 20*, 107–110.

Lesner, S. (2003). Candidacy and management of assistive listening devices: Special needs of the elderly. *International Journal of Audiology, 42*, 68–76.

Lewis, D. (1994). Assistive devices for classroom listening: FM systems. *American Journal of Audiology, 3*, 70–83.

LoPresti, E., Mihailidis, A., & Kirsh, N. (2004). Assistive technology for cognitive rehabilitation: State of the art. *Neuropsychological Rehabilitation, 14*, 5–39.

Melhuish, K., & Falloon, G. (2010). Looking to the future: M-learning with the iPad. *Computers in New Zealand Schools: Learning, Teaching, Technology, 22*, 1–15.

Peterson-Karlan, G., & Parette, H. (2007). Evidence-based practice and the consideration of assistive technology: Effectiveness and outcomes. *Assistive Technology Outcomes and Benefits, 4*, 130–139.

Pruitt, J.B. (1990). Assistive listening device versus conventional hearing aid in an elderly patient: Case report. *Journal of the American Academy of Audiology, 1*, 41–43.

Quist, R., & Lloyd, L. (1997). Principles and uses of technology. In L. Lloyd, D. Fuller, & H. Arvidson (Eds.), *Augmentative and alternative communication*. Boston, MA: Allyn & Bacon.

Rehabilitation Engineering Research Center on Communication Enhancement (AAC-RERC). (2011). *Mobile devices and communication apps: An AAC-RERC white paper*. Retrieved from http://aac-rerc.psu.edu/index.php/pages/show/id/46

Sadao, K., & Robinson, N. (2010). *Assistive technology for young children: Creating inclusive learning environments*. Baltimore, MD: Paul H. Brookes Publishing, Co.

Schlosser, R., Koul, R., & Costello, J. (2007). Asking well-built questions for evidence-based practice in augmentative and alternative communication. *Journal of Communication Disorders, 40*, 225–238.

Shah, A. (2012, September 18). Apple keeps top spot in customer satisfaction. *Computer World*.

Social Security Amendments of 2001 (PL 113-21), 42 U.S.C. §§ 1395 *et seq.*

Sohlberg, M.M. (2011, February 15). Assistive technology for cognition. *The ASHA Leader*.

Sutton, M. (2012, June 5). APP-titude: Apps to aid aphasia. *The ASHA Leader*.

Sweeney, S. (2012, August 28). APP-titude: Apps that crack curriculum content. *The ASHA Leader*.

Technology-Related Assistance for Individuals with Disabilities Act of 1988 (PL 100-407), 29 U.S.C. §§ 2201 *et seq.*

Wakefield, L., & Schaber, T. (2012, July 31). APP-titude: Use the evidence to choose a treatment app: This evidence-based practice model provides strategies for selecting an app. *The ASHA Leader*.

Welzl-Muller, K., & Sattler, K. (1984). Signal-to-noise threshold with and without hearing aid. *Scandinavian Audiology, 13*, 283–286.

Zabala, J. (1995). The SETT framework: Critical areas to consider when making informed assistive technology decisions. Retrieved from http://www.eric.ed.gov

Zabala, J. (2005). *SETT*. Retrieved from http://www.joyzabala.com

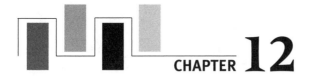

CHAPTER **12**

Family-Centered Practice

Denise LaPrade Rini and Jane Hindenlang

CHAPTER OBJECTIVES

After reading this chapter, students will be able to

- Define core terms within: *family*, *family-centered approach*, *family-centered practice*, *palliative care*
- List premises of a family-centered approach
- List premises and principles of family support
- Identify family-centered assessment and intervention resources
- Discuss and respond to sample scenarios from the perspective of a family-centered service delivery model
- List/state challenges to implementation of family-centered practice
- List several resources or organizations which stipulate family-centered practice as the approach to be used in delivering communication disorders services

Family: It is the genesis of our being. It is the primary and most powerful context for the development of our emotions, security, values, beliefs, human interactions, rules, roles, and responsibilities, goals, and ambitions—spouses, partners, mothers and fathers, daughters and sons, brothers and sisters, aunts and uncles, nieces and nephews, cousins, neighbors, and friends.

From the moment of our birth, we become members of families and function in that context. Yet, many clinicians who are first entering home- and family-based clinical situations often experience some trepidation. Traditional service delivery methods in communication disorders have centered on the needs of the client as an individual. According to those methods, the professional has assumed responsibility for decision making and is seen as the "expert." Speech-language pathologists (SLPs) have typically worked with an individual or a small group within a clinical setting, such as a speech center, a hospital, or a school. Recently, however, there is a trend toward providing services within the contexts natural to clients, such as their homes, vocational settings, or recreational settings. In the current health care climate, there is a demand to demonstrate functional changes in everyday environments. Increasingly, our roles shift from that of direct service provider to that of consultant in educating family members and facilitating their ability to support the client's growth to more functional communication. The increasing growth of an aging population, survival of the youngest early birth babies, and transformation of terminal medical conditions to chronic health conditions all predict that the incidence and prevalence of communication disorders and delays will rise, as will the need to provide services through a family-centered framework. Although communication disorders professionals feel prepared to provide treatment and have been trained in a wide range of clinician-directed, client-centered techniques, they often feel overwhelmed when faced with the multiple and personal demands of the family context.

Increasingly, a number of federal and state legislative provisions, as well as certain insurers, mandate that clients and their families assume a primary role in the decision-making process in assessment and intervention and that services be provided in a natural-environment framework. It is important to obtain input from clients and their families about their needs and desires in order to create and implement meaningful, relevant services. Programs such as the federal birth-to-3 system have required a **family-centered approach** in work with very young children. However, this approach is applicable, relevant, and important throughout the client's life span and continuum of care, and within a range of programs with the various communication disorders we encounter. As clinicians, we must ask ourselves to what extent can we draw upon our own experiences as family members in order to deliver services successfully in a family-centered context. What roles do family members assume when one of them is involved in treatment for a communication disorder? Who constitutes family? How does this influence the manner in which the clinician provides the intervention? In order to answer these questions and to effectively implement family-centered practice, we need to know something about family, family systems, and available clinical tools and resources for assessment and intervention according to this service delivery model.

WHAT IS FAMILY?

The growing recognition that family is the primary context in which we exist, as well as the expanding focus on family as the vehicle through which individual needs can be met, has led to our defining what family is. Each of us defines "family" based on our own family and experiences, but we must be aware that the term *family* is a far-ranging concept. Hanson and Lynch (2004, p. 4) cite Gelles (1995, p. 10) in stating that a family is a social group that possesses a structure in which various individuals assume roles. Those individuals carry out specific functions, and the family members identify themselves as having blood or other primary relationship ties. Thus, a family may reflect the 1950s concept of two parents with two children, with grandparents who are seen on the weekend. Or a family may be a group of close friends who live together and provide combined financial and emotional support for each other, as well as carrying out everyday activities (food shopping, transportation, etc.). A family may have three or four generations living together, with grandparents filling the role of parents to grandchildren. Aunts and uncles who live nearby may regularly have input into family decisions, such as living arrangements, number of children, or jobs to be sought.

This broader picture of family must be kept in mind as we apply a family systems approach to service delivery.

In addition, sociological and family counseling literature delineate different types of families (e.g., Goldenberg & Goldenberg, 2008), described by how their members function and what roles they assume, both individually and among each other. According to Hidecker, Jones, Imig, and Villarruel (2009), using a family paradigm framework adopted from family science professionals may be helpful in assisting clients and families in identifying their beliefs, values, and preferences to support decisions relative to goals and service options. For instance, one family may have one main decision maker with other members who follow and support that person's directive. Another family may make decisions as a group (parents, perhaps grandparents or other stakeholders) after discussion of all the information and options among all members. At best, it would be important for SLPs to educate themselves regarding these dynamics; at the least, we must be aware of these family dynamics and how they affect the therapeutic process and interaction with clinical personnel.

FAMILY SYSTEMS THEORY

When we work with clients and their families, we need to understand how families function. The shift from the individual to the family as a focus of study, and the concept of family as a functioning transactional system as an entity in itself through which individuals are viewed and understood, was considered a revolution in psychotherapy when the concept of family therapy began in the 1950s (Goldenberg & Goldenberg, 2008). Rosin and colleagues (1996) discussed the diversity of contemporary American families and the impact that this diversity has on professionals and educators who interact with them. They listed four sources of diversity that present particular challenges for clinicians:

1. The growing number of families whose ethnic, cultural, and linguistic backgrounds are different than those of service providers

2. The differences in family structure (e.g., decrease in traditional two-parent homes)

3. The impact of poverty on disability

4. The increase in the number of families that have parents or adults with disabilities

In addition, it is important to be aware that the family unit is not a static entity but, rather, a dynamic and complex system. The family may include primary relatives and secondary persons, such as more distant relatives (e.g., grandparents, aunts, uncles), significant partners and/or friends and neighbors who fulfill family roles. *Family* refers to those individuals who provide caregiving, giving emotional, physical, and/or financial support, and who affect the client's quality-of-life and well-being. Families change and develop over time. Major life experiences, such as new partnerships, the birth of a child, children leaving home, aging, illness, and death, create changes. Many situations can challenge families, such as a change in an economic situation, a change in employment, a household move, an acute or chronic illness, or an accident.

Often, the clinician enters the family system not during the system's typical functioning but during one of these challenging stages. It is important to be aware that the family may be in flux and that family member roles and responses to illness, disability, and developmental delay may be different than would be evident in noncrisis situations. Specific reactions related to the age and role of the affected family member may also occur. A family with an infant or young child recently diagnosed with a disability may react to the loss of their dreams for the child and their loss of hope regarding future experiences that they believe the child may never have. There may also be an awareness of the demands of substantial lifelong care if the disability is serious and persistent. When an adult family member experiences illness or a condition resulting in communication disorder, the effect is different because that person has held certain roles in the family that may no longer be possible to carry out. The economic status of the family may be directly and significantly affected, and there may be a reversal in caregiver roles due to the disability. The concomitant communication disorder itself further creates frustration and difficulty coping, negotiating, and exchanging important information.

KEY CONCEPTS OF A FAMILY SYSTEMS PERSPECTIVE

If we adopt a family systems perspective (Begun, 1996), these concepts provide the guidelines for our practice:

The family as a whole is greater than the sum of its parts. This concept reflects that each family has its own patterns, rules, behaviors, and boundaries. The family as a whole has meaning and its preservation may transcend the goals and interests of any one member.

Change in one part of the family affects the whole family system. The interdependence among family members will cause any change or experience that occurs to any one member to affect the entire family (e.g., member illness and concomitant communication disruption).

Subsystems are embedded within the larger family system. Different family members have their own particular relationships and systems (e.g., siblings, spouses, parent–child).

The family system exists within a larger social and environmental context. The family is a component of larger systems, such as extended families, neighborhoods, religious communities, and political and economic communities.

Families are multigenerational. Most family systems of multiple generations are also interwoven with members and ideas of past generations, along with future anticipated generations.

What implications do these concepts have for professionals in the field of communication disorders? If we acknowledge and act on these family service concepts, our approach to the family will be different than if we hold a more traditional client-centered, clinician-directed approach. For example, in a traditional approach, the clinician might consider how a specific therapeutic intervention will affect the client. In a family systems approach, however, the clinician will also consider how therapy approaches affect the other members of the family and their relationships to one another. In some instances, the family may be the focus of intervention. In a traditional approach, a clinician might make assumptions about a family member's role based on his or her position (e.g., parent, sibling), but in a systems approach, each family member's true role would be deduced through interview and observation of how members interact and how that interaction may change over time with new experiences (Begun, 1996; see also Chapter 7).

Every person is a member of a family (or families) and assumes many different family roles throughout his or her lifetime. Each clinician brings to the experience his or her own beliefs about what families are and how they "should" function, as well as the roles that the clinician and all family members should assume. Within a family-centered approach, the clinician needs to place these beliefs aside in order to be effective and clear-sighted in the service delivery process. As professionals, it is important to recognize not only what we have to offer but also what we can learn from our clients and their families or significant partners to establish more ecologically valid management paradigms.

DEFINING FAMILY-CENTERED PRACTICE

Family-centered practice has its roots in the consumer-led movements of the 1960s; consumers of health care and other human services were granted the rights to safety, to be informed, to choose, and to be heard (Goldenberg & Goldenberg, 2008). Head Start, created in 1965, mandated parent involvement and control of local programs (Johnson, 2000). One definition of family-centered practice, generated by the Beach Center on Disability (formerly the Beach Center on Families and Disability), states, "Family-centered service delivery, across disciplines and settings, recognizes the centrality of the family in the lives of individuals. It is guided by fully informed choices made by the family and focuses upon the strengths and capabilities of these families" (1997, p. 1).

The family support movement acknowledges and builds on the many strengths and resources of families and communities (Rini & Whitney, 1999). The Beach Center lists key components of family-centered service delivery (Table 12.1). In addition, core concepts indicated by the Institute for Patient- and Family-Centered

Table 12.1.   Principles of family support

Staff and families work together in relationships based on equality and respect.
Staff embrace families' capacity to support the growth and development of all family members—adults, youth, and children.
Families are resources to their own members, to other families, to programs, and to communities.
Programs affirm and strengthen families' cultural, racial, and linguistic identities and enhance their ability to function in a multicultural society.
Programs are embedded in their communities and contribute to the community-building process.
Programs advocate with families for services and systems that are fair, responsive, and accountable to the families served.
Practitioners work with families to mobilize formal and informal resources to support family development.
Programs are flexible and continually responsive to emerging family and community issues.
Principles of family support are modeled in all program activities, including planning, governance, and administration.

Source: Beach Center on Families and Disability (1997).

Care (n.d.) include respect, support, choice, flexibility, collaboration, information, and identification of family strengths. Family empowerment extends beyond support by systematically assisting family members to direct their strengths and resources toward meeting the present and future needs of their members, themselves, and their communities. Thus, it is accepted as best practice that the client's relations to both family and community should be explored when formulating and implementing an intervention plan. It makes use of family values, traditions, customs, and resources. Even though every family-centered intervention cannot address the full range of a complex set of systems, an acceptance of the family context as part of the individual's treatment is an important factor in achieving positive outcomes and best practice. For example, Gadow (1981) offers a response to the typical roles assumed by professionals when developing decision-making procedures. In her 1981 study, she proposed an advocacy model in "an effort to help individuals become clear about what they want in a situation, to assist them in discerning and clarifying their values, and to help them in examining available options in light of their values" (Gadow, 1981, p. 137). Family-centered services means that the full context of the family, assessed with the family, is taken into consideration whenever intervention occurs and/or decisions need to be made (Table 12.2).

There are legal provisions that mandate family primacy in communication assessment and intervention. The Individuals with Disabilities Education Improvement Act (IDEA) of 2004 (PL 108-446), with its birth-to-3 component, requires that parents or guardians direct the contents of the individualized family service plan (IFSP), including outcomes for the child and family, and a statement of family needs and resources around which intervention must be designed. For children ages 3–21, IDEA 2004, as this law has come to be known, requires family input for permission to assess and to target what to assess. As critical members of the child's placement and planning team, the law indicates that family work with other team members (educational staff) to develop the child's individualized education program (IEP). Although school-based services are less likely to be fully family centered, many school systems require clinicians to have contact with the family on a regular basis to discuss the course of assessment and intervention, to integrate family goals, and to share ideas for both school- and home-based intervention.

For adults in hospitals, rehabilitation centers, or long-term care settings, there is the Patient Bill of Rights, which ensures family notification and patient and family input and/or attendance at all case conferences. A patient and his or her family may also partner with professionals to set short- and long-term plans of care, as well as to formulate statements of family needs. In 2010, the Joint Commission for Accreditation and Certification of Hospitals developed and published a document entitled "Advancing Effective Communication, Cultural Competence, and Patient- and Family-Centered Care: A Roadmap for Hospitals." This was in response to studies showing these areas as critical in increasing patient satisfaction and adherence to treatment protocols. The International Classification of Functioning, Disability and Health (World Health Organization [WHO], 2002) has challenged our thinking about service delivery by considering how any disability influences an individual's ability to reintegrate into activities at home, at work, and in the community. Audiologists and SLPs need to consider limitations in communication experienced by clients within daily activities (i.e., activity

Table 12.2.   Premises of family support

The primary responsibility for the development and well-being of children lies within the family, and all segments of society must support families as they rear their children. The systems and institutions on which families rely must effectively respond to their needs if families are to establish and maintain environments that promote growth and development. Achieving this requires a society that is committed to making the well-being of children and families a priority and to supporting that commitment by allocating and providing necessary resources.

Assuring the well-being of all families is the cornerstone of a healthy society and requires universal access to support programs and services. A national commitment to promoting the healthy development of families acknowledges that every family, regardless of race, ethnic background, or economic status, needs and deserves a support system. Because no family can be self-sufficient, the concept of reaching families before problems arise is not realized unless all families are reached. To do so requires a public mandate to make family support accessible and available, on a voluntary basis, to all.

Children and families exist as part of an ecological system. An ecological approach assumes that child and family development is embedded within broader aspects of the environment, including a community with cultural, ethnic, and socioeconomic characteristics that are affected by the values and policies of the larger society. This perspective assumes that children and families are influenced by interactions with people, programs, and agencies, as well as by values and policies that may help or hinder families' ability to promote their members' growth and development. The ecological context in which families operate is a critical consideration in programs' efforts to support families.

Child-rearing patterns are influenced by parents' understanding of child development and of their children's unique characteristics, personal sense of competence, and cultural and community traditions and mores. There are multiple determinants of parents' child-rearing beliefs and practices, and each influence is connected to other influences. For example, a parent's view of his or her child's disposition is related to the parent's cultural background and knowledge of child development and to characteristics of the child. Because the early years set a foundation for the child's development, patterns of parent–child interaction are significant from the start. The unique history of the parent–child relationship is important to consider in programs' efforts.

Enabling families to build on their own strengths and capacities promotes the healthy development of children. Family support programs promote the development of competencies and capacities that enable families and their members to have control over important aspects of their lives and to relate to their children more effectively. By building on strengths rather than treating impairments, programs assist parents in dealing with difficult life circumstances as well as achieving their goals, and in doing so, enhance parents' capacity to promote their children's healthy development.

The developmental processes that make up parenthood and family life create needs that are unique at each stage in the life span. Parents grow and change in response to changing circumstances and the challenges of nurturing a child's development. The tasks of parenthood and family life are ongoing and complex, requiring physical, emotional, and intellectual resources. Many tasks of parenting are unique to the parent's point in her or his life cycle. Parents have been influenced by their own childhood experiences and their own particular psychological characteristics, and are affected by their past and present family interactions.

Families are empowered when they have access to information and other resources and take action to improve the well-being of children, families, and communities. Equitable access to resources in the community—including up-to-date information and high-quality services that address health, educational, and other basic needs—enables families to develop and foster optimal environments for all family members. When families have meaningful experiences, participate in programs, and influence policies, it strengthens existing capabilities and promotes the development of new competencies, such as the ability to advocate on their own behalf.

Source: Family Resource Coalition (1996).

level) and the emotional, psychological, and social consequences of the impairment for the individual, spouse, caregiver, and family (i.e., participation level). Under the patient-centered medical home model of care, which is supported by the Patient Protection and Affordable Care Act (PL 111-148), audiologists and SLPs will be considered subject matter experts or specialists and will be accountable and responsible for collaborating and communicating with the primary care physician and other team members, including the patient and family members, about appropriate medical and nonmedical needs.

CULTURAL AND SOCIOECONOMIC CONSIDERATIONS

Contemporary practice also requires the audiologist and SLP to consider the unique ethnic, linguistic, and cultural background of the family. When there is a discrepancy between the culture of the family and client and that of their service providers, these differences can impede the development of a positive, family-centered intervention program if the clinician is not familiar with customs and family dynamics and imposes his or her own beliefs and values onto the therapeutic situation. It is critically important for the clinician to understand how culture and tradition influence communication behavior, both at the level of clinician–family information exchange and at the level of clinician–client therapy interaction (see Chapter 10 regarding multicultural issues). Realizing that cultural considerations include a broad variety of family traditions and elements—among them customs revolving around foods; holidays; religious observances; roles of men, women, and children; and verbal and nonverbal pragmatic behaviors—is an important awareness that clinicians should develop. Direct study (i.e., reading about and consulting with people of those cultures) regarding different cultures of clients with whom a clinician regularly interfaces may be one way of learning about them; observation of and deference to customs of behavior and interaction may be another. Equally important is the awareness that membership in a certain cultural or linguistic group or emigration from a certain country of origin does not dictate that those families will automatically exhibit the customs or observations of that country or culture. Each family must be viewed individually.

In her discussion of family-centered services among the chronically impoverished, Humphrey (1995) described issues that affect parents' and clinicians' views of each other and that threaten the effectiveness of the intended partnership. She noted the influences of poverty on parenting and pointed out that the demographics between those of low socioeconomic status and the clinician are often radically different. Rini and Whitney (1999) surveyed a number of studies that illustrate the deleterious effect poverty has on families and children in particular. Poverty is often accompanied by a host of other deficits in family resources, such as inadequate food and housing (which may include toxins such as lead paint and asbestos that are directly dangerous to health); restricted access to medical care, medications, and equipment; lack of transportation; and below-standard education. Chronic illness of family members may be more common than in families of high socioeconomic status. If further complicated by substance abuse (i.e., alcohol, legal and illegal drugs), environmental or domestic violence, and/or mental illness, the family of low socioeconomic status experiences multiple stressors that threaten family function. If different cultural backgrounds are also involved, then the number of obstacles between the members of this intervention team increases greatly. When families are experiencing multiple stressors, additional resources besides those directed at remediating a communication disorder in one family member are needed.

FAMILY-CENTERED PRACTICE IN COMMUNICATION DISORDERS

Traditionally, service delivery in communication disorders has followed a model in which the professional is viewed as the authority who identifies the presence and severity of the communication disorder along with treatment recommendations, if appropriate. Intervention would include educating family members and modeling interactive intervention behaviors that family members would be expected to imitate and implement. Family members of individuals with communication disorders have often been perceived as being unsophisticated or too subjective to adequately observe or delineate the aspects of the individual's communication disorder. Cress (2004) found this perception to be inaccurate. A review of multiple sources "confirmed that parents are accurate and thorough observers of their children, although they may not convey their observations in the same terms as professionals" (Cress, 2004, p. 51). This observation has been confirmed by these authors, who have noted that in their experience, family members have been very specific regarding their family member's abilities, difficulties, and needs, even in cases in which families have been significantly negatively affected by issues disrupting family function (e.g., illness, legal or financial issues, family disintegration).

The American Speech-Language-Hearing Association (ASHA) has delineated an extensive list of professional roles and responsibilities for speech-language pathologists and audiologists in its Scope of Practice (2007). In contemporary practice, the amount of professional time directed to activities beyond evaluation and direct treatment has increased. The role of family is mentioned throughout all areas in which an SLP might engage: clinical services, prevention, advocacy, education, administration, and research. Of note are supports often provided to clients at both ends of the life span. For example, SLPs may be part of **palliative care** teams. Palliative care is an approach that improves the quality of life of patients and their families facing the problem associated with life-threatening illness, doing so through the prevention and relief of suffering by means of early identification and impeccable assessment and treatment of pain and other problems, physical, psychosocial, and spiritual (WHO, 2002). The philosophy behind this model is patient focused and family centered. It is interdisciplinary care that aims to relieve suffering, improve quality of life, optimize function, and assist with decision making. Palliative care is for patients who have advanced illnesses and may or may not be terminal, as well as for their families. Pollens (2004, p. 694) described four primary roles for the SLP in palliative treatment:

> 1) to provide consultation to patients, families, and team members in the areas of communication, cognition, and swallowing function; 2) to develop strategies in communication skills to support the patient's role in decision making, to maintain social closeness, and to assist in fulfilling end-of-life goals; 3) to assist in optimizing function related to dysphagia symptoms in order to improve patient comfort and eating satisfaction and to promote positive feeding interactions for family members; 4) to communicate with members of the interdisciplinary team in order to provide and receive input related to overall patient care.

During the 1990s, particularly with the initiation of birth-to-3 services across the country (Individuals with Disabilities Education Act Amendments of 1997, PL 105-17) and the expansion of home health care services for adults, there has been an increasing movement toward true inclusion of family members in the decision-making process. Families are now involved in planning and conducting assessment tasks, identifying and prioritizing desired intervention outcomes if delays are diagnosed, developing intervention objectives, and implementing intervention activities. Wahrborg and Bornstein (1989), in investigating family attitudes and rehabilitation outcomes, suggested that an important positive relationship exists between active family support and stroke rehabilitation outcomes and, conversely, a nonsupportive family may interfere with stroke recovery, resulting in physical and emotional deterioration of the client.

There are no prescriptive procedures to family-based approaches, but the tenets of this practice suggest that both assessment and intervention are dynamic and collaborative, occur over time in several different contexts, and include relevant stakeholders. Functional communication and social relevance are embraced, particularly in our work with persons with complex communication needs. Outcomes and goals focus on improving individuals' quality of life by enabling them to become participating members in their families and communities and to experience a sense of personal competence, as well as to achieve, or resume, levels of functional independence. Client and family education contributes to achieving improved outcomes, and clients tend to fare better when their families and partners are involved. Thus ASHA (2005) has adopted evidence-based practice (EBP) as a systematic approach to clinical decision making. The goal of EBP is to provide high-quality services reflecting the interests, values, needs, and choices of the individuals we serve by integrating clinical expertise, best current evidence, and client values. When interpreting best current evidence, the clinician and team must consider family preferences, environment, culture, and values.

The nature, content, and methods of interpersonal communication are critically important in the overall service delivery process. In particular, the ways in which service providers relay information and suggestions may be key to how the clinician's communication is important. Effective communication includes five significant characteristics:

1. *Clarity:* Information should be provided in language that is familiar and understandable to the family.

2. *Succinctness:* Information needs to be directed at the specific areas being discussed.

3. *Redundancy:* Information should be provided frequently to allow family members to process, internalize, and consider it.

4. *Respect:* Information should be provided in a manner that acknowledges the contribution of the family.

5. *Genuineness:* The clinician must present him- or herself as a sincere human being and be perceived as such in order for necessary trust to develop among the people involved.

Family-Centered Assumptions and Attitudes

Our frame of reference includes the following family-centered assumptions and attitudes:

- Any circumstance that affects one family member (the client) affects other members, as well as the family as a whole.

- The family has a right to establish its own priorities.

- The family must be accepted as being the experts concerning their family member.

- The clinician must evidence genuine listening in collaboration with family members to obtain assessment information and in developing intervention goals.

- The family must be acknowledged as having the right to form their own approach to raising their child or caring for an older family member, as long as health and safety are not at issue.

- The clinician must acknowledge any personal bias regarding preconceived notions of expected role behavior in approaching a family and must place these notions aside in order to assess the function of the specific family and client.

- In situations in which a family report appears to differ significantly from a clinician's observation (particularly in situations in which communication behaviors are underreported), it is the responsibility of the clinician to explore with the family the situations in which they may perceive the client differently or to assist them in identifying behaviors that help them become aware that the client may have expanded skills.

Family-Centered Assessment

Best practice suggests that we view assessment as a dynamic process that is ideally completed over time and in a variety of contexts in order to sample a representative set of communication behaviors (Lidz & Pena, 1996; see also Chapter 4). Naturalistic contexts are also emphasized (Lund & Duchan, 1993). These contexts include places where clients are comfortable and familiar, places containing objects that are salient and immediate for them, and places in which typical social and communication exchanges occur. Linder (1993) discussed the limitations of traditional assessment in communication disorders, which has often required that the client be evaluated out of context (e.g., in an unfamiliar office or clinic setting, separated from family, individually rather than in a setting with peers or siblings) and presented with tasks that are often unrelated to any immediate activity, interest, or communication exchange. For example, federal and state birth-to-3 guidelines ensure that developmental assessment takes place within a natural environment and with family as key team members.

A number of family factors must be included in the assessment process. Knowledge of the cultural and linguistic contexts and characteristics of the family is primary in developing a preliminary understanding of the communication expectations and style of the environment (Halpern, 1993; Lund & Duchan, 1993; Shipley & McAfee, 2009). Size of the family, educational and socioeconomic backgrounds, and family members' expectations of each other all have an influence on what clinicians will see and what families perceive as areas of competence and need. One of the greatest challenges involves obtaining a representative sample of client and family communication behavior within the constraints of time and materials set by the agencies that govern the provision of services. A clinician must also conduct a comprehensive family assessment in such a way that the family does not feel that its privacy is violated (Donahue-Kilburg, 1992) and that is consistent with how they prefer to be included.

Utilizing intensive family interviews and observing family–client interactions are aspects of family-centered assessment. **Ethnographic interviewing** refers to information that is gained from observations made of a family in context and told from a family's perspective (Hammer, 1998; see also Chapter 7). These techniques are applied in such a way that families are not assessed for their adequacy; rather, they are valued for engaging in a dialogue to obtain valid information about the client's behavior (Hanson, 2004). Family and/or caregiver interviews are the typical means by which information is obtained, often in the absence of a preestablished relationship between the clinician and the family. It is obviously important for the clinician to be perceived as trustworthy and responsive to the concerns voiced by the family. At times, these concerns may go beyond communication to include illness, housing, coping issues, education, domestic issues, substance abuse, and so forth. At other times, the family may need to focus solely on communication problems; in which cases, trust revolves around the clinician's ability to hone in on the important communication issue.

Family-Centered Assessment Questions

In evaluating a client, the clinician may consider a number of questions, among them these:

1. Is there a communication difference in this client in comparison to peers of his or her chronological and/or mental age and linguistic or cultural community?

2. Is this difference interfering with daily interactions within the family unit?

3. Is the client's communication functional for the purposes of attending to safety issues, expressing needs, negotiations, coping, planning, and developing literacy skills?

4. If the client's communication appears adequate within the immediate family context, is it sufficient for the larger context of the world outside of the family and for purposes that the family and the client intend (school, workplace, social settings)?

5. Do issues with the client's communication indicate areas of need, such as medical, economic, or mental health, to be addressed by and for the entire family?

Infants, Toddlers, and School-Aged Children For children younger than 3 years of age, there are a number of instruments and procedures that enable the clinician to obtain information regarding speech-language development from the parent. The Vineland Adaptive Behavior Scales, Second Edition (Sparrow, Balla, & Ciccietti, 2005) include a communication scale that provides parent report about receptive and expressive language as one component of a comprehensive developmental assessment tool. The MacArthur-Bates Communicative Development Inventories, Second Edition (Fenson et al., 2007) assesses receptive and expressive vocabulary size and early grammatical production. These two instruments provide results in terms of standard scores, which are often required to determine eligibility for intervention services. In addition, these scales are also available in Spanish, under the names Vineland-II and the MacArthur Inventarios del Desarrollo de Habilidades Communicativas (Jackson-Maldonado et al., 2003), respectively. Among other available parent-report format instruments are the Language Use Inventory (O'Neill, 2007), Receptive-Expressive Emergent Language Scale, Third Edition (Bzoch, League, & Brown, 2003), the Rossetti Infant–Toddler Language Scale (Rossetti, 2005), and the Early Language Milestone Scale, Second Edition (Coplan, 1993). These scales include areas of specific speech-language milestones rated by parents. Wetherby and Prizant's Communication and Symbolic Behavior Scales: Developmental Profiles (2002) include two tools in which parents provide information about the child's communication status, the Infant-Toddler Checklist and the Caregiver Questionnaire.

Although the assessment of communication disorders among school-age children usually includes background information provided by parents, there are few published assessment tools for older children that rely on parent report. One exception is the Children's Communication Checklist–2 (Bishop, 2003), a well-standardized measure that examines semantic, syntactic, and pragmatic aspects of language function. When assessments are completed within the school system, it is easy for the family to become separated from the assessment experience. Yet, special education laws require that parents be notified in writing and give signed consent for assessment, so presumably parents are aware of an upcoming evaluation and have the opportunity to initiate input into the process. Incumbent on the clinician is the obligation to obtain information from family members and to verify assessment results with the family. It is interesting to note that a number of well-established evaluation tools for school-age children have included, in their most recent editions, sections that allow for specific parent input regarding the child's communication behavior. Clinicians must also recognize that the child's wishes, perceptions, and input are critical components in the assessment process.

Adults   In the case of adults or adolescents with acquired and chronic disabilities, clinicians can gather information through the use of questionnaires and rating scales that rely on client, family, and/or significant others' observations and knowledge. Some of these questionnaires and scales can be administered to the client and family via interviews, or the family members can administer or complete them independently. Access to families or partners who know the client well can be helpful in determining the reliability of normative test scores. Family members can provide a window into a client's premorbid functioning that can assist in assessment. For example, the clinician can consider how a person's low score on a reading comprehension test might be interpreted differently once it is revealed the person was illiterate preinjury. Two published tools are available to clinicians: The General Health and History Questionnaire (Kreutzer, Leininger, Doherty, & Waaland, 1987) asks for information on current levels of functioning as well as premorbid status, as does the Preinterview or Referral Form for Collecting Family and Medical History and Status Information (Chapey & Patterson, 2008). For this age population, it is important to gain the perspective of the client by taking the time and effort to provide appropriate materials as opposed to only gaining the information by proxy.

There are several family-needs assessments that provide insight into the relative strengths of the family and its need for information or resources. These tools are useful for developing communication goals, educational programming, and referrals. One example is the Everyday Communicative Needs Assessment (Worrall, 1992). There are also partner skill and attitudinal surveys that assist in providing information for creating comprehensive management plans. The Quality of Communication Life Scale (Paul et al., 2004) is a tool that is used to attain information about the influence of a person's communication disorder on his or her relationships; communication interactions; participation in social, leisure, work, and education activities; and overall quality of life. Lubinski's Communication/Environment Assessment and Planning Guide (2008) may be used to identify opportunities for communication, barriers to successful communication, and overall effectiveness of communication interactions. The Communication Effectiveness Index (CETI; Lomas et al., 1989) is an index of 16 daily situations in which the family member rates the partner's performance. Similar in scope to CETI is ASHA's Functional Assessment of Communication Skills for Adults (Frattali, Holland, Thompson, Wohl, & Ferketic, 1995). In addition, assessments may look at conversational interactions between partners using conversational discourse measures where not only is the client's discourse is measured but also the partner's. Social Networks (Blackstone & Berg, 2012), intended for people with complex communication needs and their communication partners, is an inventory that assists clients and families in identifying their own everyday communication supports and contexts. There are three other published assessment tools that are useful for assessing the communication environment for individuals with severe developmental disabilities. The Communication Supports Checklist (McCarthy et al., 1998) includes a section about environmental support for communication. *Achieving Communication Independence* (Gillette, 2003) and *Analyzing the Communication Environment* (Rowland & Schweigert, 1993) both include items related to communication opportunities during daily routines.

The Life Interests and Values Cards (Haley, Womack, Helm-Estabrooks, Caignon, & McCulloch, 2010) were developed to use with adults with aphasia. They consist of three sets of cards depicting activities in four different categories. They can be used to facilitate conversations about previous and current interests to help with goal-setting targeting activity and participation. Included is a questionnaire for friends and family to complete, and the results when compared to persons with aphasia responses can provide "constructive dialog about new priorities, possible misunderstandings, and ways to overcome barriers to activity participation" (2010, p. 14).

Family-Centered Intervention

One of the guiding principles of ASHA's preferred practice patterns includes recognition that communication is an interactive process; the focus of intervention should include training of communication partners, caregivers, family members, peers, and educators. As with assessment, family-centered intervention implies that family members have key decision-making power in all aspects of intervention and that their personal styles, as well as linguistic, cultural, and traditional values, will be respected and incorporated into intervention. Styles of interaction between the family and the client may, to a large extent, dictate how directly involved with intervention the family may actually be. Within the framework of family-centered practice, there is a continuum of family involvement with intervention. On the one end, the family and the client identify communication goals and the mode of service delivery, but designated professionals provide intervention, and family members focus indirectly on communication goals during daily interactions. On the other end, family members function directly as interventionists, assuming responsibility for intervention strategies and selecting techniques and materials according to collaboratively selected communication goals. For example, one of the authors worked with the family of a 33-month-old boy with a severe speech sound disorder who chose to make the goal of the intervention for him to use family names, say yes and no, and attempt to repeat some words of other family members. Through consultation with the clinician, the child's mother constructed specific pictorial material and games that were of particular interest to the child (e.g., his favorite animals and characters), and they reviewed these daily. After 3 months, the established objectives were achieved. Not all families are able and willing to assume this role, however. Some clients resist their families' efforts to assume the role of instructor. Some clients reject any activities that are structured and perceived as focusing directly on their own difficulty. Between these two poles is a range of family involvement that includes both family-directed and client-directed activities along with clinician input.

Infants, Toddlers, and School-Age Children   IDEA 2004 provides mechanisms for parents and other family members to have direct input into the intervention process for children, adolescents, and young adults, ages 0–21. From birth to 3 years of age, the IFSP is family directed and the family states the specific outcomes that are the priority issues they wish to have addressed. Issues related to economic circumstance (i.e., education, employment, child care, respite, housing), medical issues (i.e., health of the child or other family members), substance abuse, and/or behavioral health issues may be addressed on the IFSP. Examples of exercises that early intervention team members may conduct with family members while developing a child's IFSP for birth-to-3 services include construction of an "Eco-map," through which family can depict persons who are part of the family's system (http://www.birth23.org/IFSP). Communication outcomes are expected to project long-term goals and are generated by parents in their own words. Interim objectives for a specific period of time (e.g., 3–6 months) are developed by parents and the providing professionals. The materials and techniques included are chosen for their desirability and comfort for the parents as well as appropriateness.

A well-established program that focuses on the parents' or family's role as model and interventionist in their children's communication development is the Hanen Centre's It Takes Two to Talk Program I (Pepper & Weitzman, 2004; also in Spanish and French), which focuses on training and support of parents as they assume direct responsibility for their child's learning. There are other parent programs for communication skills development available commercially, published under the titles *Hickory Dickory Talk* (Johnson & Heinze, 1990), *HELP...at Home* (Parks, 1990), *Parent Articles* (Schrader, 1988), and *Help Me Talk* (Eichten, 2000). Another online tool directed to parents to assist them in facilitating their children's communication development is "Teach Me to Talk" (Mize, 2012). These tools, and others like them, provide family members with suggestions for activities and materials that can be adapted to suit the family's needs. Many families are eager to learn about various intervention approaches and techniques. Curricula and materials devised for overall early childhood education, such as included in *The Crosscultural, Language, and Academic Development Handbook* (Diaz-Rico & Weed, 1995), can provide ideas and sequences of activities that parents can implement and individualize to their own family context. The advent of the Internet has enabled families to locate and explore information regarding every possible type of medical and communicative condition and materials and suggestions for intervention. This immediate access has provided families with knowledge and a degree of empowerment heretofore not possible. However, a new role for SLPs and audiologists is to present criteria to parents to judge which sources are most reliable and accurate, and which reflect sound scientific principles as well as best practice.

For school-age children, adolescents, and young adults, the planning and placement team is the mechanism that provides for parent input. Intervention is outlined through the IEP, which should be developed by all team members, including the student and his or her parents. Within the public schools, however, family-centered intervention may be difficult to achieve because of several factors: parent access to classrooms, availability of school staff and activities to working parents, school accessibility to parents without transportation or child care services, and strict time demands that minimize the possibility of authentic family–staff discussion and team goal development. In addition, service delivery often focuses on academic and social communication goals pertaining only to the school setting. School personnel must strive to have ongoing contact and flexible activities to be responsive to family needs.

In providing support for the adolescent or young adult with a communication disorder, clinicians can include family members. For example, in areas of articulation and fluency, family members can review lists of specific practice materials with the client. Carryover activities require the involvement of the family to provide contexts in which the client can practice new communication behaviors. The client, family, and clinician may devise specific contracts or procedures jointly. For higher level language skills, a number of commercially available workbooks and computer-based programs can provide basic stimuli for client–family work sessions.

Adults   Although there is no legislated mechanism to ensure family input to intervention plans for adults with disabilities, many facilities follow a Patient Bill of Rights in administering adult care. This document provides for the patient's right to have his or her family involved with every case conference and aspect of planning, as well as family input about the services to be provided. A central issue relative to family involvement with an adult with disabilities is the willingness of the patient to have that involvement. This will be partially dependent on preexisting family relationships, the degree of independence the patient previously had in self-care, and medical determination of whether the patient is capable of being responsible for his or her own decisions and future care. Family involvement cannot be mandated because the integrity of the adult's right to decide must be protected. This can present a challenge for the clinician when there is a disagreement between patient and family members about who is in charge of the patient's care. Often, when such conflicts exist, mediation may be needed to explore possible resolutions and special personnel (e.g., a social worker) may need to take the lead in the situation.

The individual who experiences significant communication loss due to neurological illness or trauma presents a different challenge to the family. As an adult, the client has held a specific position and role in the family. A style of communication and interaction has developed between the person and his or her family, friends, and social or work associates. Loss of communication is devastating because it affects all these areas. In addition, the client often experiences other medical difficulties, which may include loss of mobility, decrease in sensory or cognitive function, coronary and vascular fragility, and so forth. Communication disorders superimposed on preexisting medical conditions will significantly affect the person's overall function and degree of independence and quality of life, which has a consequent influence on the family. Still, much can be done to facilitate and broaden communication among the client, the family, and the community. For example, these individuals can participate in client-directed group therapy in which each client works on individualized goals but within a social context. At the same time, family members can participate in a parallel group therapy activity focused on family support and carry-over strategies (Johannsen-Horbach, Crone, & Wallesch, 1999).

Much of the information derived from the interview portion of the assessment may help establish goals related to activity and participation levels in collaboration with family partners. There are interventions that focus on family education, communication skills training for both the client and the partners, and counseling programs that offer support for the partners. The professional can work with families to develop realistic goals and match them to functional outcomes (Burns, 1996). Partners of people with acquired brain injury not only may participate in the therapy but also may be the primary focus of therapy. Several authors have developed approaches that coach or co-construct conversation between the client and significant other. The spouse or partner serves as clinician, while the clinician assumes the role of facilitator. Kagan's (1999) Supported Conversation for Adults with Aphasia (SCA) trains volunteers to interact with individuals with aphasia. The Family Based Intervention for Chronic Aphasia (FICA; Alarcon, Hickey, Rogers, & Olswang, 1997) focuses on treating the disability within naturally occurring interactions. Sorin-Peters, who works with couples living with aphasia using adult learning approaches and incorporating education, skills training, and counseling within an experiential learning cycle, found that the result of her 2003 study "suggests a relationship in which the speech-language pathologist and couple are active collaborators in the process" (p. 415). Purdy and Hindenlang (2005) developed a family education and training program using these same adult learning principles, but rather than working with the couples individually, they created classes of five to six couples. Benefits for both the client and partner included joint problem-solving opportunities as well as a chance to view and discriminate different communication impairments. Ylvisaker and Feeney (1998) suggested collaboration within everyday contexts among all people who interact with individuals with disability caused by acquired brain injury.

For individuals with a chronic disability and their families, the need for education and training is lifelong. The Self-Anchored Rating Scale (SARS) has recently been applied to aphasia treatment as a method to enhance quality of life. It is based on a family systems therapy model and is solution focused by helping clients and their families identify realistic long- and short-term goals and selecting approaches to achieve them (Fox, Andrews, & Andrews, 2012).

Professional Collaboration

To achieve a more comprehensive and family-centered approach, interdisciplinary collaboration is necessary. First, it is important that professionals become familiar with the cornerstones of each other's disciplines and how these relate to family-centered and transdisciplinary practice. Typically, when one discipline learns the scope of practice and professional language of another, the opportunities to collaborate expand. Second, it is helpful when each discipline is able to incorporate a broader perspective into evaluations and interventions. For example, the SLP who recognizes that a client has fine motor issues can call on the expertise of a colleague in occupational therapy. A psychologist may recognize that a client or his family experience challenges in treatment because of hearing impairments and will therefore consult with the audiologist. Collaborating professionals can offer a broader spectrum of insight and support to the family being served. This is particularly important when service is provided through a single transdisciplinary professional who must address a range of needs within the family as well as the client. Professionals can work together to assess the level and types of needs that exist in a family and then help families identify and secure community resources. In addition, professionals may find opportunities to partner with families to advocate for additional resources as a result of their joint assessment of the community.

Family-Centered Service Provision in Natural Environments

Family-centered service provision in natural environments (e.g., home, child or adult care center, classroom, workplace) can immediately address the specific communication requirements of the context, including appropriate objectives and stimuli. Family members can immediately be part of communication services and help the client use skills in daily routines. There are, however, also challenges that the clinician may face in working within the natural environment. Distractions of a typical environment, such as noise, extraneous activity, and the comings and goings of the family members or other people, as well as the client's own impulses to respond to his environment, may be factors. Natural environments may not always be safe, secure, healthy, supportive, or facilitative of development or rehabilitation. Although an important element in family-centered service delivery, the natural environment may not be a necessary or logical element for the provision of that service. In other words, family-centered practice can be the goal regardless of the location of client and family members.

Challenges

There may be barriers to advancing family-centered practice. According to the Institute for Patient- and Family-Centered Care (2010), these include attitudinal barriers on the part of the professional (e.g., fears, beliefs, perceptions), educational barriers (e.g., lack of understanding among all parties, lack of preparation for training), and organizational barriers (e.g., inability to gain consensus, limited resources, lack of leadership).

In identifying attitudinal and personal challenges, Ensher and Clark (2011) insightfully discuss the needs and ideals that may motivate us to seek family-centered practice. These may also lead us to assume roles in those relationships that are extraneous or inappropriate to our purpose as professionals. It is important for us to be aware of these factors and to address them in our professional lives so that they do not interfere with our work with families.

In terms of professional training, Luterman (2008) refers to data indicating that few SLPs and audiologists have specific training in working with families and providing the quality and nature of information required by them during intervention or counseling. Training programs in communication disorders will need to evolve to include both classroom and, most important, context experience for students to prepare them for different service approaches of the future.

Organizational or administrative issues may present themselves in a number of ways. For example, services may be obstructed by the demands of time management, commuting from site to site, and managed care and economic realities (e.g., quotas on client contacts). In many states, consultation (i.e., the time spent conferring with other professionals, the family, or physicians that is not direct treatment time) is not compensated by insurance and therefore is not billable or eligible for qualifying as "client contact," despite the necessity for fulfilling this function.

In the experiences of these authors, because communication is such an important priority for a majority of clients and their families, and because a focus on communication often is less intimate than a focus on personal relationships and family function, the SLP is often the first professional who is approached when there is a developmental-communicative or medical-communicative issue with a family member. As the clinician–family relationship develops, the family may confide in the clinician, at times revealing highly sensitive or complex situations and emotions. It is imperative at these times that the SLP involve a colleague within an appropriate discipline, either directly if the family so desires or in a consultant role to guide the clinician's response to the situation. Most often, the work of the SLP or audiologist occurs in the context of a voluntary program, so at some level, clients and their families have expressed a willingness to seek and participate in such services. This fact can minimize the degree of conflict often present in crisis situations faced by other professionals, who may be dealing with disagreements in implementation of critical medical care, identifying and responding to criminal activity, removing a family member from the home, and so forth. However, in cases where serious issues arise, it is critical that the clinician know what laws and regulations are in regard to mandatory reporting of health, safety, and legal or life-threatening situations and will act on them.

CONCLUSION

The benefits for family-centered practice appear compelling. Building capacity in families may assist with developing realistic functional and social goals, enhance the functioning of the individual, and help with transferring skills to daily life. In addition, working within the family framework may provide an authentic context from which to view a person's strengths and weaknesses. Family-centered practice is not merely a theoretical construct or philosophical position. Its practical implementation dictates collaboration and partnership among the family, the client, and the clinician and other involved service providers in ways that are based on the needs and wishes of the family. Possessing and using knowledge and tools available for involving, or following, family in the assessment and treatment of their loved ones is very important. Most important, however, are the clinician and family members themselves. In discussing the process of counseling as implemented by the audiologist or SLP, Luterman describes the crucial role and characteristics that must be conveyed by these professionals: "Very often we have to let go of our preconceived notions.... We can facilitate the growth (of the family) by not overhelping and by at all times respecting the dignity and the capacity of our clients to grow" (2005, p. 180). For the clinician who embraces the concept that communication assumes immersion in human interactions, a family-centered approach to service provision will prove to be a vital element of practice.

PROBLEM-SOLVING SCENARIOS

These are examples of actual situations. What is consistent or not consistent within the scenarios with family-centered practice? What and how could you make changes? What arguments would you advance to administrative service delivery decisions?

A. A clinician working in birth-to-3 visits a home to work with the family's speech-delayed 2-year-old. She has specific objectives to work on and specific ways to work. She insists on having the child sit at a table to do picture work but becomes exasperated when the child cries and wants his mother, who comes home from work right before the session.

B. At a school district's placement and planning team meeting for an incoming 3-year-old, family members are asking the SLP if they can remain with the child for his first session because he frequently becomes anxious during separations. The SLP responds that she is "very strict" about the separation rule and that she will just come out and get the child to remove him from his family to bring him to her speech group, saying he will stop crying eventually.

C. A high school student who is diagnosed with intellectual disability has begun participating in off-grounds vocational training. Work supervisors report that she has become increasingly noncompliant and exhibits a negative attitude. Her parents had signed her IEP because they had been told that this was the course of action that all such students followed. When asked about her behavior, the student expressed that she didn't like to be forced to do things she didn't want to do.

D. A center-based early intervention program has an open door policy for parents and other family members. The families involved in the program come from poor communities where there is frequent crime, safety problems with their homes, and other distractions. At the program site, they discuss their problems, hopes, dreams, and activities with other parents. They participate in program planning and implementation, organize activities, create materials, and learn about medical and developmental issues. In addition, food and family supplies are often provided to the parents. Home visits are a component of the program. To the great distress of the families, the administrative entity that operates this program shuts it down, saying it does not comply with requirements to provide service in a natural environment.

E. For 6 months, a 31-year-old man has resided in a long-term care facility, where he has received physical therapy and occupational therapy services for his first 6 weeks and speech therapy for approximately 4 months. He remains nonambulatory and uses a customized wheelchair for mobility and positioning. His speech is significantly dysarthric, and he has swallowing difficulties. He has been discharged to his parents' home and referred for home health care. The SLP begins services following the assessment. He schedules his client twice weekly visits at the same time each week; family members are not present due to work responsibilities.

F. You have been asked to participate in an evaluation of a 2-year-old child from another country. You are not sure of the family's language, and you know you have no familiarity with it. When you arrive at the designated location, the family does not want to admit you to the premises, but they express great concern about the child. A community member who is somewhat familiar with the family's language is present to serve as interpreter but has never participated in this type of professional activity before. What are some issues you might be facing? What questions need to be answered? What information should be provided to the family?

G. A child you have been seeing for intervention at home has begun making gains and attending to the activities in your sessions. The child's mother, who has been present for most of each session's duration, decided to begin to work at home part time. During your visit, she holds an exercise session in a neighboring room. There are eight women who come in and out of the home over the period of 90 minutes. Your client is naturally curious and restless and having difficulty remaining with you. What issues exist? What conversation, if any, should you have with the mother? What alternatives for intervention do you have?

H. A 50-year-old woman had a stroke 4 weeks prior to your evaluation of her in her home. She lives with her husband and 16-year-old son. Her daughter, age 20, is a sophomore at a college 3 hours away. During your first visit, you observed the client to be tired and easily frustrated. Her husband observed your visit; he said that he had been told by a speech-language pathologist in the hospital that his wife had global aphasia. During your second visit the following week, the client again appeared fatigued and was reluctant to participate in therapy. She also refused to have her husband present at the therapy session, and you observed her "yelling" at him. At the time the client had her stroke, she and her family were getting ready to take a trip to Florida to visit family. What issues exist? Who are the relevant stakeholders in this scenario? What information is needed, and how might it be obtained?

STUDY QUESTIONS

1. What is family-centered practice?
2. What are the key concepts of family systems theory?

3. In what ways is family-centered practice different than traditional practice?
4. What are some ways in which assessment and intervention services can be provided in a family-centered manner?
5. What role does collaboration have in family-centered practice?
6. Name situations or professional demands that might pose challenges to providing true family-centered services?
7. Name some issues that create different considerations between family-centered service delivery for adults and family-centered service delivery for children.

REFERENCES

Alarcon, N., Hickey, E., Rogers, M., & Olswang, L. (1997, March). *Family-based intervention for chronic aphasia (FICA): An alternative service delivery model.* Paper presented at the Non-Traditional Approaches to Aphasia Conference, Yountville, CA.

American Speech-Language-Hearing Association. (2007). *Scope of practice in speech-language pathology.* Retrieved from http://www.asha.org/policy

American Speech-Language-Hearing Association. (2005). *Evidence-based practice in communication disorders.* Retrieved from http://www.asha.org/policy/PS2005-00221

Beach Center on Families and Disability. (1997). *Families and Disability Newsletter, 8*(2), 1. Lawrence: University of Kansas.

Beach Center on Families and Disability. (2013). *Family research tool kit.* Retrieved from http://www.beachcenter.org/families/family_research_toolkit.aspx?JScript=1

Begun, A.L. (1996). Family systems and family-centered care. In P. Rosin, A.D. Whitehead, L.I. Tuchman, G.S. Jesien, A.L. Begun, & L. Irwin (Eds.), *Partnerships in family-centered care: A guide to collaborative early intervention* (pp. 33–63). Baltimore, MD: Paul H. Brookes Publishing Co.

Bishop, D. (2003). *Children's Communication Checklist—2.* London, England: Harcourt Assessment.

Blackstone, S., & Berg, M. (2012). *Social networks: A communication inventory for individuals with complex communication needs and their communication partners.* Verona, WI: Attainment.

Burns, M. (1996). Use of the family to facilitate communication changes in adults with neurological impairments. *Seminars in Speech and Language, 17,* 115–122.

Bzoch, K., League, R., & Brown, V.L. (2003). *The Receptive-Expressive Emergent Language Scale* (3rd ed.). Austin, TX: PRO-ED.

Coplan, J. (1993). *Early Language Milestone Scale* (2nd ed.). Austin, TX: PRO-ED.

Chapey, R., & Patterson, J. (2008). Assessment of language disorders in adults. In R. Chapey (Ed.), *Language intervention strategies in aphasia and related neurogenic communication disorders* (5th ed., pp. 64–160). Philadelphia, PA: Lippincott Williams & Wilkins.

Cress, C. (2004). Augmentative and alternative communication and language: Understanding and responding to parents' perspectives. *Topics in Language Disorders, 24,* 51–61.

Diaz-Rico, L.T., & Weed, K.Z. (1995). *The crosscultural, language, and academic development handbook.* Boston, MA: Allyn & Bacon.

Donahue-Kilburg, G. (1992). *Family-centered early intervention for communication disorders.* New York, NY: Aspen Publishers.

Eichten, P. (2000). *Help me talk: Parent's guide to speech & language stimulation techniques for children 1–3 years* (2nd ed.). Richmond, VA: Pi Communication Materials.

Ensher, G.L., & Clark, D.A. (2011). *Relationship-centered practices in early childhood.* Baltimore, MD: Paul H. Brookes Publishing Co.

Family Resource Coalition. (1996). *Guidelines for family support practice.* Chicago, IL: Author.

Fenson, L., Marchman, V.A., Thal, D., Dale, P.S., Bates, E., & Reznick, J.S. (2007). *MacArthur-Bates Communicative Development Inventories: User's guide and technical manual* (2nd ed.). Baltimore, MD: Paul H. Brookes Publishing Co.

Fox, L., Andrews, M., & Andrews, J. (2012). Self-anchored rating scales: Creating partnerships for post-aphasia change. *Perspectives on Neurophysiology and Neurogenic Speech and Language Disorders, 22*, 18–27.

Frattali, C., Holland, A., Thomson, C., Wohl, C., & Ferketic, M. (1995). *The American Speech-Language-Hearing Association Functional Assessment of Communication Skills for Adults* (ASHA FACS). Rockville, MD: American Speech-Language-Hearing Association.

Gadow, S. (1981). Advocacy: An ethical model for assisting patients with treatment decisions. In C.B. Wong & J.P. Swazey (Eds.), *Dilemmas of dying: Policies and procedures for decisions not to treat*. Boston, MA: G.K. Hall Medical Publishers.

Gelles, R.J. (1995). *Contemporary families: A sociological view*. Thousand Oaks, CA: Sage.

Gillette, Y. (2003). *Achieving communication independence*. Eau Claire, WI: Thinking Publications.

Goldenberg, I., & Goldenberg, H. (2008). *Family therapy: An overview* (7th ed.). Belmont, CA: Thomson Brooks/Cole.

Haley, K., Womack, J., Helm-Estabrooks, N., Caignon, D., & McCulloch, K. (2010). *The Life Interests and Values Cards*. Chapel Hill: University of North Carolina.

Halpern, R. (1993). Poverty and infant development. In C.H. Zeanah (Ed.), *Handbook of infant mental health* (pp. 73–86). New York, NY: Guilford Press.

Hammer, C.S. (1998). Toward a "thick description" of families: Using ethnography to overcome the obstacles to providing family-centered early intervention services. *American Journal of Speech Language Pathology, 7*, 5–22.

Hanson, M.J. (2004). Ethnic, cultural, and language diversity in intervention settings. In E.W. Lynch & M.J. Hanson (Eds.), *Developing cross-cultural competence: A guide for working with children and their families* (4th ed., pp. 3–18). Baltimore, MD: Paul H. Brookes Publishing Co.

Hanson, M.J., & Lynch, E.W. (2004). *Understanding families: Approaches to diversity, disability and risk*. Baltimore, MD: Paul H. Brookes Publishing Co.

Hidecker, M.J., Jones, R., Imig, D., & Villarruel, F. (2009) Using family paradigms to improve evidence-based practice. *American Journal Speech Language Pathology, 18*, 212–221.

Humphrey, R. (1995). Families who live in chronic poverty: Meeting the challenge of family-centered services. *American Journal of Occupational Therapy, 49*, 7.

Individuals with Disabilities Education Act Amendments of 1997 (PL 105-17), 20 U.S.C. §§ 1400 *et seq.*

Individuals with Disabilities Education Improvement Act of 2004 (PL 108-446), 20 U.S.C. §§ 1400 *et seq.*

Institute for Family-Centered Care. (2010). *Partnering with patients and family*. Retrieved from http://www.familycenteredcare.org/faq.html

Institute for Family-Centered Care. (n.d.). *Patient- and family-centered care core concepts* [Data file]. Retrieved from http://www.familycenteredcare.org/faq.html

Jackson-Maldonado, D., Thal, D.J., Fenson, L., Marchman, V.A., Newton, T., & Conboy, B. (2003). *MacArthur Inventarios del Desarrollo de Habilidades Comunicativas: User's guide and technical manual*. Baltimore, MD: Paul H. Brookes Publishing Co.

Johannsen-Horbach, H., Crone, M., & Wallesch, C. (1999). Group therapy for spouses of aphasic patients. *Seminars in Speech and Language, 20*(1), 73–82.

Johnson, B. (2000). Family-centered care: Four decades of progress. *Family Systems and Health, 18*, 137–156.

Johnson, K., & Heinze, B. (1990). *Hickory dickory talk: A family approach to infant and toddler language development*. East Moline, IL: LinguiSystems.

The Joint Commission. (2010). *Advancing effective communication, cultural competence, and patient- and family-centered care: A roadmap for hospitals*. Oakbrook Terrace, IL: Author.

Kagan, A. (1999). Supported conversation for adults with aphasia: Methods and resources for training conversation partners. *Aphasiology, 12*, 851–864.

Kreutzer, J., Leininger, B., Doherty, K., & Waaland, P. (1987). *General Health and History Questionnaire*. Richmond, VA: Medical College of Virginia, Rehabilitation Research and Training Center on Severe Traumatic Brain Injury.

Lidz, C., & Pena, E. (1996). Dynamic assessment: The model, its relevance as a non-biased approach, and its application to Latino American preschool children. *Language, Speech, and Hearing Services in Schools, 27*, 367–384.

Linder, T.W. (1993). *Transdisciplinary play-based intervention: Guidelines for developing a meaningful curriculum for young children*. Baltimore, MD: Paul H. Brookes Publishing Co.

Lomas, J., Packard, L., Bester, S., Elbard, H., Finlayson, A., & Zogharth, C. (1989). The Communicative Effectiveness Index: Development and psychometric evaluation of a functional communication measure for adult aphasia. *Journal of Speech and Hearing Disorders, 54*(1), 113–124.

Lubinski, R. (2008). Environmental systems approach to adult aphasia. In R. Chapey (Ed.), *Language intervention strategies in aphasia and related neurogenic communication disorders* (5th ed., pp. 269–296). Philadelphia, PA: Lippincott Williams & Wilkins.

Lund, N., & Duchan, J. (1993). *Assessing children's language in naturalistic contexts* (3rd ed.). Upper Saddle River, NJ: Prentice Hall.

Luterman, D. (2008). *Counseling persons with communication disorders and their families*. Austin, TX: PRO-ED.

McCarthy, C.F., McLean, L.K., Miller, J.F., Paul-Brown, D., Romski, M.A., Rourk, J.D., & Yoder, D.E. (1998). *Communication supports checklist: For programs serving individuals with severe disabilities*. Baltimore, MD: Paul H. Brookes Publishing Co.

Mize, L. (2012). *Teach me to talk therapy manual*. Retrieved from http://www.teach metotalk.com

O'Neill, D. (2007). The Language Use Inventory for Young Children: A parent-report measure of pragmatic language development for 18- to 47-month-old children. *Journal of Speech, Language, Hearing Research, 50*(1), 214–228.

Parks, S. (Ed.). (1990). *HELP... at home*. Palo Alto, CA: VORT.

The Patient Protection and Affordable Care Act of 2010 (PL 111-148), 42 U.S.C. §§ 300gg *et seq.*

Paul, D., Frattali, C., Holland, A., Thompson, C., Caperton, C., & Slater, S. (2004). *Quality of Communication Life Scale*. Rockville, MD: American Speech-Language-Hearing Association.

Paul, R., & Norbury, C. (2012). *Language disorders from infancy through adolescence* (4th ed.). St. Louis, MO: Mosby.

Pepper, J., & Weitzman, E. (2004). *It takes two to talk: A practical guide for parents of children with language delays*. Toronto, Canada: Hanen Centre.

Pollens, R. (2004). Role of the speech-language pathologist in palliative hospice care. *Journal of Palliative Medicine, 7*(5), 694–702.

Purdy, M., & Hindenlang, J. (2005). Educating and training caregivers of persons with aphasia. *Aphasiology, 19*(35), 377–388.

Rini, D., & Whitney, G. (1999). Family-centered practice for children with communication disorders. In R. Paul (Ed.), *Child and adolescent psychiatric clinics of North America: Language disorders* (pp. 153–174). Philadelphia, PA: W.B. Saunders.

Rosin, P., Whitehead, A.D., Tuchman, L.I., Jesien, G.S., Begun, A.L., & Irwin, L. (1996). *Partnerships in family-centered care: A guide to collaborative early intervention*. Baltimore, MD: Paul H. Brookes Publishing Co.

Rossetti, L. (2005). *The Rossetti Infant–Toddler Language Scale*. East Moline, IL: LinguiSystems.

Rowland, C., & Schweigert, P. (1993). *Analyzing the communication environment*. Tucson, AZ: Communication Skill Builders.

Schrader, M. (1988). *Parent articles: Enhance parent involvement in language learning*. Tucson, AZ: Communication Skill Builders.

Shipley, K.G., & McAfee, J.G. (2009). *Assessment in speech-language pathology* (4th ed.). Clifton Park, NY: Delmar Cengage Learning.

Sorin-Peters, R. (2003). Viewing couples living with aphasia as adult learners: Implications for promoting quality of life. *Aphasiology, 17*(4), 405–416.

Sparrow, S., Balla, D., & Ciccetti, D. (2005). *Vineland Adaptive Behavior Scales* (2nd ed.). Circle Pines, MN: AGS Publishing.

Trivette, C., & Dunst, C. (2007). Capacity-building family-centered helpgiving practices. *Winterberry Research Reports, 1*(1), 1–10.

Wahrborg, P., & Bornstein, P. (1989). Family therapy in families with an aphasic member. *Aphasiology, 3*, 93–98.

Wetherby, A.M., & Prizant, B.M. (2002). *Communication and symbolic behavior scales: Developmental profile*. Baltimore, MD: Paul H. Brookes Publishing Co.

World Health Organization. (2002). *International Classification of Functioning, Disability and Health* (ICF). Retrieved from http://www.who.int/classifications/icf/en

Worrall, L. (1992). *Everyday communicative needs assessment*. Queensland, Australia: Department of Speech and Hearing,

Ylvisaker, M., & Feeney, T. (1998). *Collaborative brain injury intervention: Positive everyday routines*. San Diego, CA: Singular Publishing Group.

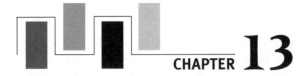

CHAPTER 13

Research in Clinical Practice

Procedures for Development
of Single-Case Experimental Designs

Geralyn R. Timler and Michelle S. Bourgeois

Geralyn R. Timler and Michelle S. Bourgeois

CHAPTER OBJECTIVES

After reading this chapter, students will be able to

- Define the components of single-case experimental designs
- State the importance of continuous and reliable measurement of client progress
- Describe elements of a comprehensive treatment protocol
- Discuss procedures for implementation of single-case experimental designs in clinical settings

---

Brooke is a speech-language pathologist (SLP) employed in a nonprofit community speech and hearing clinic. Her caseload primarily consists of preschoolers and school-age children with a variety of communication needs, many of whom have autism spectrum disorder (ASD). To keep current about the latest trends in autism research, Brooke and her colleagues meet monthly to discuss one or more journal articles related to interventions for children with ASD. Brooke uses knowledge obtained from these readings and discussions as well as her own experiences with past clients to develop, implement, and modify assessment and intervention plans for her current caseload. She regularly reports assessment and intervention data to family members, health care and educational agencies, and insurance companies.

Brooke's daily professional activities are typical of many practicing SLPs. Brooke regularly treats multiple clients with similar communication needs. She strives to develop effective and time-efficient assessment and intervention protocols. Brooke also must provide valid and reliable clinical data in her diagnostic and progress reports to concerned family members and interested third-party payers. Although Brooke sees herself primarily as a clinician, many of the daily professional activities that Brooke performs parallel those of clinical researchers who investigate assessment and intervention practices in communication sciences and disorders. Brooke (and you, the reader) may be surprised to learn that with careful thinking and planning, something that many conscientious clinicians already do daily, research activities can be integrated into clinical practice. Integration of these activities can provide important contributions to one's own clinical knowledge and to the evidence base for clinical practice via publication in professional journals.

In this chapter, we describe how clinicians can apply research evidence and their own clinical experience to develop *replicable* **single-case experimental design** studies. A study is replicable when the implementation of the study's protocol can be repeated by other clinicians or by the same clinician with a new client and similar outcomes or results are demonstrated. Replicable single-case studies are characterized by explicit description of **assessment** procedures, one or more **target behaviors,** and treatment procedures, as well as consistent measurement of the client's progress. The primary objectives of single-case experimental designs are to determine whether a treatment is effective and how much treatment is needed to reveal the desired effectiveness (Robey, 2004). When measurement and treatment procedures are implemented consistently and systematically, the data obtained from these designs can be used to inform clinical decision making. For example, these designs address such important clinical questions as "Did the treatment change my client's performance?" "Should I 'tweak' one or more of the treatment procedures for my next client?" "How many treatment sessions were needed before my client demonstrated the new behavior outside of therapy?" The ultimate goals of creating explicit, systematic, and therefore replicable clinical procedures and measures are threefold: 1) to provide valid and reliable **evaluation** and documentation of a client's progress; 2) to replicate the assessment and **treatment protocol** with other clients who have similar communication goals; and 3) to provide evidence of data-based "effective" treatments for you, your colleagues, and a wider clinical community. In short, replicable assessment and treatment protocols facilitate more effective and efficient services for our clients.

In the discussion that follows, we describe the components of single-case experimental designs and provide strategies for implementing these designs in clinical settings. First, the phases, or time components, of single-case experimental designs are explained. Second, procedures for continuous measurement of behavior change are outlined. Third, we advocate for developing treatment manuals so that the treatment is delivered consistently and systematically, increasing the likelihood that the treatment effects will be replicated with other clients or behaviors. Finally, we return to Brooke, the SLP in the community clinic, to describe how she used a single-case design to implement a treatment protocol for a 6-year-old with ASD. We also provide an example of a single-case experimental design developed for an adult with a degenerative memory disorder. These examples illustrate how to develop and implement single-case experimental designs for support of **evidence-based practice** and clinical decision making.

SINGLE-CASE CLINICAL EXPERIMENTAL DESIGNS

Clinical researchers in communicative sciences and disorders use group and single-case experimental designs to evaluate the efficacy of a treatment. Within group approaches, the researcher compares the performance of one group to one or more other groups of research participants. By randomly assigning participants to treatment and comparison groups, the groups should be equivalent, varying in similar ways for characteristics such as age, gender, income level, developmental level, and severity of the disorder. In many group design studies, the researcher implements a treatment protocol that already has some support in the research literature, perhaps from published single-case design studies. In fact, group studies are usually attempted only after the feasibility and effectiveness of the treatment protocol has been demonstrated in single-case or small-sample studies (Robey, 2004). One group receives a particular type of treatment while the other group(s) receives no treatment or a different treatment. Pretreatment and posttreatment measures are administered to evaluate changes in group performance. Data from the groups are analyzed. If significant posttreatment differences are detected among the groups, the results provide evidence for the efficacy of the treatment. Group design studies require much time and effort for the activities of participant recruitment and matching, treatment implementation, measurement, and analysis. Therefore, group studies are attempted only after evidence for the effectiveness of the treatment has been demonstrated by single-case studies.

Single-case experimental designs focus on a small sample of participants and the changes observed within each participant rather than differences among groups of participants. In single-case designs, the clinician documents changes in an individual participant's performance by measuring behaviors repeatedly and periodically over time. This documentation parallels the practices of routine clinical data gathering. In particular, the clinician observes whether one or more behaviors change in response to the treatment procedures within and across treatment sessions. The clinician also monitors the degree of the client's change over time to determine if this change is sufficient to warrant the termination of treatment.

The phrase *single-case design* is somewhat of a misnomer. Although some single-case studies document the performance of a single individual, it is the repeated measurement of an individual's performance, rather than the analysis of a group's performance at one time point, that provides specific information about the target behavior. Most published single-case studies include replication of the treatment effects with a minimum of three or more participants or for several different target behaviors in one or more individuals. Only if desired behavior changes are demonstrated repeatedly with other clients or target behaviors when and only when treatment is implemented can one be confident that the treatment is responsible for the observed behavior changes. Treatment effects must be replicated with another client or target behavior before the treatment is considered to be responsible for the observed behavior changes.

The first step in single-case research is to ask two clinical questions: "Will this specific treatment protocol improve the target behaviors of a client with these specific characteristics?" and "Will these improvements maintain over time?" To answer these questions, the clinician must understand well the clients for whom the specific treatment has a reasonable expectation to effect the target behavior. He or she must have had some success with the treatment improving the target behavior with similar clients, or some reasonable expectation, from learning about the treatment's success with other clients, that the treatment will improve the current client's behavior. Essentially, clinicians ask these questions and make these clinical decisions every day for their "single cases." For each individual client, clinicians identify treatment targets through assessment procedures, gather **baseline** performance data on the targets, apply the treatment procedures, evaluate performance change during treatment, and decide when the target has improved sufficiently to terminate treatment. If successful, the treatment is then applied to another target behavior, monitored throughout treatment, with the expectation that the treatment effects seen on the first target will be replicated with the second behavior. To gather evidence of a treatment's effectiveness, clinicians can accumulate examples of several successful replications of this process with multiple clients and share these results with other clinicians who may want to replicate these treatment outcomes with their own clients. For this replication process to occur, clinicians need to have well-defined assessment, treatment, and measurement protocols in written form (i.e., a treatment or protocol manual) to share with others.

There are many types of single-case experimental designs. We highlight one basic design here, the AB(A) design. Resources for more in-depth discussion of other single-case designs are provided at the end of this chapter. The AB(A) design is a relatively common single-case design in clinical research. Each of the letters represents a specific time, or phase, in the research study. The first *A* in AB(A) designs represents the baseline phase, or the pretreatment phase. The second phase, *B*, is the treatment phase; this phase begins as soon as a stable baseline has been documented and treatment is initiated. The last *(A)* is the return to baseline or treatment withdrawal phase; this phase includes all measurement sessions of the target behavior after the treatment for that behavior has been terminated. During each phase, data are collected continuously on the target behavior, that is, the behavior that the treatment protocol is designed to change. The target behavior is the focus of the short-term **behavioral objectives** that clinicians develop when a client's treatment goals are identified. The target behaviors are operationally defined to include the context and method of measurement and observation for that behavior (see the measurement section for details about development of operational definitions). Some examples of target behaviors include increased sentence length, elimination of off-topic comments, reduction in temper tantrums, and correct /s/ production. In clinical research designs, the target behavior is the **dependent variable** because this behavior is hypothesized to change as a result of the treatment. The treatment is the **independent variable** because this is the variable manipulated by the clinician. Further details about each of the ABA phases follow.

Baseline Phase

Kazdin (2011) suggests that the baseline A phase serves two purposes. First, the baseline phase provides descriptive information about the client's existing level of performance for one or more target behaviors. In other words, how frequently or how adequately does a client demonstrate the behavior of interest? Second, baseline data can be used to predict the client's immediate and future performance of the target behavior. Baseline data that demonstrate a consistent increase (e.g., a toddler producing more two-word sentences each subsequent session) or decrease of the target behavior (e.g., an adult demonstrating fewer perseverations or repetition of the same words over time) suggest that the client may be changing without intervention.

The stability and the trend of baseline data provide descriptive and predictive information. A *stable baseline* is characterized by little, if any change in the frequency or duration of the behavior of interest. The client may be performing the behavior of interest at very high levels (e.g., a large number of correct /r/ productions at the word level) or at very low levels (e.g., number of labels produced by an adult with aphasia during a word retrieval task), but minimal change is observed across the baseline sessions. *Trend* refers to the slope or pattern of change in the target behavior based on multiple measures over time (Kazdin, 2011). Ideally, measures of the target behavior should be stable or demonstrating a trend in the undesired direction during the baseline phase (e.g., fewer instances of the target behavior). Stable or undesirable trends in performance support the need for treatment of the target behavior. The stability and trend in observations of the target behavior are related to the *variability* of the behavior. In some cases, observations of a target behavior may be so variable, with no discernible upward or downward trend, that more baseline data must be taken to reveal a pattern in the variability. In this case, the goal of treatment may be to reduce the variability rather than to eliminate the behavior altogether. One example of a communicative behavior that can be highly variable is the number of stuttered syllables per minute in an adult with a fluency disorder. The goal of the treatment might be to reduce the number of stuttered syllables to an acceptable range (thus, reducing the variability of the behavior), rather than to eliminate the behavior altogether.

The graphs in Figure 13.1 illustrate various types of baseline trends. The data in these graphs represent the number of two-word utterances produced by three toddlers during 10-minute play samples with their mothers. The first graph in Figure 13.1 demonstrates baseline data that can be described as stable with little trend for change. In the second graph, the baseline data are not stable because the target behavior appears to be increasing, thus demonstrating a trend toward more two-word productions over time. For this child, more baseline data sessions are needed to determine if the target behavior will increase without intervention over time. If the trend continues, this child does not need intervention for two-word sentence production. In the third graph, the client's behavior is highly unstable and variable. Due to the instability, it is difficult to determine the trend of the behavior, that is, whether it will continue to increase or decrease over the next few baseline sessions. If the client's performance is highly variable, the clinician may want to delay treatment on this target behavior to examine possible causes for the variability. In the case of the toddler moving into two-word sentence production, it may be that the child has learned several two-word phrases for a particular activity or play set. When the favored play activities are available, the toddler produces more two-word utterances than when less preferred activities are used. Thus, the context of the activity influences the toddler's expressive language production. Identification of context variables that contribute to increases or decreases in a client's performance can be helpful information for treatment planning.

The graphs in Figure 13.1 (particularly the graphs for Toddlers 2 and 3) underscore an important question for the clinician: "How many baseline data points should I collect before beginning the treatment phase?" Most experts recommend a minimum of "several" baseline data points, usually at least three or more (Barlow, Nock, & Hersen, 2009; Kazdin, 2011). In some published research

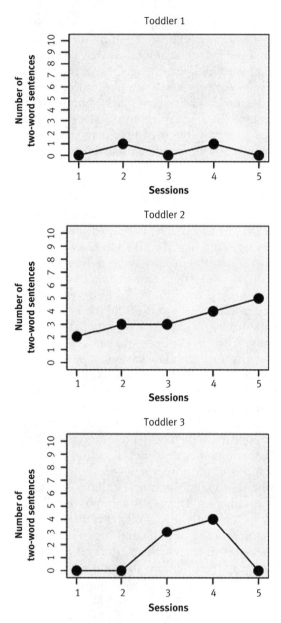

Figure 13.1.   Various trends in baseline data.

studies, the baseline phase consists of 10 or more measurement sessions before the clinical researcher is satisfied with the stability and trend of the target behavior. Clearly, it would be difficult to justify such a lengthy baseline phase in clinical practice settings. Most clinicians begin treatment immediately after one or two diagnostic sessions with their clients. One practical and creative method to collect sufficient baseline data is to have multiple activities for data collection within one treatment session. For example, if a child has multiple sound targets, data could be collected on a set of /r/ stimuli (e.g., picture cards), then during a conversation sample, followed by data collection on a set of /f/ stimuli, then a set of /r/ stimuli, then a play session, and then a set of /f/ again, and so forth. Alternating data collection on the relevant targets within a single session allows the clinician to collect multiple data points per session on the target behavior. Multiple measures of the target behavior may seem counterintuitive because clinicians are eager to begin treatment as soon as possible on all problematic communicative behaviors; however, it is important to remember that baseline data contribute important information for clinical decision making. Documentation of positive changes in a target behavior suggesting that treatment could be delayed on that behavior preserves clinical and client resources for other communicative behaviors that are unlikely to change without treatment. As such, baseline data are an important tool for assessment and intervention.

Treatment Phase

The treatment B phase begins when the target behavior is at a stable level (i.e., either not occurring or occurring infrequently or very frequently depending on the desired direction of the behavior). In clinical settings, the treatment phase usually continues until the target behavior is observed at the desired level of performance; this is referred to as a *performance-based termination criterion*. Treatment is provided until the client has achieved a predetermined level of accuracy or performance (e.g., correct production of /r/ 80% of the time in spontaneous conversation across three sessions). The treatment is terminated when the client meets the criterion.

One alternative to performance-based termination is time-based criteria. Time-based criteria are used in some published treatment protocols (e.g., a predefined number of sessions and weeks for a published literacy program or voice program). In these cases, treatment is terminated based on the number of sessions rather than client performance. If the client continues to require treatment, the clinician might change to a different treatment protocol or add more sessions to the treatment than originally planned. In most clinical settings, treatment is usually not terminated until the client's performance of the target behavior is at acceptable levels. Thus, performance-based termination criteria are preferable to time-based criteria.

Whether the termination of treatment is based on performance or time, treatment data are examined carefully and continuously throughout the treatment phase. Effective treatments facilitate an increase (or decrease) in the target behavior over time. If the clinician does not see a change in the desired direction, the treatment protocol may be modified. Treatment data inform clinical decision making about the efficacy of treatment procedures.

Withdrawal Phase

The final (A) phase of an AB(A) design is the return to baseline or treatment withdrawal phase. Data collected during this phase may be described differently depending on the clinician's hypotheses about potential changes in the target behavior after treatment has ended. If the clinician hypothesizes that the frequency or duration of the target behavior will return to baseline levels when treatment is terminated, the data from this phase are sometimes called "withdrawal" data. In this case, the return to baseline levels supports the hypothesis that the treatment—and not something else such as maturation or a new medication— was responsible for the change in the target behavior. For example, one of the treatment strategies for a child learning to interact with his peers might include a picture checklist to remind him about the steps for starting a conversation. During the withdrawal phase, the checklist is removed, and subsequently the child's peer interactions decrease. The clinician interprets this reduction as preliminary evidence for the efficacy of the checklist in supporting the child's conversation behaviors. Clinicians who implement a withdrawal phase and are looking for a return to baseline performance frequently include a second treatment phase (i.e., the ABAB design) to reinstate the desired behavior. The expectation is that the target behavior will return to levels observed during the first treatment phase. Such findings also support the efficacy of the treatment because the effects of the treatment are replicated in the second treatment phase. Replications document treatment efficacy and provide better and stronger evidence than does an ABA design alone. Replications with a multiple-baseline design with baselines staggered in length provide even much stronger evidence than repeated AB designs (an example of a multiple-baseline design study is provided in the adult **case study** at the end of this chapter).

Alternatively, if the researcher hypothesizes that the target behavior will remain at levels similar to those observed in the treatment phase or if the behavior will continue to improve, the data may be described as *maintenance data*. In this case, the clinician hypothesizes that the treatment has changed the client (or the client has learned a new skill), so the target behavior is mastered and treatment is no longer needed for that target. For example, a treatment protocol for an adult with a voice disorder may include strategies to reduce abusive vocal behaviors. The adult learns to use these strategies independently during the treatment phase and subsequently, the maintenance data from the withdrawal phase reveal improved voice production.

Target behaviors that interfere with learning, such as hitting, hand flapping, and interrupting, are behaviors that frequently require ongoing treatment in the forms of environmental supports to sustain desirable levels of the behavior. Treatments that provide positive support for alternative "replacement" behaviors are used to reduce negative target behaviors (Halle, Ostrosky, & Hemmeter, 2006). For example, temper tantrums and hitting observed in some individuals with disabilities may be reduced when the individual is offered a choice of activities or a picture schedule to help the individual prepare for transitions to a new activity. If the treatment is removed (in this case, the treatment is the environmental supports), undesirable levels of the target behavior may return.

Many treatments in communication sciences and disorders are designed to change the individual by teaching the individual a new skill or behavior. For example, clinicians expect clients to "learn" phoneme and language targets. Removal of the treatment does not eliminate the client's behaviors because the treatment changes the clients in ways that cannot be reversed. As such, the client's level of the target behavior is maintained even after the treatment is withdrawn. The data obtained in the treatment withdrawal phase is then referred to as maintenance data; sometimes this phase is then called the *maintenance phase* (instead of the withdrawal phase although the withdrawal of the treatment is implied here). In clinical settings, many clinicians use the time after treatment to assess whether the maintenance of the target behavior remains at levels observed during the treatment phase. A clinician may monitor the client's progress on the target behavior and simultaneously begin treatment on a new target behavior. Alternatively, a clinician might dismiss a client from the caseload because the client has met all treatment goals but asks the client to return for periodic reassessments to monitor that the client's progress is maintained over time.

MEASUREMENT IN SINGLE-CASE EXPERIMENTAL DESIGNS

In single-case research, the individual's performance of the target behavior is compared, not to the performance of others in a specific group but to the individual's own performance over time. Therefore, a necessary element of single-case experimental design is continuous and reliable measurement of the target behavior. There are several important steps in this process. First, the client is assessed and the target behavior is identified. Next, an operational definition for the target behavior is developed, including a method to measure this behavior in the baseline, treatment, and posttreatment phases (Kazdin, 2011). Finally, the **reliability** of the measurement method is examined.

Assessment and Identification of the Target Behavior

A variety of assessment methods have been developed to diagnose, assess, and inform treatment planning for individuals with communication disorders. Clinicians use **norm-referenced tests** to describe a client's overall abilities and to identify the presence or absence of a communication disorder. In clinical research, it is important to use the same norm-referenced test(s) for all clients who will receive the treatment being evaluated in order to document potential differences in client characteristics. Examination of client characteristics is particularly important when two or more clients demonstrate very different responses to the same treatment.

Although norm-referenced scores provide a picture of the client's overall abilities, these scores usually provide limited information for treatment planning because multiple samples of the behavior of interest are needed (Paul & Norbury, 2012). Moreover, scores from norm-referenced tests may not be sensitive to changes in the specific treatment targets because norm-referenced tests focus on a broad base of skills. Additional assessment tools are therefore required for treatment planning. Some frequently used tools for treatment planning include **criterion-referenced assessments** (e.g., conversation samples); developmental checklists; informal clinical protocols; dynamic assessment protocols; parent, teacher, and self-report measures; and behavioral observations. The information obtained from these tools is used to identify behaviors to be addressed in treatment. For example, administration of a norm-referenced articulation test might identify that a client has an articulation disorder. Item analysis of the client's responses on this test reveals that the client has difficulties with /r/ production. The clinician collects more samples of the client's /r/ production across various tasks and settings, including a conversation sample, an informal clinical task comprised of

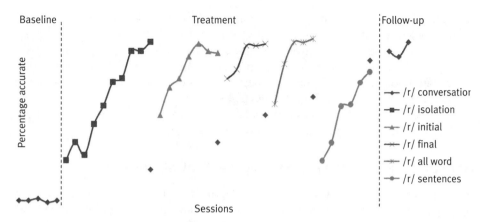

Figure 13.2. An ABA study for treatment of /r/ production. Treatment and probe data (i.e., /r/ production in a 5-minute conversation with a peer) are presented. Note that the client first demonstrates generalization of correct /r/ production in Session 15.

10 pictured /r/ words, and an observation of the child in a small-group interaction activity in the classroom. Through these multiple procedures, the clinician documents that the child has a persistent problem with /r/ production. Thus, correct /r/ production in conversation is identified as a treatment target. Baseline data collection will consist of multiple repetitions of these assessment procedures in order to document the stability of the target behavior in different conversations. Figure 13.2 illustrates a useful way to graph assessment and treatment data for an /r/ treatment program.

Operational Definition of the Target Behavior

After initial identification of the target behavior, an operational definition of this behavior, including the methods to measure the behavior, must be developed (Kazdin, 2011). This definition clearly describes the target behavior, so observers would readily agree that the behavior was present or not present (or accurate or inaccurate as dictated by the behavior). The operational definition also includes details about the context and method of observation of the target behavior, including how and when the behavior will be observed and measured. Returning to the example of /r/, an operational definition of correct /r/ production might be "Spontaneously correct /r/ production in words and sentences during a 5-minute conversation with a peer." This definition informs observers that only spontaneously correct productions of /r/ will be counted and only when those productions occur during a conversation with a peer. What if the client corrects an /r/ production after the clinician provides tongue placement cues during the conversation? According to the operational definition set for this particular client, a corrected production will not be included in the tally of correct responses. Is it useful to know that the placement cues facilitated correct production? Yes, changes in client performance in response to treatment prompts and cues reveals whether the implemented treatment strategies are effective. If the client's performance during treatment does not change, it is unlikely that changes will be observed in the operationally defined target behavior when these prompts and cues are not present. As such, clinicians use treatment data to modify and refine aspects of the treatment protocol as needed.

In clinical research, the ultimate goal of treatment is that the client performs the target behavior without clinician prompts or cues. Often, the operational definition also specifies that the target behavior must be observed when the client interacts with a set of activities, materials, or communication partners or in settings that differ from those presented in the treatment sessions. **Generalization** is the term used to describe when a client performs newly acquired skills across other materials, people (e.g., family members, teachers, peers), and settings such as home, school, recess, and workplace (Stokes & Baer, 1977). Most treatment studies report some form of *generalization probe data*, that is, data collected without prompts and cues and with generalization materials, partners, or settings. In our /r/ example in Figure 13.2, we note that correct /r/ production has begun to generalize to conversation probes with the child's peer by Session 15 of the treatment phase.

To summarize, in the treatment phase of single-case designs, two types of data are collected. Treatment data are collected during every treatment session; these are the data that reflect client performance when treatment prompts, cues, and feedback are provided. Generalization probes are also collected during the treatment phase. Generalization probes are collected less frequently than treatment data, perhaps one time per week or every other treatment session. Both treatment and probe data sets are important to examine because these data sets inform the clinician about the client's response to the treatment and the client's ability to generalize this response to nontreatment activities, settings, and partners.

Measurement Reliability

Operational definitions of target behaviors must be both accurate and reliable. An operational definition is accurate if the measure reflects all variations of the desired target behavior. If the clinician has defined the target behavior as "production of novel two-word sentences during a 10-minute play session with the caregiver," then only new two-word sentences should be counted, and two-word sentences that were produced in response to the caregiver's model should not be counted.

Reliability refers to the consistency or agreement in labeling repeated observations of the target behavior (Hegde, 2003). When observations of the presence, absence, or appropriateness of target behaviors are completed by the same person, it is called *intraobserver reliability*. For example, the clinician may count the number of novel two-word combinations during the therapy session and again later while viewing a video recording of the session to determine that the same observations were made each time. If there is good agreement (i.e., 80% or more), the clinician can be confident that the operational definition includes sufficient detail about how and when the target behavior occurs and that adequate "self" reliability is achieved.

Intraobserver reliability is important but not sufficient to document measurement reliability. *Interobserver reliability*, or agreement among two or more observers, is needed to document that the target behavior is occurring as described in the operational definition (Kennedy, 2005). In fact, treatment research cannot be published in respected journals without reporting interobserver reliability. Interobserver reliability of the dependent measures is established prior to the start of the study. This is done by developing and piloting the operational definition, including the methods for scoring or coding the behavior, and then recruiting a second observer to learn the definitions and independently count or code the behaviors. One simple way to examine agreement between two observers is to compare the datasheets from both observers and mark any disagreements in red ink on the second observer's sheet. To calculate the interobserver agreement, the total number of agreements is counted and this number is divided by the sum of the total number of agreements plus disagreements, and then multiplied by 100 (Rosenthal & Rosnow, 2008). This formula yields a percent agreement figure; percent agreement less than 80% is typically considered inadequate. Inadequate agreement indicates that more coding practice is needed or that the operational definition must be clarified. Problems with the specificity and completeness of the operational definition need to be resolved prior to collecting any study data. This often necessitates collecting additional pilot data until the observers consistently achieve 80% or above agreement.

When both observers achieve adequate agreement, the baseline phase of the study begins. Reliability checks need to be continued throughout the study on a minimum of 20% of the data collected from all phases of the study.

Reliability of the treatment delivery is also important, to ensure that treatment is being applied consistently and as planned. Is the treatment delivered in the same manner during each treatment session and for each participant? To facilitate consistent treatment delivery, treatment manuals and treatment delivery checklists are used before and during treatment.

DEVELOPMENT OF TREATMENT MANUALS AND TREATMENT CHECKLISTS

Increasingly, clinical researchers are recognizing that unclear or conflicting treatment outcomes might be related to inconsistencies in how a treatment protocol was implemented across clients (Warren, Fey, & Yoder, 2007). Therefore, it has become important to convince journal readers that the evaluated assessment and treatment protocol were standardized. *Standardization* involves explicit written description of all assessment, measurement, and treatment procedures so that these procedures can be replicated. The written protocol should include a description of all the following elements: assessment and measurement tools, the treatment schedule and dose, treatment stimuli and tasks, clinician instructions, models, prompts and feedback for correct and incorrect performance, and the criteria for the termination of treatment. Finally, a method for examination of treatment fidelity, or how closely the delivery of the treatment matches the standardized treatment protocol, must be developed. Treatment fidelity checklists are used to score the individual components of the treatment as applied by the clinician during a session. Interrater reliability of treatment application is conducted by having two observers score the session and compare their checklists for agreement (as described above). Agreement reliability below 90% would necessitate reviewing the procedures manual with the clinician and discussing treatment inconsistencies. An example of a treatment fidelity checklist is presented in Figure 13.3.

Treatment Schedule and Dose

Most clinicians are familiar with the schedule of treatment (i.e., two times a week for 30 minutes), but they may be less familiar with *treatment dose*. Treatment dose

Treatment procedures	Teacher behavior		Child behavior	
Teacher reminds Brian about report card.	Circle: Yes/No		Tally the following behaviors:	%
Teacher gives praise for sitting.	Tally: Yes IIII	Tally: No I	Sitting: IIIII	4/5 80%
Teacher gives praise for good listening.	Yes	No	Good listening:	
Teacher gives praise for hand raising.	Yes	No	Hand-raising:	
Teacher ignores inappropriate turns.	Yes	No	Inappropriate turns:	
Teacher completes Brian's report card.	Circle: Yes/No			
Teacher provides appropriate consequence for Brian's performance.	Circle: Yes/No			

Figure 13.3. Treatment fidelity checklist for Brian's treatment sessions. (*Source:* Riley-Tillman, Chafouleas, & Briesch, 2007.)

refers to the number of teaching episodes within one treatment session (Warren, Fey, & Yoder, 2007). A teaching episode is broadly defined as the clinician behavior or treatment task that is intended to elicit the target behavior. Common "teaching" episodes in speech and language interventions include strategies such as modeling, direct instruction (e.g., "Say X"), placement cues, time delay (to wait for a client response), and picture cues. Dose specification, or explicit criteria for number of teaching episodes, is important because intensity of treatment affects treatment outcomes. Recall the earlier example of the target behavior for /r/: "Spontaneously correct /r/ production in words and sentences during a 5-minute conversation with a peer." Suppose two clients of similar age and developmental level are receiving treatment for /r/ production at school. Probe data reveal that one client achieves correct /r/ production much earlier than the second client does. Potential reasons for differences in client progress could include client characteristics (e.g., attention), attendance (e.g., missed sessions), and differences in treatment dose within each session. Close examination of the treatment delivery reveals that the first client received 40 teaching episodes within each 20-minute treatment session, whereas the other client received only 20 teaching episodes within each 20-minute session. These data suggest that the first client's rapid progress, in comparison to the second client's progress, may be due to differences in treatment intensity within each of the treatment sessions. As this example illustrates, it is important for clinicians to specify the number (or approximate range) of teaching episodes within a treatment session.

How many teaching episodes should be included in a session? The answer to this question varies according to the target behavior that is to be changed. It is likely that more teaching episodes can be delivered for articulation targets than for targets related to language, particularly in the area of pragmatics (Warren, Fey, & Yoder, 2007). Some assistance for informing clinical decisions about treatment dose can be found in recently published treatment efficacy studies because study authors are now more likely to include details about treatment dose in their manuscripts.

Treatment Stimuli and Tasks

Clinicians use a variety of materials and activities to teach communicative behaviors. In order to replicate a treatment protocol, the specific materials and activities to be implemented during the treatment must be described. Does this mean that all clients who receive the treatment must receive identical materials and activities in the same sequence? No! Client preference should be taken into consideration so that the client is actively engaged in the treatment activities. If a client is not interested in an activity, limited progress will be observed. Therefore, most treatment protocols include a set of equivalent materials and activities to allow for client preferences. For replication purposes, it is necessary to describe the procedures used for identification of client preference. Does a nonverbal client choose an activity from a set of pictures? Does a toddler's caregiver identify favorite toys? Does the adult with aphasia initiate a topic of conversation for the day from current news? Does the child with a learning disability select which textbook he or she will use to review a lesson about identification of main ideas in a paragraph? Systematic replication of the protocol is facilitated when clinicians provide explicit details about the procedures for selection and the set of potential activities and materials.

Clinician Directions, Models, Prompts, and Feedback

The instructions, models, prompts, and feedback that a clinician is to provide within and across the treatment sessions should be described. Teaching episodes in speech and language treatments frequently include a number of clinician prompts and feedback to elicit and facilitate a client's performance. When multiple types of prompts are used, it is important to describe the hierarchy of the prompts. For example, many treatment protocols for teaching turn-taking skills in preschoolers call for the clinician to provide an indirect model (e.g., "I think Steve has the crayon that you need"), followed by a direct request if the client does not respond to the indirect model (e.g., "Say, Steve, could I have the crayon?"). Treatment protocols for speech sound and articulation targets frequently use a series of prompts, from placement cues, to visual cues, to requests for direct imitation of a model. Recall that the ultimate goal of treatment is that the client produces the target behavior without prompts and cues. As such, it is important to deliver the prompts in such a way that a client does not become *prompt dependent*, or unable to produce a correct response until a prompt is given. Systematic delivery of prompts from least supportive to most supportive may prevent or reduce prompt dependency (Timler, Vogler-Elias, & McGill, 2007). The type and order of prompts, including the feedback to be provided if the client is nonresponsive or incorrect, should be described in the treatment manual.

Criterion for Termination of Treatment

Clinicians must decide whether to use a performance-based or time-based criterion for termination of the treatment. In clinical practice settings, the performance-based criterion is preferred because clinicians usually treat clients until communication skills are mastered. The treatment protocol should include descriptions of potential scenarios for early termination of treatment. For example, if a treatment protocol calls for 6 weeks of implementation, but the client's performance of the target behavior reaches the desired level at Week 2 of the treatment, the treatment protocol should allow for early termination of the treatment. Similarly, the treatment protocol should also include recommendations for terminating the treatment earlier than anticipated if the client is not responsive to the treatment or if the client's level of performance actually decreases during the treatment. For example, if a nonverbal toddler does not produce words or imitate vocalizations within the early sessions of a verbal modeling treatment, the clinician might decide to terminate the treatment or modify the treatment protocol to include addition of other treatment procedures such as the introduction of an augmentative communication system.

Treatment Fidelity

Treatment fidelity, or how closely a standardized treatment protocol is implemented, can be examined using a written checklist of the procedures in the protocol. An observer views the treatment session and notes whether each procedure was observed and implemented correctly. The percentage of correctly implemented procedures is calculated; at least 90% treatment fidelity across multiple treatment sessions is desired. The procedures in the checklist are usually scored as observed or not observed; treatment fidelity is then tallied in a manner similar to the procedures described in the reliability section. As with reliability of the target behavior, reliability of treatment fidelity needs to be established prior to beginning the treatment phase. Clinicians usually spend ample time learning the treatment procedures, but often they do not measure how well they actually adhere to the protocol during the study. The more explicit the treatment descriptions and reliability checks, the more likely it is that the clinician and the wider clinician community will be persuaded that changes in the target behavior are due to the treatment rather than to some extraneous factor.

HYPOTHETICAL CHILD CASE STUDY

Brooke serves children with autism in small-group and individual settings. She conducts an intensive summer social language program for young school-age children with high-functioning autism (HFA). One summer, she meets Brian, a 6-year-old with HFA, who with two other boys is enrolled in a thrice-weekly 2-hour conversation group. Unfortunately, Brian's behaviors keep him from participating fully in the program. During large-group instruction time at the beginning of each session, Brian often disrupts the attention of his peers by shouting out answers and ignoring Brooke's requests to wait his turn to speak. Whereas his peers find this entertaining, Brooke does not. Brooke consults with Brian's school **psychologist,** and the two of them decide to implement a treatment to improve Brian's turn-taking skills in the summer program.

Assessment Protocol

When Brooke met Brian, he already had a confirmed **diagnosis** of an ASD. Brooke's assessment protocol focused on tools to describe his language abilities, social skills, and problem behaviors. The protocol included a comprehensive language battery to identify his overall abilities in expressive and receptive language; conversational language sampling to document functional communication abilities in syntax, semantics, and pragmatics; and parent- and teacher-report measures to describe his social skills and problem behaviors. These tools revealed that Brian's language skills were generally within normal limits in syntax and semantics. Analysis of conversation samples and a parent-report measure indicated Brian had a pragmatic **language disorder.** Parent- and teacher-report measures revealed significant levels of behavioral concerns at home and school.

Operational Definition of the Target Behavior

Brian's behavioral goal focused on increasing appropriate turn-taking skills. One of the target behaviors for this goal was to replace Brian's "shouting out" behaviors with raising his hand when he wanted to say something during the opening activity in the conversation group. The operational definition of the target behavior was as follows: "Brian will decrease the number of times that he takes a turn inappropriately during large-group instruction to one time per activity. Brian will raise his hand to signal that he wants to answer or ask a question in the small group." Note that this operational definition does not focus on the content of Brian's answers and questions. The target behavior is observed whenever Brian raises his hand even if his comment or question is not correct. This operational definition required that data be collected for both the inappropriate behavior of shouting out as well as the replacement behavior of hand raising. Accordingly, both behaviors were tracked during the baseline, treatment, and treatment withdrawal phases.

Treatment Protocol

The treatment for the target behavior consisted of two major components: clinician praise and child reinforcement. The list of implemented treatment procedures within each session are found in the treatment fidelity checklist in Figure 13.3. Clinician praise focused on attending to and praising group members who demonstrated good listening and turn-taking skills. For example, when the clinician asked a question, she would state the names of the children who were quietly listening and who raised their hands. If Brian commented without raising his hand, she ignored his response. The child reinforcement component included use of a daily behavior report card (Riley-Tillman, Chafouleas, & Briesch, 2007). The report card was developed by Brooke and Brian together, and the card focused on three task compliance behaviors. For example, one behavior was stated as "Brian raised his hands two times or more during the opening activity." Each behavior was rated by Brooke as yes or no at the end of a treatment session. If all behaviors were rated as a yes, Brian received a small prize.

The treatment termination criterion was defined by Brooke and the school psychologist as "Brian will demonstrate one occurrence or less of inappropriate turn-taking and Brian will raise his hand at least two times during the opening activity for three consecutive treatment sessions."

Results

The graph in Figure 13.4 displays the results of the ABAB design. Detailed instructions for graph construction can be found in Dixon et al. (2009). The operational definition of the target behavior necessitated tracking two behaviors: inappropriate turns and the replacement behavior of hand raising. The baseline phase was comprised of five sessions. Baseline probes revealed a flat and stable trend for hand raising; Brian did not raise his hand at all during the opening activity of the 2-hour

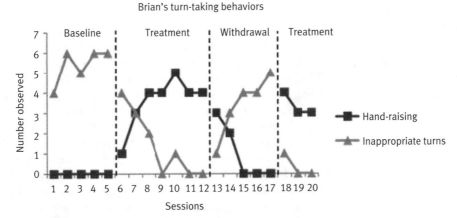

Figure 13.4. Hypothetical results for an ABAB single-case experimental study implemented to change turn-taking behaviors. Note that in the withdrawal phase, the target behavior returned to baseline levels. The treatment effects were then replicated in the second treatment phase because the target behavior once again improved in the desired direction. (*Source:* Riley-Tillman, Chafouleas, & Briesch, 2007.)

conversation session. The number of Brian's inappropriate turns was somewhat variable because his talkativeness varied from session to session. The treatment was initiated during Session 6. Treatment phase data revealed that Brian raised his hand for the first time as soon as the treatment was initiated. Brian met the termination by Session 11 because Brian had three consecutive sessions of one or no inappropriate turns and raised his hand multiple times during these sessions. Note that treatment was delivered during Session 12 and that the withdrawal phase began with Session 13. Treatment withdrawal included elimination of the daily report card. Treatment withdrawal probes revealed that Brian's use of the target behavior began to return to pretreatment levels; that is, at Session 13 he began to take inappropriate turns with an upward trend in the number of inappropriate turns and stopped raising his hand to signal that he wanted a turn. Brooke and the school psychologist decided to reinstate use of the daily report card for a second treatment phase (the second B of an ABAB design) during Session 18. Treatment data from this second treatment phase revealed a return of Brian's hand-raising behaviors with a simultaneous decrease in the number of inappropriate turns. The replication of the treatment effects in the second B phase provided support for the efficacy of this behavior treatment for Brian. The school psychologist intended to replicate the treatment in a new setting in September when Brian returned to school.

HYPOTHETICAL ADULT CASE STUDY

Robin was providing clinical services to senior adults in an assisted living facility where the staff were concerned that John was not making friends and adjusting to his new living arrangements. John's diagnosis of vascular dementia was thought to be the reason for his reluctance to join in group activities or to have a conversation with other residents of the facility. The director of nursing asked, "Can the conversation skills of individuals with dementia be improved?" Robin decided to evaluate a treatment she had recently read about for improving the specific conversational behaviors of persons with dementia: the use of a memory book during conversational interactions.

Assessment Protocol

Robin first reviewed John's medical chart to confirm the dementia diagnosis. She determined that John had not received any previous services from an SLP, nor had he had a comprehensive neuropsychological assessment. In order to plan treatment to improve conversation skills, she needed to assess John's hearing, vision, cognitive status, conversation, and reading skills. An informal communication **screening** measure of functional hearing and functional vision, as well as a 5-minute structured conversation sample (Bourgeois, Dijkstra, Burgio, & Allen-Burge, 2001), was administered to determine his responsiveness to conversational situations. Cognitive testing documented the severity level of John's dementia. A reading screening test (Bourgeois, 1992) confirmed his ability to read sentences in a memory aid. In addition, he produced content words (i.e., nouns, verbs, adjectives) on a picture description subtest of an aphasia battery, confirming his responsiveness to visual stimuli in a memory aid.

Operational Definition of the Target Behavior

The goal of John's intervention was to improve his conversation skills. The operational definition of the target behavior was that "John will increase the number of unambiguous on-topic statements of fact (Novel statements) when using a memory aid in conversations with a familiar partner." The criterion for treatment success was an increase in level and trend in the frequency of the statements compared to baseline levels of the target behavior upon visual inspection of the graph. In order to track this target behavior, Robin developed codes and definitions for appropriate and inappropriate verbal behaviors (e.g., novel statements of fact, utterances comprised of "empty speech") and codes for verbal behaviors related to the memory book (Memory book statements read aloud). A sample of some of the codes is presented in Table 13.1.

Baseline Phase

Before treatment began, baseline sessions were conducted to determine the frequency of the target behavior. The clinician met with John on a daily basis and conducted a 5-minute conversation with the following prompts: "Tell me about your family," "Tell me about your life," or "Tell me about your day." She

Table 13.1.   Sample of verbal behavior codes used in memory book treatment

M	Memory aid statements: Must be one of the thirty memory aid items; must be intelligible, unambiguous, and use exact wording
N	Novel statements: Must be an intelligible and unambiguous statement of fact contributing additional content related to one of the training topics and/or training stimuli
A	Ambiguous utterances: Must be an intelligible utterance that is ambiguous because of one or more of the following: • Empty phrase: A phrase or common idiom contributing no content to the discourse • Indefinite term: Utterances containing highly nonspecific nouns (e.g., *stuff*, *thing*, *something*) • Deictic terms: Utterances containing deictic terms with unclear referents (e.g., *this*, *that*, *here*, *there*) instead of content nouns • Pronouns without antecedents: The use of pronouns without referents specified previously
U	Unintelligible utterances: Sentence fragments, grammatically incomplete phrases, non-English phrases, multiple joined sentence fragments

From Bourgeois, M. (1992). *Conversing with memory impaired individuals using memory aids: A memory aid workbook*. Gaylord, MI: Northern Speech Services, Inc.; adapted by permission.

tape-recorded the conversation and counted the number of each target behavior (i.e., Novel statements and Memory book statements), and she then graphed them. See Figure 13.5 for the graph of the baseline, treatment, and follow-up maintenance data for this treatment program. When she determined that John had a low and stable rate of the target behavior, "Novel statements of fact," treatment began.

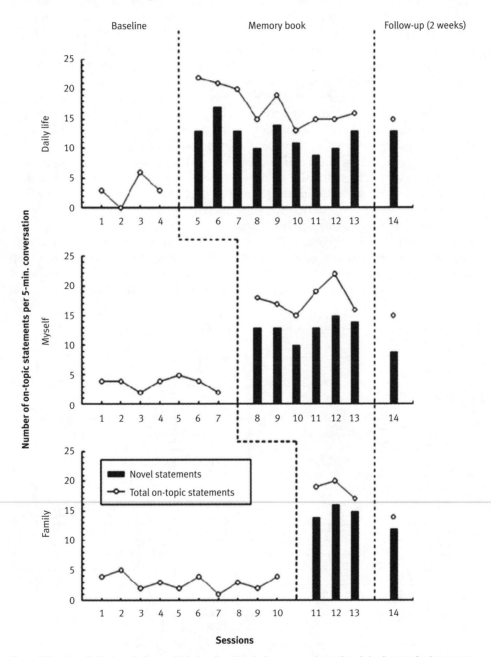

Figure 13.5. Hypothetical results for a multiple-baseline ABA single-case experimental study implemented to increase on-topic statements in a memory book treatment. Note that the implementation of the treatment phase was staggered across conversation topics to demonstrate experimental control and replication of the treatment effects.

Treatment Protocol

The method for improving conversation skills was to train the patient to use a memory aid as a compensatory strategy during conversations. Specific treatment behaviors included reading aloud sentence stimuli, describing familiar pictures, and turning pages of the memory aid. The memory aid was developed with the assistance of John's daughter, who completed a Memory Book Information form and provided photographs from the family album. The clinician made a book containing 10 pages of content, each page illustrated with a family photo, for each of three topics (My Day, My Life, My Family), with a total of 30 pages. A systematic procedure was developed for training sessions to ensure uniformity of the treatment and to enable other "therapists" to conduct the treatment. Consistent procedures were identified for introducing the session, prompting John to engage in the treatment behaviors (reading, describing, and turning pages), responding to and reinforcing correct behaviors, and correcting inaccurate behaviors. The clinician practiced these procedures, with another person role-playing a patient, until she obtained a satisfactory criterion level of performance on delivery of all program steps. The Treatment Procedures Data Sheet (Figure 13.6; Bourgeois, 1992) was used to ensure that each step of the treatment program was conducted uniformly by the clinician. The Training Data Sheet (Figure 13.7; Bourgeois, 1992) was developed to collect data on John's responses during training sessions and to ensure that he practiced each step of the program during each treatment session. Training sessions were recorded (audio or video) for reliability coding at a later time. The clinician and a second

Name:			Trainer:						Topic:		
Date:											
Topic prompt:											
"Tell me about. . ."											
Correct response:											
Reinforce											
Repeat / expand											
"What does this remind. . ?"											
+ Reinforce											
Repeat / expand											
− Model											
Incorrect: "Wait, read this"											
+ Reinforce											
Repeat / expand											
− Model											
"What else about . . . (topic) . . .?											
Record response:											

Figure 13.6. Treatment procedures data sheet to examine treatment fidelity. (From Bourgeois, M. [1992]. *Conversing with memory impaired individuals using memory aids: A memory aid workbook*. Gaylord, MI: Northern Speech Services, Inc.; reprinted by permission.)

Name:_____   Topic:_____

| | | | | | | | | |
Date:

1. My name is John Doe.
2. I am from Somerset, PA.
3. I live with my son Bob.
4. His house is in Clairton, PA.
5. Bob's wife is Marion.
6. Their oldest son is Bobby.
7. Their daughter is Misty.
8. The cat's name is Rover.
9. I spend the day with Clyde.
10. I like to read the newspaper.

"Tell me about_____(topic)_____."

Correct: "Good, your name is John Doe."
Incorrect: "Wait, read this."
No Response:
        "Say, my name is John Doe."
            "Good."

"What else does this remind you of?"

Correct: "Good, your middle name is Francis."
Incorrect / No Response:
        "Well, it reminds me that your middle
        name is Francis."

"What else about_____(topic)_____?"

Figure 13.7. Training sheet used in the memory book treatment to document client behavior during each treatment session. (From Bourgeois, M. [1992]. *Conversing with memory impaired individuals using memory aids: A memory aid workbook.* Gaylord, MI: Northern Speech Services, Inc.; reprinted by permission.)

trained coder rescored the session using the Treatment Procedures Data Sheet and the Training Data Sheet to calculate reliability of both the clinician's and John's behaviors during treatment. This procedure ensured uniformity of treatment delivery across training sessions.

Results

Robin was pleased with the results of John's treatment program for improving his conversation skills. As shown in Figure 13.5, John produced very few statements of content in baseline for any of the three topic prompts, but each time Robin added pages to his memory book on one of the three topics, he immediately read the statement and provided novel information about the picture. She was also pleased to note that John maintained his ability to converse using his memory book 2 weeks after treatment ended.

CONCLUSIONS

The components of single-case experimental designs include well-defined, explicit, and detailed descriptions of assessment, treatment, and measurement procedures. Table 13.2 provides a summary of these procedures. Clinicians who follow these procedures and who write explicit protocols will find it easier to replicate effective protocols across clients and across other treatment targets. The commitment to develop replicable protocols requires organization and planning. Although this advanced planning takes time and effort, this effort will be rewarded with data-based clinical practices that clinicians will be proud to share with colleagues, educational and health care agencies, and most important, to clients and their family members (Bourgeois, 1992). Clinicians who desire to disseminate the results of their replicated protocols by publishing in clinical research journals are strongly encouraged to find a research mentor at a local university or teaching hospital

Table 13.2.   Overview of steps for developing single-case experimental studies

A. Develop the assessment protocol.[a]

    1. Identify tools to determine client's overall communication abilities.
    2. Identify procedures for collecting multiple samples of the target behavior.

B. Develop operational definition of the target behavior.

    1. Identify the context and method for measurement of the target behavior.
    2. Train the observers.
    3. Establish adequate interobserver reliability.

C. Develop the treatment manual.[b]

    1. Determine the treatment schedule and dose, treatment stimuli and tasks, clinician instructions and models, and clinician prompts and feedback.
    2. Develop the treatment fidelity checklist to be used during each treatment session.
    3. Define criterion for termination of treatment.

D. Collect baseline probes.

    1. Monitor baseline data to determine when to begin treatment.
    2. Examine interobserver agreement of baseline data.

E. Begin the treatment phase.

    1. Record treatment data to monitor effectiveness of treatment procedures.
    2. Monitor treatment fidelity.
    3. Collect generalization probes.
    4. Continue to examine interobserver agreement for measurement of the target behavior.
    5. Monitor treatment data and generalization probes to identify when treatment termination criterion is met.

F. Begin the treatment withdrawal phase.

    1. Collect withdrawal probes; monitor data to determine whether these data reveal reversal or maintenance of the progress observed in the treatment phase.
    2. Reinstate a second treatment phase if needed.

G. Replicate the assessment and treatment protocol by doing one or more of the following:

    1. Implement the treatment protocol during a second treatment phase (i.e., ABAB design) for the same target behavior.
    2. Implement the treatment protocol for another target behavior with the same client.
    3. Implement the treatment protocol with another client who has similar communication needs.

H. Share your results with the client, family members, and colleagues.

    [a]Chapter 4 provides an overview of assessment issues.
    [b]Chapter 3 provides suggestions for how to use the evidence base to search for treatment information.

for assistance and collaboration. We provide only the basics of single-case experimental designs here. Comprehensive information about single-case experimental designs can be found in the resources listed below and by enrolling in a clinical research design course at a local university.

STUDY QUESTIONS

1. Describe the information that should be included in a comprehensive treatment manual.

2. What is the purpose of observing and documenting the target behavior multiple times during the baseline phase of a single-case experimental design?

3. In AB(A) single-case experimental design, what purpose(s) does the baseline phase serve?

   a. Baseline data provide descriptive information about the client's existing level of performance.

   b. Baseline data can be used to predict the client's immediate performance.

   c. Baseline data can be used to examine variability in client performance and possible reasons for this variability.

   d. All of the above are true.

4. In the treatment withdrawal phase of an ABA design study aimed at teaching strategies for word retrieval, a clinician hypothesizes that the target behavior will remain at levels similar to those observed in the treatment phase. The data from this phase might be called

   a. Treatment fidelity data

   b. Reversal data

   c. Maintenance data

   d. All of the above

5. When observations of the presence, absence, or appropriateness of target behaviors are completed by the same person, it is called

   a. Interobserver reliability

   b. Personal reliability

   c. Intraobserver reliability

   d. None of the above

6. Interobserver reliability should be established

   a. Prior to the start of the study

   b. During the treatment phase of the study

   c. After the treatment phase of the study

   d. None of the above

7. What are probe data?
    a. Data collected during the first phase of the ABA design
    b. Data collected during the second phase of the ABA design
    c. Data collected during all three phases of the ABA design
    d. Data collected when treatment prompts and cues are provided

8. The number of teaching episodes within one treatment session is the
    a. Treatment schedule
    b. Treatment dose
    c. Generalization probe
    d. Fidelity check

FURTHER READING

Barlow, D., Nock, M., & Hersen, M. (2009). *Single case experimental designs: Strategies for studying behavior change* (3rd ed.). Boston, MA: Pearson Education.
Hegde, M. (2003). *Clinical research in communicative disorders: Principles and strategies* (3rd ed.). Austin, TX: PRO-ED.
Kazdin, A. (2011). *Single-case research designs: Methods for clinical and applied settings* (2nd ed.). New York, NY: Oxford University Press.
Kennedy, C. (2005). *Single-case designs for educational research*. Boston, MA: Allyn & Bacon.
Kratochwill, T.R., Hitchcock, J., Horner, R.H., Levin, J.R., Odom, S. L., Rindskopf, D.M., & Shadish, W.R. (2010). *Single-case designs technical documentation*. Retrieved from What Works Clearinghouse web site, http://ies.ed.gov/ncee/wwc/pdf/wwc_scd.pdf

REFERENCES

Barlow, D., Nock, M., & Hersen, M. (2009). *Single case experimental designs: Strategies for studying behavior change* (3rd ed.). Boston, MA: Pearson Education.

Bourgeois, M. (1992). *Enhancing the conversations of memory-impaired persons: A memory aid workbook*. Gaylord, MI: Northern Speech Services.

Bourgeois, M., Dijkstra, K., Burgio, L., & Allen-Burge, R. (2001). Memory aids as an AAC strategy for nursing home residents with dementia. *Augmentative and Alternative Communication, 17*, 196–210.

Dixon, M., Jackson, J., Small, S., Horner-King, M., Lik, N., Garcia, Y., & Rosales, R. (2009). Creating single-subject design graphs in Microsoft Excel 2007. *Journal of Applied Behavior Analysis, 42*, 277–293.

Halle, J., Ostrosky, M., & Hemmeter, M. (2006). Functional communication training: A strategy for ameliorating challenging behavior. In R. McCauley & M. Fey (Eds.), *Treatment of language disorders in children* (pp. 509–546). Baltimore, MD: Paul H. Brookes Publishing Co.

Hegde, M. (2003). *Clinical research in communicative disorders: Principles and strategies* (3rd ed.). Austin, TX: PRO-ED.

Kazdin, A. (2011). *Single-case research designs: Methods for clinical and applied settings* (2nd ed.). New York, NY: Oxford University Press.

Kennedy, C. (2005). Single-case designs for educational research. Boston, MA: Allyn & Bacon.

Paul, R., & Norbury, C. (2012). *Language disorders from infancy through adolescence: Listening, speaking, reading, writing, and communication*. Philadelphia, PA: Elsevier Health Sciences.

Riley-Tillman, T., Chafouleas, S., & Briesch, A. (2007). A school practitioner's guide to using daily behavior report cards to monitor student behavior. *Psychology in the Schools, 44*, 77–89. doi:10.1002/pits.20207

Robey, R. (2004). A five-phase model for clinical-outcome research. *Journal of Communication Disorders, 37*, 401–411.

Rosenthal, R., & Rosnow, R. (2008). *Essentials of behavioral research: Methods and data analysis* (3rd ed.). New York, NY: McGraw-Hill.

Stokes, T., & Baer, D. (1977). An implicit technology of generalization. *Journal of Applied Behavior Analysis, 10,* 349–367.

Timler, G., Vogler-Elias, D., & McGill, F. (2007). Strategies for promoting generalization of social communication skills in preschoolers and school-age children. *Topics in Language Disorders, 27*(2), 163–177.

Warren, S., Fey, M., & Yoder, P. (2007). Differential treatment intensity research: A missing link to creating optimally effective communication interventions. *Mental Retardation and Developmental Disabilities Research Reviews, 13,* 70–77.

Glossary

accent   Pronunciation of a language variety.

advocacy   Steps taken by individuals or groups to understand, implement, or influence public policy.

Alzheimer's disease   A progressive disease of the brain that is characterized by impairment of memory and a disturbance in at least one other thinking function (e.g., language, perception of reality).

American Sign Language   A symbolic communication system making use of manual signs, used by deaf people to communicate.

aphasia   A language disorder resulting from brain damage and characterized by impairment of comprehension, formulation, and language use.

apraxia of speech   A disorder characterized by difficulty in performing voluntary motor acts in the absence of paralysis.

assessment   The process of collecting and analyzing data about an individual in order to make clinical decisions.

assistive technology   Tools that help an individual overcome limitations related to a disability by either enhancing the skills the individual has or by compensating for absent or nonfunctional skills.

atrophy   A wasting of tissues, organs, or the entire body.

audiogram   A graphic representation of a hearing test.

auditory brainstem evoked response audiometry   A type of electro-physiological testing designed to measure an individual's neural responses to sound. This is an objective hearing test that does not require the client's participation.

auditory brainstem response   An electrophysiological response to sound, consisting of five to seven peaks that represent neural function of auditory pathways.

augmentative and alternative communication   An area of practice that attempts to compensate temporarily or permanently for the impairment and disability patterns of individuals with severe communication disorders.

baseline   Frequency of a behavior or level of functioning prior to the initiation of treatment.

behavioral audiological test   Measure that pertains to the observation of the activity of a person in response to some stimuli.

behavioral objective   Intervention goal that specifies an action a client is to perform, the conditions under which the action will be performed, and how well the action must be performed for the objective to be achieved.

Blisssymbols   A set of visual symbols developed to serve as an alternative communication system for individuals with severe speech disorders.

bound morpheme   Unit of meaning that does not appear unless attached to another morpheme (e.g., plural /s/, past tense -*ed*).

case conference   Formal meeting involving service providers, clients, and family members in which evaluation findings, treatment outcomes, and necessary support services are discussed.

case history questionnaire   A written set of questions used as a tool to gather and organize information regarding the nature of a client's speech, language and hearing concerns, general developmental and health history, educational background, and history of related support services.

case law   Court decisions regarding disputed interpretations of laws that influence how policies are implemented in the disputed case and that also set a precedent for future practice.

case series   A collection of case studies in which several participants receive the same treatment and their outcomes are measured following the intervention.

case study design   A design in which a single individual, event, or context is intensively studied using both qualitative and quantitative data.

cerumen   Earwax; the waxy secretion in the external auditory meatus.

cleft palate   A cleft palate is an opening in the roof of the mouth in which the two sides of the palate did not fuse while the fetus was developing in utero.

closed question   Question that elicits only a yes or no or a one-word answer (e.g., "Do you have a dog?" "What did you eat for lunch?").

cluttering   A fluency disorder characterized by a rapid, irregular rate of articulation, a high frequency of dysfluencies, and reduced intelligibility.

cochlear implant   Device that enables persons with profound hearing loss to perceive sound. Consists of an electrode array surgically implanted in the cochlea, which delivers electrical signals to the eighth cranial nerve, and an external amplifier, which activates the electrodes.

code of ethics   American Speech-Language-Hearing Association and American Academy of Audiology guidelines that define clinically acceptable conduct and conscientious judgment that members are expected to internalize and apply in clinical settings.

code switching   Alternations between languages at the word, phrase, or sentence levels.

cognitive-communication disorder Any aspect of communication (e.g., listening, speaking, reading, writing, pragmatics) that is affected by disruption of cognition.

coherence The relationship of the meaning or content of an utterance to the content of previous utterances and to the overall content of the discourse.

cohesive ties Words used to mark the coherence among the parts of a message.

Commission of the Accreditation of Rehabilitation Facilities A regulatory body that oversees the quality of care provided to patients in rehabilitation facilities.

competent practice Clinician actions that include effective diagnostic procedures, an accurate prognosis, appropriate therapy strategies for the particular disorder, and ongoing analysis of client outcomes.

complex communication needs Individuals with significant speech, language, and/or cognitive impairment with limited means of conventional communication.

complex sentence Sentence that contains more than one main verb phrase. Includes sentences containing conjoined, embedded, and subordinate clauses.

conflict of interest A compromise in professional judgment in which a clinician loses his or her sense of objectivity because of personal or financial gains.

conductive hearing loss Diminished sound sensitivity due to middle ear, outer ear, or tympanic membrane pathology.

conjunction Linking word that tie ideas within and across sentences. Both coordinate (e.g., *and, but, or*) and subordinate (e.g., *when, if, because*) conjunctions are in this category.

consultative or collaborative Relates to the provision of communication services through models of both direct and indirect formats.

continuing education The act of updating clinical skills and keeping abreast of the latest trends and advances, achieved through reading textbooks and journal articles, attending workshops, shadowing professional colleagues, and participating in research activities.

continuum of care (COC) Levels of rehabilitation through which patients pass based on need and intensity of services.

continuum of naturalness The range of intervention activities, from the most highly structured to the most naturalistic.

criterion-referenced test/assessment Test or procedure that measures an individual's performance in terms of absolute levels of mastery.

criterion-related validity A measure of the extent to which performance on a test can be correlated with performance on another instrument believed to measure the same skill or behavior.

cultural sensitivity Attuning to and adjusting for the culturally determined characteristics of communication in various communities when engaging in interactions with culturally or linguistically different clients.

cystic fibrosis A genetic disease in which the body produces a thick, sticky mucus that clogs the lungs, leading to serious and life-threatening lung infections.

dedicated communication devices Assistive technology devices used solely for the purpose of communicating.

dependent variable The particular outcome of a treatment.

diagnosis Identification of a disease or disorder based on symptoms presented.

diagnostic evaluation report A written report used to summarize information obtained in both audiological and speech-language evaluations. This report serves as a legal record of assessment findings, diagnoses, and recommendations.

dialect Rule-governed and mutually intelligible form of a language characterized by social, ethnic, and geographical differences in its speakers.

differential diagnosis The process of distinguishing a disorder or condition from others with similar symptoms.

digitized speech Prerecorded speech that is digitally stored.

direct selection Device activation through the use of pointing or touching. Most commonly used by individuals with intact motor functioning.

direct services Working with a client in a hands-on format.

discharge summary A written report of a client's cumulative progress from the initiation of therapy to the discharge from service.

durable medical equipment A piece of equipment that meets criteria for coverage under Medicare and Medicaid.

dynamic display A computer screen that electronically presents symbols. Symbols are typically stored in folders. Once a folder is activated, symbols in that folder appear.

dysarthria of speech Motor speech disorder resulting from nervous system impairment.

dysfluency An interruption in the smoothness of the flow of speech (e.g., stuttering).

effect-size estimate The magnitude of a treatment's effect in standard deviation units.

electrolarynx A battery-operated instrument that makes a humming sound to help people who have lost their larynx to talk.

electronic medical records Creation, storage, and retrieval of patient/client records in digital format used to standardize documentation format and provide greater authorized access.

electronystagmography A method of measuring eye movements, especially nystagmus, to assess the integrity of the vestibular mechanism.

electrophysiological test Audiological testing procedure that measures involuntary responses to sound within the auditory nervous system.

endoscopy Visual examination of the vocal apparatus by means of a long, slender medical instrument used for examining the interior of hollow organs.

ethics The moral and/or civil codes of conduct for a particular person, situation, community, religious group, organization, or society that evolve from a philosophy of human interaction that values behaviors personally or collectively regarded as good, honest, proper, and respectable.

Ethics Calibration Quick Test A series of questions to enable clinicians to analyze the ethical propriety of a situation.

ethnographic interviewing Information gained from observations made of a family in context and told from a family's perspective.

evaluation The formal and informal procedures conducted as part of an assessment.

evidence-based practice The use of current high-quality research-based data to make clinical decisions.

experimental design Research in which the researcher randomly assigns participants to treatment groups and places rigorous control on all known variables that might influence the outcome variable so that direct influence of the intervention on a particular outcome can be assessed.

exposition facilitative play A client-centered method of intervention in which the clinician provides indirect language stimulation by modeling language forms that are related to client-initiated actions.

family-centered approach The provision of assessment and intervention from the family's point of view, taking into account family goals, dynamics, and circumstances.

fixed display Displays in which the symbols, objects, or pictures are attached to the device in a particular location.

fluency The smooth, uninterrupted flow that is typical of speech.

follow-up letter Letter written to referral sources discussing the status of the individual referred for clinical services, evaluation finding, and/or treatment outcomes.

frequency modulation amplification system An assistive listening device designed to enhance signal-to-noise ratio, in which a remote microphone–transmitter worn by a speaker sends signals via FM to a receiver worn by a listener.

functional assessments An assessment that takes into account how well an individual uses communication in activities of daily living.

functional disorders   Problems resulting in impaired communication that are derived from the way the client uses or misuses the voice and are not as a result of neurological or anatomical change or damage.

functional maintenance plan   A written plan developed by a speech-language pathologist or other rehabilitation specialist working in a Medicare-funded health care facility outlining rehabilitation supports to be provided by noncertified support staff and other caregivers.

generalization   Carryover of trained behavior into settings other than the training context.

gloss   A clinician's interpretation of the intended meaning of a client's word or utterance.

guidelines   Suggestions for implementing and monitoring public policies, which do not have the weight of law.

health maintenance organization   A type of managed care organization that provides a range of care on a prepayment basis.

hearing conservation   A program designed to protect the ears from hearing loss due to exposure to noise.

home care services   Nursing and rehabilitation services provided to patients confined to their homes.

hypernasality   Speech produced with excessive resonance in the nasal cavity.

hyponasality   Speech produced with too little resonance in the nasal cavity.

idiolect   Every individual's unique way of speaking.

independent variable   A manipulated variable in an experiment or study whose presence or degree determines the change in the dependent variable.

indirect services   Consultation with family members, teachers, and/or medical personnel about a client's communication needs.

individual transition plan   An integrated component of an Individualized Education Program for students ages 16 to 21 developed to facilitate their transition from an educational environment to an appropriate vocational or supported adult service setting.

individualized education program   A federally mandated written plan developed by an interdisciplinary education team identifying services and supports for children ages 3 to 21 who have been determined to be eligible for special education services.

individualized family service plan   A written plan outlining family-centered supports and services for children birth to 3 years of age who are eligible for early intervention services based on the presence of significant developmental delays or disabilities.

informativeness   The degree to which a client's discourse is relevant, truthful, not redundant, and reflects plausible inferences and interpretations.

intelligibility   The degree to which a client's speech can be understood.

intensive care unit   A specialized unit in a general medical hospital for patients in critical condition who require close monitoring.

interdisciplinary   A team approach in which professionals perform tasks within their own disciplines while sharing information and coordinating services with each other.

internal consistency   A measure of the degree to which items on a test correlate with each other.

interrater reliability   The extent to which two or more independent scorers are in agreement about a test score.

intervention   A planned clinical program to change client behavior.

interviewing   A process by which a clinician gathers information related to an individual's communication disorder through direct verbal exchange and through which a clinician begins to establish trust with a client while educating him or her about issues related to communication impairment.

intraoperative monitoring   Continuous assessment of integrity of cranial nerves during surgery.

Joint Commission on the Accreditation of Health Care Organizations   A regulatory body that oversees the quality of care provided to patients in a variety of health care facilities.

language difference   Expected community variations in syntax, semantics, phonology, pragmatics, and the lexicon.

language disorder   Communication that deviates significantly from the norms of the community.

language interference   The influence of one language on another.

laryngectomy   A surgical procedure in which the larynx (and possibly connecting tissues) is removed, usually due to cancer. An individual who has undergone this procedure is referred to as a laryngectomee.

laws   Actions taken by legislative bodies and signed into law by executive officials who are responsible for their implementation and the enforcement of penalties for violations.

letter of justification   Written letter to other service providers, program administrators, insurance companies, and other agents advocating for services, supports, and equipment needed for effective client management.

listening device   Personal (e.g., hearing aid) or community (e.g., audio loop) enhancement system for individuals with hearing impairment.

local norms   The administration of standardized tests to typically developing individuals in the community in which the clinician is working and noting the scores they receive and the quality of their responses.

long-term goal   The relatively broad change in communicative behavior to be achieved during a course of therapy.

managed care   Approach to the delivery of health care that attempts to control quality while containing costs.

managed care organization   An agency that manages or controls health care expenditures by closely monitoring how service providers (e.g., hospitals, physicians) treat their patients and by evaluating the necessity, appropriateness, and payment efficiency of health services.

maze behavior   A type of disfluency involving repetitions, revisions, and false starts in the flow of speech.

mean   The arithmetic average of scores.

measure of central tendency   Description of where the center of a distribution of scores lies. Reported as the mean, median, and/or mode.

Medicaid   A program jointly funded by the states and the federal government that reimburses hospitals and physicians for providing care to qualifying individuals who cannot finance their own medical expenses.

Medicare   Prepaid hospital insurance (Part A) and optional additional medical insurance (Part B) available to individuals over age 65 who are eligible for benefits or disability based on their employment before retirement and administered by the federal Health Care Financing Administration (HCFA).

Medigap   Supplemental hospital insurance designed to cover what Medicare does not.

misrepresentation   A type of dishonesty that occurs when truth is distorted or falsified.

mobile technology   Commercially available devices designed for mainstream usage, including cell phones, tablets, and MP3 players.

Möbius syndrome   A rare birth defect caused by the absence or under-development of the sixth and seventh cranial nerves, which may result in swallowing problems, crossed eyes, lack of facial expression, and speech difficulties.

modal verb   Auxiliary verb used to express the subjunctive mood or future tense (e.g., *can, will, shall, may, could, would, should, must, might*).

modifiability   The process of change through mediation or teaching.

morpheme   The smallest unit of meaning in a language. Can be free-standing words, inflections (bound morphemes, such as plural /s/ or past tense *-ed*), prefixes (e.g., *re-, un-*) or suffixes (e.g., *-ly, -ness*).

multidisciplinary   An approach to service provision in which professionals from different disciplines work independently and report to the team.

multiple baseline across behaviors design   A form of single-case design where intervention begins on a subset of goals while performance on nontreated goals is monitored. Once criterion on treated goals is reached, intervention begins on a new subset of goals.

multiple sclerosis A progressive inflammatory disease in which the myelin sheath of the nerves of the central nervous system (i.e., brain and spinal cord) degenerates, resulting in problems with vision, speech, walking, writing, and memory.

narration A recital of events, especially in chronological order.

nares The nostrils or nasal passages.

nasogastric tube A feeding tube inserted through the nose and ending in the stomach.

neonatal intensive care unit A specialized intensive care unit for newborn infants who need intensive medical management.

normal distribution A symmetrical bell-shaped curve representing the scores of a normal population on a test. In a normal distribution, most scores fall in the middle and fewer scores are found at the high and low extremities.

norm-referenced test Test designed to compare a client's score results against a normed basis; also called formal test.

oncology A division of medicine specializing in diagnosis and management of cancer.

open-ended question A remark that encourages an elaborated reply rather than a one-word answer (e.g., "Tell me more about that"); also called open-ended comment.

otoacoustic emissions Low-level sounds produced by the cochlea that can be measured. Absence of otoacoustic emissions suggests hearing loss.

otolaryngology Branch of medicine specializing in the diagnosis and treatment of diseases of the ear, nose, and throat.

otoscopic Relates to inspection of the external auditory meatus and tympanic membrane with an otoscope.

ototoxic Having a poisonous action on the ear, particularly the hair cells of the cochlear and vestibular end organs.

outpatient facility Designated location where therapy can be provided to patients who live at home and are transported to a rehabilitation center.

overdiagnosis Labeling individuals with communication disorders who, instead, are typically developing.

palliative care Addressing the physical, intellectual, emotional, social, and spiritual needs of both patients and families and facilitating patient autonomy, access to information, and choice throughout the continuum of illness.

paralinguistics Information that accompanies a speech signal to enhance its meaning, including tone of voice, facial expressions, and gestures.

Parkinson's disease A neurological condition characterized by tremors, rigidity, droopy posture, and masklike face.

percentile rank A derived score that indicates the percentage of individuals whose score falls at or below a given raw score.

phonetic inventory A list of all speech sounds (often restricted to consonant sounds) that are produced by a client in a speech sample.

phonology System for developing an appropriate clinical question.

PICO Acronym standing for *patient, patient group,* or *problem; intervention* being considered; *comparison intervention;* and desired *outcome.* System for developing an appropriate clinical question.

planning and placement team An interdisciplinary team consisting of educators, therapists, family members, and educational support personnel charged with the development and implementation of an Individual Educational Plan for students ages 3 to 21 who receive special educational services.

play audiometry A technique used for testing the hearing of preschool children. The child is conditioned to perform an action, such as putting a block in a bucket, when he or she hears a sound.

posttest A pretest readministered after a course of therapy to assess client progress.

pragmatics Study of the appropriate use of language in context.

pretest A baseline measurement taken before the initiation of treatment on a goal.

professional ethics Right and wrong actions in the workplace.

professional relationship Collegial behavior characterized by an open communication style and a climate of mutual respect and cooperation.

prognosis A statement that describes the likelihood that a benefit will be gained from treatment.

prosody The rhythm and melody of speech expressed by intonation, stress, pause, and juncture.

psychiatrist A physician who specializes in the psychiatric needs of patients.

psychologist A professional who evaluates and manages the psychological and/or psychosocial needs of the patient.

public policy Any action (or lack thereof) taken by local, state, or federal officials to address a given problem or set of problems.

pure tone audiometer A device that emits tones at different frequencies and intensities to assess the hearing threshold of an individual.

quasi-experimental study An empirically based research design aimed at evaluating the effect of an intervention on a specific outcome but lacking one or more key features of a true experimental design.

radiologist A physician specialized in radiology, the branch of medicine that uses ionizing and nonionizing radiation for the diagnosis and treatment of disease.

randomized control trial A research design in which the investigator assigns participants randomly to two or more groups who then receive systematic treatment (or, in some cases, no treatment), and the outcomes for each group are compared.

referral Sending a client to another professional whose area of expertise better matches the client's needs.

referral letter Letter written to doctors, therapists, or other service providers referring an individual for medical or clinical evaluation and/or treatment.

registers The varieties of a language that depend on the context and conversational participants.

regulations Detailed rules for interpreting and implementing a particular law.

reliability The consistency of a test or a procedure over repeated administrations and by different examiners.

repetition A sound, syllable, or word repeated more than twice. One of the core behaviors in stuttering.

representativeness How well a sampling of behavior resembles a client's true behaviors and level of functioning.

resonance The modification of laryngeal tone by altering the shape of the oral and nasal cavities.

scanning Either through the use of a facilitator or specialized software, unwanted items are discarded until the user reaches the desired item. The user then indicates the selection through an alternative means such as an eye blink, switch, or other device.

screening Initial assessment procedure that allows individuals who require a complete evaluation to be identified.

secondary dysfluency behaviors Extraneous movements of the face or other body parts associated with dysfluent speech.

self-contained classroom A service provision model in which the speech-language pathologist is the primary educator, providing both academic and intense speech-language remediation.

semantics Study of the way in which words and ideas are combined and expressed.

sensorineural hearing loss Diminished sound sensitivity due to cochlear and auditory nerve pathology.

service delivery model The system that is used to organize speech-language and hearing programs.

SETT Acronym standing for *student, environment,* the *tasks* a student needs to accomplish before attempting to determine what *tools* will be required. A framework that assists a planning and placement team in goal setting and maintenance.

signal-to-noise ratio   The ratio of intensities of foreground to background noises, often used as a measure of vocal quality.

single-case experimental design   A research design in which the investigator systematically manipulates variables so that a relationship between the treatment and the outcome can be inferred, usually on one or a small number of participants.

skilled nursing facility   Previously known as a *nursing home*. Include a percentage of residents who require services from such trained professionals as nurses and rehabilitation specialists.

SOAP note   Acronym standing for *subjective, objective, assessment,* and *plan*. A commonly used format in medical and other service delivery settings to record and analyze data specific to a client's ongoing medical status and/or performance in therapy.

sociolinguistic factors   Verbal and nonverbal characteristics that might influence interaction with a client and his or her family.

speech-generating device   An electronic aid that produces speech output.

standard deviation unit   Measure of the degree of variation in a distribution.

standard error of measurement   The standard deviation of error around an individual's true score.

standard score   A derived score that has been transformed into a distribution with a known mean and standard deviation.

statistical significance   The probability that differences between groups observed over a course of treatment resulted from the manipulation of the independent variable.

stimulability   The degree to which a nonmastered skill or behavior can be elicited.

stuttering   A type of fluency disorder. Speech usually marked by repetitions, prolongations, and/or pauses.

syntax   Study of the rules that govern the internal structure of language, including grammar and word order.

synthesized speech   Algorithms included as part of special software on a device that generate synthetic speech. An example of synthetic speech is the text-to-speech function on a computer or iPhone.

target behavior   The verbal or nonverbal behavior that is to be changed during an intervention or treatment.

task analysis   The breakdown of an intervention goal into a series of prerequisite skills and the ordered steps that must be followed to achieve it.

task sequence   An ordered series of steps through which a clinician plans to help a client progress toward an intervention goal.

test–retest reliability A measure of a test's consistency or stability over time.

tinnitus Sensation of ringing or other sound in the head, without an external cause.

transdisciplinary A team approach in which members from different disciplines work collaboratively to focus on shared goals. Team members work together and may cross discipline lines.

treatment protocol A planned clinical program designed to change client behavior.

T-unit Terminal unit of production used to segment utterances of school-age children and adults. Consists of an independent clause and all the dependent clauses associated with it.

underdiagnosis The process of not diagnosing a true communication disorder because all aspects of an individual's communication skills are believed to be dialect or second-language features.

validity The extent to which a test measures what it claims to measure.

verbosity Excess speech; the use of more words than is necessary to convey an idea. Often exhibited in acquired aphasia.

videofluoroscopic swallowing study A radiographic examination of swallowing performed while the patient drinks liquids and eats solid food.

visual reinforcement audiometry A technique for testing the hearing of very young children in which the child's looking toward a sound is reinforced with lights or moving toys.

voice output communication aides Mid-technology devices with fixed displays that produce a message upon activation.

World Health Organization An international organization that developed the International Classification of Functioning, Disability and Health, which provides a model for evaluating the interactions among an individual's health condition, level of functioning, and contextual factors.

Answer Key

CHAPTER 1

1. Answers may vary.

2. Testing hearing, fitting hearing aids, counseling clients and families on hearing habilitation, and working with cochlear implants.

3. Working with parents of premature infants on feeding and communication, developing language in preschool children, helping school-age children who stutter, and retraining adults who lose language due to stroke.

4. *Similarities:* Degree from program accredited by Council on Academic Accreditation in Audiology and Speech-Language Pathology is required; the applicant must have demonstrated knowledge of the biological sciences, physical sciences, statistics, and the social/behavioral sciences. *Differences:* Master's degree required for speech language pathology, doctoral for audiology; areas of required knowledge differ.

CHAPTER 2

1. Consumer protection and client welfare are safeguarded.

   The professional reputation of the discipline is maintained.

   Professional behavior is regulated.

   Objective guidance is available for ethical dilemmas and deliberation.

   Practitioners can rely on an external code in addition to their own values.

   Clients have an objective standard against which to evaluate their clinician's actions.

2. Answers may vary.

3. Continuing education, reading textbooks and journal articles, attending workshops, taking a course at a local university, shadowing professional colleagues, and participating in research activities.

4. Competition, service eligibility, discharge, resources, managed care, scope of practice. Answers may vary.

5. *Misrepresentation:* Type of dishonesty that occurs when truth is distorted or falsified.

   Conflict of interest: Occurs when a speech-language pathologist or audiologist receives personal or financial gain from clients or manufacturers that compromises professional judgment.

   Nondiscrimination: Refraining from excluding clients from professional practice for reasons other than the person's potential to benefit from our services.

   Infection control: Safeguarding clients from infectious diseases.

   Informed consent: Having clients participate in clinical practice only when they are told about their speech-language or hearing condition and are informed about the relative strengths, weaknesses, and risks (i.e., side effects) associated with a recommended plan of action or inaction.

   Referral: Safeguarding a client's right to appropriate clinical services by sending a client to another professional when a client presents a communication disorder beyond the clinician's level of expertise.

6. To model ethical behavior.

7. To handle the adjudication process when violations are alleged.

8. Answers may vary.

CHAPTER 3

1. The conscientious integration of clinical experience, theoretical knowledge, and knowledge of the scientific literature.

2. b

3. P, patient, patient group, or problem; I, intervention being considered; C, comparison intervention; O, outcome that is desired. This is the first step in EBP decision making, used to identify the clinical question.

4. 1. Develop a four-part clinical question.
   2. Find the internal evidence and answer the clinical question based solely on this evidence.
   3. Find the external research evidence.
   4. Critically appraise the external evidence.
   5. Integrate the internal and external evidence.
   6. Evaluate the decision by documenting the outcomes.

5. 1. *Research design:* Identifying which design was used for a particular study because each design answers different types of questions and varies according to the level of evidence
   2. *Methodological quality:* Determining whether the researcher took adequate steps to avoid bias and subjectivity.
   3. *Consistency and strength of observed effects:* Examining the statistical significance, effect-size estimates, and consistency of study effects on identified outcomes.

CHAPTER 4

1. a

2. c

3. b

4. b

5. d

6. d

CHAPTER 5

1. Language sample analysis allows for increased sensitivity in diagnosing disorders, has strong face validity (ecologically valid), allows for assessment of clients who are difficult to test, and provides guidance for treatment planning. Speech and language sampling also serves to supplement standardized testing results as well as provide a clinical measure of speech and language performance when no formal tests are available in a given language.

2. What can the client respond to during a linguistic interaction? In other words, what are the client's functional comprehension skills like? What types of communicative intentions can the client express? Is a range of intentions available, or is the range very limited? How frequently does the client attempt to communicate? Can the client initiate communication as well as respond? By what means does the client attempt to get messages across? Does he or she use gestures, gaze, vocalizations, words, behaviors, or some combination of these? Does the client have any ability to associate pictures, printed symbols, or written language with their communicative intents? Does the client show the cognitive-linguistic correlates of communication, such as attentiveness to the communications going on around them; visual scanning of pictures, computer screens, or other media; behaviors that reveal their recall of past events; choice making; manual sequencing of steps to complete a task; and simple cause-and-effect behaviors?

3. Any number of low-cost video recorders may be used to video language sampling for later analysis. It is important that the environment be as free from noise as possible prior to recording the sample. For nonverbal clients, it is important that the client be fully visible in the recording (not obstructed by environmental objects or the clinician).

4. Answers may vary. What is important to consider is in which natural contexts a particular client has the need to communicate. Any number of communication contexts may be used as long as it is a context in which the client has a need to function.

5. The main advantage of using computer-assisted language analysis is the ability to perform multiple analyses on the same transcript. It is still important that the clinician elicit a representative sample and that the sample is transcribed correctly. Manual methods may be performed during the evaluation

process and do not always require transcription of the sample. Yet any complex analysis will have to be completed using a transcribed sample rather than attempting to analyze speech or language during the evaluation.

6. For preschoolers, it is recommended that utterances are segmented using either rising or falling intonation. For school-age children and adults, T-units are often used.

7. Analysis of language samples from adults with acquired impairments should include analysis of phonological errors, syntax, morphology, semantics, and pragmatics.

8. Answers may vary.

9. Answers may vary.

10. Answers may vary.

11. Analysis of voice quality, resonance, and prosody are typically assessed perceptually when performing speech sampling. A perceptual assessment of voice use (such as the Consensus Auditory-Perceptual Evaluation of Voice) may be used to guide the clinician's perceptual assessment. Further, client–report assessments (such as the VHI) may be used to assess the impact a client's voice has on his or her daily life. Instrumental analysis gives the clinician objective voice data with which to monitor a client's progress in therapy, especially when a clinician becomes "acclimated" to a client's voice quality and perceiving small changes in the client's voice is difficult to reliably accomplish.

CHAPTER 6

1. Eliminate the disorder; provide compensatory strategies; modify the disorder.

2. Do statement, condition, criterion.

3. The goal is broken down into small steps by examining the input and output prerequisites necessary to complete the task.

4. *Clinician-directed:* Clinician controls all aspects of the intervention.

   Hybrid: Blended approaches that are naturalistic but still controlled by clinician.

   Client-centered: Responsive approaches that emphasize the provision of communication therapy in authentic settings.

5. Answers may vary.

6. Self-talk, parallel talk, expansions, extensions, and recasts.

7. Arrange the environment.

   The client initiates the interaction.

   The clinician selects the target response.

The clinician uses cues and prompts to obtain a more elaborated response.

The clinician provides confirmation that the communicative intent was achieved.

8. Answers may vary.

9. To track the client's progress from one session to another.

To provide documentation of the efficacy of the intervention.

To maximize clinician effectiveness.

10. When they are more likely promote the use of the newly acquired target behavior in everyday speaking situations.

CHAPTER 7

1. Principles of effective oral and written communication include organizing information in a logical manner, clearly introducing topics, avoiding using technical language, explaining technical terms when necessary, using objective terms instead of vague or subjective terms, avoiding redundancy, using "people-first" language.

2. Advantages of using an in-person interview rather than a written case history include the opportunities to establish a trusting relationship, demonstrate respect for cultural interaction styles, adjust interview topics, and clarify questions.

3. Cultural factors that may influence a person's response to interview questions include differing perceptions of formality versus informality during an interview, different willingness to respond to direct versus indirect questions, differing interpretations of silence, and different degrees of willingness to disagree with an interviewer.

4. Follow-up counseling after a diagnostic evaluation is important in order to summarize initial assessment findings, answer client/patient questions, reduce uncertainty and anxiety caused by a lack of information, provide additional education regarding communication disorders, and discuss appropriate follow-up actions.

5. A topic is appropriate to be addressed by an audiologist or speech-language pathologist if it involves feelings, attitudes, and questions relating to the presenting communication disorder and its impact on that person's life.

6. An *individual education plan* for speech-language therapy includes a section for identifying team members and background information about the student, as well as summaries of the student's present level of educational performance, long-term goals and short-term educational objectives, the type and frequency of special services, service providers, adaptive equipment, classroom accommodations, instructional sites, modifications to academic schedules, and specialized instructional strategies.

7. An individual intervention plan, SOAP note, progress report, and discharge summary document a continuum of information related to speech-language services. The individual intervention plan documents the goals, objectives, activities, and materials needed for a therapy session. A SOAP note documents the progress a client has made in meeting therapy goals and objectives, as well as recommendations for subsequent sessions. A progress report summarizes therapy outcomes across a set period of time and makes recommendations for continued intervention, whereas a discharge summary documents progress at the completion of a term of therapy.

Test Answer Key

1. b

2. d

3. b

4. a

5. c

CHAPTER 8

1. Answers may vary.

2. Answers may vary.

3. Answers may vary.

4. Answers may vary.

5. Answers may vary.

CHAPTER 9

1. Answers may vary.

2. Answers may vary.

3. Answers may vary.

4. Answers may vary.

5. Answers may vary.

6. Answers may vary.

7. Answers may vary.

8. Answers may vary.

CHAPTER 10

1. Answers may vary. Answers should include a distinction between the respondent's culture and language and those of the individual to whom he or she is providing clinical services.

2. Answers may vary. Answers might include, but are not limited to, topics such as mother–child interaction, types of child-directed speech, narrative genres, and dialects.

3. Answers may vary. Examples include, but are not limited to, dynamic assessment, observation, testing beyond the ceiling on a standardized test, criterion-referenced testing, parent report, and teacher report.

4. Answers may vary. Q1: Examples include, but are not limited to, child-directed speech, mother–child interaction, amount of talk, type of talk, pragmatics, and appropriate conversational partners. Q2: Examples include, but are not limited to, dynamic assessment, observation, testing beyond the ceiling on a standardized test, criterion-referenced testing, parent report, and teacher report.

5. Answers may vary. Examples include, but are not limited to, 1) establishing contacts and hiring bilingual speech-language pathologists (SLPs) as consultants or diagnosticians to provide clinical services; 2) establishing cooperative groups in which groups of school districts or programs might hire an itinerant bilingual SLP; 3) establishing networks such as forging links between university settings and work settings to help recruit bilingual speakers into the workforce; 4) establishing clinical fellowship year and graduate student practica sites; 5) establishing interdisciplinary teams in which monolingual SLPs are teamed with bilingual professionals from other fields; and 6) training support personnel such as bilingual aides, students, family members, or members of the community.

6. Answers may vary.

7. Answers may vary. Go to http://census.gov.

8. Answers may vary.

9. a

10. c

11. b

12. c

13. b

CHAPTER 11

1. Clinicians, both speech-language pathologists and audiologists, use assistive technology as part of their clinical practice in a number of different ways and with diverse populations. Technology can be used to augment communication

for individuals with complex communication needs through the use of dedicated communication devices or it can be used to teach a specific skill through the use of specialized applications available for consumer-based electronics. Technology can also be used to create optimal listening environments through the use of assistive listening devices.

2. Evidenced-based decisions incorporate clinical knowledge, scientific evidence, and client values into the clinical decision process. There are several methodologies that assist clinicians when making evidenced-based decisions regarding technologies, such as the SETT framework. These frameworks ensure that clinicians utilize their clinical expertise, evaluate the available scientific evidence, and include the client's values during the technology assessment process.

3. An assistive technology assessment has several basic components; however, they may vary depending on your client and his or her individual needs. A comprehensive record review is typically the first step in the assessment process. The information collected during this initial step will likely determine subsequent steps in the assessment procedure. Direct observation of the client is completed to gain cursory information on the individual's cognition, motor functioning, and current means of communication. An interview with the client's caregiver is also conducted to collect information that cannot readily be obtained through clinical observation or direct assessment. Formal assessment of the client's present level of functioning will typically be completed in a collaborative fashion with other professionals, including physical therapists, occupational therapists, and special education teachers. The final step of the technology assessment includes synthesizing and disseminating the data collected to the client's caregivers and other support personnel.

4. Assistive listening devices were initially thought to help only those with hearing impairment. Through continued research in the field, however, these devices are now known to be useful for those with even minimal hearing loss. Although assistive listening devices are commonly used in school environments for children with hearing impairment, other groups of people such as the elderly may also benefit from similar technology. There are a range of devices that have been designed for home use including infrared television amplifiers and vibrating alarms built into bed pillows that support listening for those with hearing loss.

5. The primary purpose of all augmentative and alternative communication (AAC) devices is to provide the user with a means of communication. The main difference between low-, mid-, and high-tech AAC systems is the amount of technology that is utilized by each group of devices. Low-tech devices use little or no technology—for example, tapping a picture of a cookie to request a snack. Mid-tech devices include voice output switches with fixed displays. These devices allow the user to communicate through the use of prerecorded messages. Last, high-tech devices are those with dynamic displays and synthesized speech. Computers, tablets, and those devices with computer-like screens are typically classified as high-tech AAC systems.

6. The use of mobile technology can be observed in populations with and without communication disorders. Given its popularity in today's culture, this technology has changed how individuals communicate with one another. For those with and without communication impairments, the portability and connectivity of these devices enable the user to communicate through a range of modalities, including text messages, e-mail, and even video messaging. For those with communication disorders, these devices can also be used as dedicated communication systems. These devices may be more sought after as dedicated communication systems given their social acceptability, portability, and limited expense.

7. There are three main issues related to the use of mobile technology for individuals with communication disorders. Although much less expensive than traditional AAC systems, these devices are not considered durable medical equipment and are not covered by Medicare or Medicaid. Since these products were not designed specifically for individuals with special needs, their durability in this application is not well known. What is known is that these devices are more fragile than traditional, dedicated AAC systems and may not withstand dropping, exposure to moisture, or repeated rough handling. Tech support is another issue that should not be overlooked when considering consumer-based electronics. Many traditional AAC companies provide extensive technical support, whereas mobile technology may not offer that level of support. Whereas Apple and other manufacturers of mobile technology will provide hardware-related assistance, it is unlikely they will provide support for third-party-designed applications.

CHAPTER 12

1. The provision of assessment and intervention from the family's point of view, taking into account family goals, dynamics, and circumstances.

2. The family as a whole is greater than the sum of its parts.

   Change in one part of the family affects the whole family system.

   Subsystems are embedded within the larger family system.

   The family system exists within a larger social and environmental context.

   Families are multigenerational.

3. The main difference between traditional practice and family-centered practice is that in the latter the family is always considered as a primary partner in selecting approaches and making decisions regarding assessment and treatment goals and directions for a client, rather than a preselected set of conditions that are imposed on every client who is in treatment.

4. Answers may vary.

5. Families and professionals have equal partnerships; thus, collaboration is the core of this approach.

6. Answers may vary.

7. Differences in the role of the client in the family based on age, prior life experience, whether or not responsibilities are assumed by the client within the family, level of financial conditions, and many other factors are involved that may create different considerations in service delivery for adults and children.

CHAPTER 13

1. The treatment manual should include a description about how often the treatment will be delivered across sessions (e.g., two times a week) and within a session (e.g., 20 models per 30-minute session). The manual should also include a description of the treatment stimuli (materials) and tasks as well as the specific instructions, prompts, and feedback that the speech-language pathologist (SLP) will use to deliver the treatment. A description of the target behavior(s) addressed by the treatment is needed, including examples of acceptable and unacceptable responses.

2. The target behavior is observed multiple times to examine the stability and trend of the behavior. When the behavior is not changing or is changing in an undesired direction during the baseline phase, the SLP has evidence to support initiation of treatment to change the target behavior.

3. d

4. c

5. c

6. a

7. c

8. b

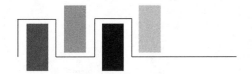

Index

Page references to figures and tables are indicated by *f* and *t*, respectively.